Pediatric Cytopathology

ASCP Theory and Practice of Cytopathology 4
William W Johnston, MD, Series Editor
Duke University Medical Center

The ASCP Theory and Practice of Cytopathology Series
Cytopathology of the Uterine Cervix • Volume 1
Cytopathology of the Endometrium • Volume 2
Cytopathology of the Central Nervous System • Volume 3

Teaching Slide Sets in the ASCP Theory and Practice of Cytopathology Series
Cytopathology of the Uterus Teaching Slide Set
Cytopathology of the Endometrium Teaching Slide Set
Cytopathology of the Central Nervous System Teaching Slide Set

Pediatric Cytopathology

Kim R Geisinger, MD
Professor, Department of Pathology
Director of Anatomic Pathology
Wake Forest University Medical Center
Bowman Gray School of Medicine
Winston-Salem, North Carolina

Jan F Silverman, MD
Professor, Department of Pathology and
    Laboratory Medicine
Director of Cytology
East Carolina University School of Medicine
Greenville, North Carolina

Paul E Wakely, Jr, MD
Associate Professor, Department of Pathology
Director of Cytopathology
Medical College of Virginia
Virginia Commonwealth University
Richmond, Virginia

Contributor
Michael B Kodroff, MD
Clinical Associate Professor
Department of Radiology
East Carolina University School of Medicine
Greenville, North Carolina

American Society of Clinical Pathologists
Chicago

Publishing Team

Andrea Blumenfeld (design/production)

Jeffrey Carlson (series design)

Renee Kastar (marketing)

Beena Rao (editorial)

Joshua Weikersheimer (editorial/publishing direction)

Notice

Trade names for equipment and supplies described herein are included as suggestions only. In no way does their inclusion constitute an endorsement or preference by the American Society of Clinical Pathologists. The ASCP did not test the equipment, supplies, or procedures and, therefore, urges all readers to read and follow all manufacturers' instructions and package insert warnings concerning the proper and safe use of products.

Library of Congress Cataloging-in-Publication Data

Geisinger, Kim R.
     Pediatric Cytopathology/Kim R. Geisinger, Jan F. Silverman, Paul E. Wakely, Jr.;
contributor, Michael B. Kodroff.
        p. 368 cm.   (ASCP theory and practice of cytopathology; 4)
     Includes bibliographical references and index.
     ISBN 0-89189-378-4
     1. Children—Diseases—Diagnosis. 2. Cytodiagnosis. 3. Pathology, Cellular. I. Sil-
verman, Jan F. II. Wakely, Paul E. III. Title. IV. Series.
     [DNLM: 1. Cytodiagnosis—in infancy & childhood. 2. Cells—pathology. W1
AS126 v. 4 1994/QY 95 G313p 1994]
     RJ51.C88G45 1994
     618.92'007582—dc20
     DNLM/DLC   94-30542
     for Library of Congress   CIP

Printed in Hong Kong

98 97 96 95 94   5 4 3 2 1

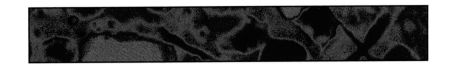

▣ Contents

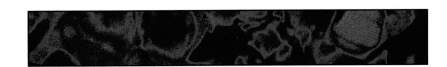

◙ Tables

◙ Figures

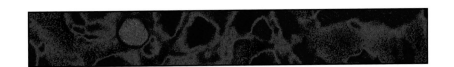

Acknowledgments

We would like to thank our colleagues and former residents and fellows who made us aware of cases of diagnostic interest and continue to teach and inspire us. We are indebted to the following individuals for sharing specimens with us: M Akhtar, MD, Riyadh, Saudi Arabia; M Almeida, MD, Lisbon, Portugal; R Craver, MD, New Orleans, LA; P Day, MD, Chandigarh, India; A Dejmek, MD, Malmö, Sweden; H Ehya, MD, Philadelphia, PA; J Georgitis, MD, Winston-Salem, NC; J Goeken MD, Iowa City, IA; A Chauvenet, PhD, MD, Winston-Salem, NC; B Naylor, MBBS, Ann Arbor, MI; C Powers, MD, PhD, Syracuse, NY; G Thomas, MD, Richmond, VA; B Wasilauskas, PhD, Winston-Salem, NC; S Woodhouse, MD, Lenoir, NC; and NA Young, MD, Philadelphia, PA.

We wish to acknowledge the help of T Holbrook, MD, and VJ Joshi, PhD, MD, both of Greenville, NC. The Document Preparation Center, Bowman Gray School of Medicine, Winston-Salem, NC, provided invaluable assistance in manuscript preparation.

Our appreciation is expressed to Joshua Weikersheimer and others from the ASCP Press for their efforts in making this book possible.

Preface

This text has been divided into two main sections, exfoliative and fine needle aspiration cytopathology. It has been written with the general cytopathologist in mind who infrequently encounters cytologic preparations from children, and for specialists in pediatric pathology who use cytology in their practice.

Our goal is to provide detailed descriptions of the cytologic morphology of many of the entities that are either unique to or are more prevalent in children and adolescents. A large number of photographs illustrating the diverse and sometimes subtle cytologic features of these lesions are used to accomplish this. We have exercised a histocytologic correlation format in many cases to assist the reader in appreciating the "pattern" of the smear in cases of aspiration cytology. Where helpful, the application and results of ancillary studies are given and pertinent clinical and laboratory findings are highlighted. Although we have tried to cover the most common lesions of children, not all pediatric entities are included because of their rarity and the gaps in our knowledge regarding their cytopathology.

The Papanicolaou stain, which is used by nearly all laboratories in this country, has been adhered to in exfoliative cytology. We have tried to balance the use of the alcohol-fixed, Papanicolaou stained smear in aspiration cytology with the air dried Romanowsky stained smear. These preparations are complementary to one another emphasizing different features of the aspiration smear, and should not be viewed as competitive stains. We encourage cytopathologists to use both because we believe this facilitates cytologic interpretation. That said, the advantages of the Romanowsky method are far preferable for hematopoietic lesions, and we bias the number of slides made with that method in those sites. Where available, tissue fragments obtained during the aspiration procedure and processed as paraffin embedded hematoxylin & eosin stained cell blocks are shown.

No attempt has been made to discuss in detail and illustrate the technique of fine needle aspiration biopsy (FNAB) which has been done in several general texts on that subject. For those unfamiliar with this technique, and the appearance of cells from pediatric lesions, aspiration and preparation of smears from pediatric specimens at the surgical bench or autopsy table is one way to gain confidence and skill. In each of our clinical practices we are allowed the opportunity to see the child, and perform the FNAB rather than having the procedure performed and smears made by someone who does not interpret the cytology. We prefer this arrangement because we are able to combine our clinical judgment with what we see on the slide. A practice that allows for *close* communication with clinicians who are adept in performing FNAB and smearing of the cellular material can be just as satisfactory.

As neoplasms and other mass lesions are much less frequent in children, the utilization of cytopathology in children is not as widespread as it is in adults. Perhaps because of this infrequent use of cytopathology in children, many of the specialists in pediatric pathology have expressed reluctance (and sometimes resistance) to use cytologic techniques, particularly FNAB, in the pediatric clinical setting. Even so, we have witnessed many instances in which FNAB cytopathology has improved the care of individual children. Our impression is that this attitude is slowly changing, and hope to encourage through this monograph a greater, more thoughtful utilization of cytopathology in children.

To our teachers; to WJF, friend and mentor; and especially to our spouses – Lori, Mary, and Anna – and children – Kristen, Brian, Mischell, Jeff, Laura, Byron, and Alexis

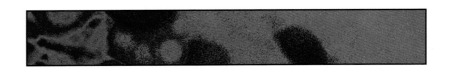

CHAPTER ONE

Introduction

The stature of cytopathology has been greatly elevated in this country as the numerous advantages of this diagnostic discipline have become much more widely acknowledged and the limitations better defined. This greater level of recognition has occurred among pathologists, the medical profession as a whole, and the general public. However, this awareness is due almost exclusively to applications in adult patients.[1-3] With regards to diagnostic cytopathology, children have been sorely neglected, except perhaps for cerebrospinal fluid cytology.[4-6] We believe that a much broader utilization of exfoliative, intraoperative and fine needle aspiration (FNA) cytology in the pediatric population will lead to an improvement in patient care.[6-25] Our purpose is to present and illustrate the cytologic morphology and diagnostic criteria for pediatric lesions. By demonstrating the advantages and disadvantages of cytology in children, we hope to stimulate others (both clinicians and pathologists) to incorporate cytopathology into their diagnostic repertoire in order to better serve pediatric patients and their families.

In the United States, only 2% of patients with cancer are infants and children, for fewer than 7,000 children under the age of 15 develop a malignant neoplasm each year.[26,27] Yet, cancer is a leading cause of death in children, some 2,000 to 3,000 dying annually. Despite this, we believe that both exfoliative and especially aspiration cytology are underutilized in the pediatric population as a diagnostic procedure.

There are a number of important differences between malignant neoplasms in adults and children. When making a diagnosis of cancer in a child, pathologists and cytotechnologists need to adhere to the same general clinical and morphologic principles which underlie a cytologic diagnosis of cancer in an adult. Throughout this book we will emphasize a systematic, clinicopathologic approach which embodies several different parameters. First, demographic data in the individual patient are important. The incidence rates of many childhood neoplasms have characteristic differences with respect to age, sex and race.[5,27] For example, most neuroblastomas occur within the first few years of life, whereas osteosarcomas are almost unheard of in those years. Ewing's sarcoma is exceedingly rare in blacks; thus, one should avoid making such a diagnosis in a black child with a small round cell tumor unless the pathologic evidence is overwhelming.

It is important to review briefly the annual incidence rates of the more frequent pediatric malignancies.[26,27] Leukemia is not only the most common form of cancer in children, it is also the most lethal type. The closely related lymphomas comprise the third most frequent type of malignancy in children. Lymphoreticular neoplasms account for nearly half of cancer-related deaths in the pediatric population. Primary brain tumors are the most common solid neoplasms in children, followed by neuroblastoma and the soft tissue sarcomas, predominantly rhabdomyosarcoma. The sixth most common form of cancer and the second most frequent intra-abdominal visceral malignancy is nephroblastoma (Wilms' tumor). Bone sarcomas occur next in frequency with two-thirds or more being osteosarcomas. Ewing's sarcoma accounts for nearly all the other primary bone cancers in children. As is obvious, many of these neoplasms are exceedingly uncommon or even rare in adults. Others, such as retinoblastoma, which comprises the eighth most frequent type of childhood cancer, is almost unheard of in adults. Germ cell tumors, as in adults, arise predominantly within the gonads.

As in adults, careful scrutiny of clinical data is important. This information may be acquired from reading the accompanying specimen requisition forms and by reviewing prior materials from laboratory files at the time of specimen sign-out. Communication with pediatricians and radiologists is the best source of pertinent information. In our experience, this is most likely to occur at the time of an FNA biopsy in which clinician, radiologist and pathologist are all functioning together as a closely integrated team. The importance of recognizing an earlier diagnosis of a specific tumor type is essential. Yet, some children with cancer will develop a second primary neoplasm, either spontaneously or in relation to therapy for the first tumor. An example of the latter includes the greatly increased incidence of osteosarcoma following curative treatment for retinoblastoma.

Knowledge concerning the exact type of specimen being reviewed and the exact site from which the specimen was obtained is exceedingly important. In the performance of FNA biopsies in adults, it is, of course, important to know what site is being sampled. We believe it is just as important to know the exact needle placement location in a diagnosis of mass lesions in children. This, and the ability of the pathologist to triage properly the specimen, are important reasons for a pathologist to be in attendance at an FNA biopsy of either superficial or deep organs whenever possible. It is also important to know which neoplasms in children metastasize to various body sites with different

Leukemia is not only the most common form of cancer in children, it is also the most lethal type

propensities; this affects diagnostic exfoliative cytology.[4,5] For example, the most likely type of exfoliative specimen in which a metastatic osteosarcoma might be recognized is pleural fluid in that the lungs are the most common site for metastases of this bone tumor.

Malignant neoplasms in the pediatric population differ significantly in several respects from those of adults. These include their histogenesis, pathogenesis and organs of origin.[26] Whereas the most frequent neoplasms in adults are epithelial in nature and are derived from external or luminal surfaces, such as the lungs, intestines and skin, which are exposed to potential exogenous carcinogens, over 90% of childhood tumors are nonepithelial and almost never arise in these sites. Furthermore, many tumors in adults arise in organs such as the breast and prostate which are under direct endocrine control; such is not the case in children.

In many childhood cancers, the responses to specific antineoplastic therapies has yielded dramatic positive results.[26,27] For example, the acute leukemias were once uniformly fatal in children. Today, the majority of children with acute lymphoblastic leukemia are survivors. Such is not the case in adults with acute leukemia. Another example involves renal neoplasms. 90% of children with nephroblastoma are now considered survivors, whereas less than half of all adults with renal cell carcinoma will survive for 5 years. Thus, it is important in children to identify specific cancer cell types so that specifically tailored therapy is provided to each patient. Supplemental diagnostic procedures, especially electron microscopy (EM) and immunocytochemistry, are often crucial in these differential diagnostic decisions in children and will be discussed and illustrated throughout the text.[12,20,28-32]

From a cytomorphologic viewpoint, pediatric neoplasms can be roughly divided into two groups based predominantly on the size of the malignant cells, their uniformity and patterns of arrangement

The majority of children with acute lymphoblastic leukemia are survivors

Table 1.1
Characterization of Childhood Neoplasms By Cell Size

Small Cell Neoplasms	Large Cell Neoplasms
Acute Leukemias	Osteosarcoma (conventional)
Non-Hodgkin's Lymphomas, Small Cell Type	Astrocytoma
Ewing's Sarcoma	Ependymoma
Neuroblastoma	Glioblastoma Multiforme
Medulloblastoma	Hodgkin's Disease
Pineoblastoma	Non-Hodgkin's Lymphomas, Large Cell Type
Retinoblastoma	Hepatocellular Carcinoma
Nephroblastoma	Germinoma
Hepatoblastoma	Embryonal Carcinoma
Primitive Neuroectodermal Tumor	Endodermal Sinus Tumor
Pancreatoblastoma	Rhabdomyosarcoma
Rhabdomyosarcoma	Pancreatoblastoma

(Table 1.1).[5] The much more common small cell tumor group is composed of neoplastic cells with uniform appearances and small sizes. They generally have diameters up to 3 times that of a small mature lymphocyte. They have a solitary, hyperchromatic nucleus with finely granular, evenly distributed chromatin. Small nucleoli may or may not be apparent but at times may be quite prominent. Generally scanty volumes of cytoplasm result in high nuclear-cytoplasmic ratios. Cytologic appearances are quite homogenous among the cells of the same tumor, as well as between tumors of the same histologic type. Classic examples of the small cell tumor group include neuroblastoma and the acute leukemias.

The much less frequent large cell tumor group is composed of malignant cells with ample cytoplasm and that contain ≥1 nuclei. The latter may be quite uniform or highly variable among the cells of the same tumor. Coarse clumps of chromatin in irregular distribution may be seen throughout the nuclei. Prominent huge nucleoli are also typical. It is not unusual to find marked pleomorphism within this category. The prototypic example of large cell malignancies is the conventional osteosarcoma.

Most pediatric tumors can be classified into one of these two categories; however, no one classification is perfect and exceptions and overlap occur between these 2 groups. For example, although rhabdomyosarcoma is often considered a small cell tumor, many neoplastic cells have moderate volumes of cytoplasm and multinucleation is common. Conversely, although the neoplastic cells of ovarian dysgerminomas may attain a rather large size and have ≥1 prominent nucleoli, these cells are characteristically highly uniform.

Some readers may wonder as to why we should consider cytology a valuable diagnostic technique in children except perhaps for smears of the uterine cervix, cerebrospinal fluid (CSF) and possibly urine, when the diagnostic mainstay of pediatric pathology has been the tissue biopsy (or even autopsy).[6] We fully agree that histologic examination of tissue is highly desirable or sometimes even indispensable. There are, however, a number of situations in which aspiration or exfoliative cytology is preferable. It is important to recognize and to accept that these two related morphologic modalities are not in competition with each other but rather frequently complement one another in the workup of diseases in children and adults.

Pediatric intraoperative cytopathology (IOC) is a topic that is either completely ignored in some medical centers and children's hospitals, or is used solely for imprints of suspicious hematopoietic lesions. Though IOC has been documented as beneficial for adult lesions, little has been written regarding its application in children.[33-36] One of us recently had the opportunity to examine our experience with pediatric IOC for a variety of lesions.[25]

Upon review of consecutive pediatric cases in which intraoperative pathologic consultation was performed, 55 cases were found in a recent 5-year period that utilized cytology. Intraoperative diagnoses were issued using either cytology alone (27 cases) or combined frozen tissue section and cytology (28 cases). In the cytology-only group, a correct interpretation distinguishing benign from malignant lesions was made in 26 of 27 cases (96%). In 56% of the cytology-only

There are a number of situations in which aspiration or exfoliative cytology is preferable

group, the amount of tissue submitted by the surgeon was ≤2 cm in greatest dimension.

IOC is an easily performed and useful supplement to the histologic frozen tissue section. It gives the pathologist a general (and sometimes a specific) idea of the nature of the lesion without actually processing the specimen. Tissue preservation is critical particularly when the amount is limited, and the pathologist needs to make a decision toward optimal triaging of tissue for various ancillary diagnostic studies (culture, immunochemistry, gene rearrangements, cytogenetics, electron microscopy, etc.), and for requests of tissue for research material. Other advantages of IOC include: avoidance of cryostat contamination with tissue from HIV-positive children, use in specimens that do not cut well or at all in a cryostat such as fat and bone fragments and superior cytologic images as compared to a frozen tissue section.

Relatively new on the American scene is the application of FNA as a diagnostic modality in children.[6-24] FNA may provide very rapid diagnostic results for mass lesions. As clinicians may invoke watchful waiting for long periods of time, particularly in a child with lymphadenopathy, to avoid a potentially unnecessary surgical procedure, FNA aids in management. The aspiration procedure itself requires only a few minutes to perform, and when coupled with at least a preliminary morphologic interpretation, overall care of the patient is generally expedited. Certain diagnostic procedures may actually be eliminated by the rapid turnaround time of aspiration cytology, and similarly, the relatively trauma-free FNA, which does not require anesthesia, may prevent unnecessary surgery for some patients, such as those with unre-

Table 1.2
Fine Needle Aspiration (FNA) Biopsy Cytology in Children

Author	# of FNA (% Malignant)	Sensitivity (%)	Specificity (%)	Inadequate
Jereb et al[7]	60 (68)	100	97	4
Schaller et al[8]	32 (59)	100	100	0
Taylor and Nunez[10]	64 (30)	98	100	7
Diament et al[11]	25 (68)	86	100	3
Wakely et al[14]	112 (35)	97	97	1
Cohen et al[17]	92 (36)	97	95	6
Rajwanshi et al[16]	245 (100)	NR*	NR	NR
Shakoor[18]	81 (58)	97	100	NR
Silverman et al[21]	135 (21)	91	100	5
McGahey et al[24]	128 (38)	NR	NR	8
Verdeguer et al[15]	70 (51)	95	80	12
Howell et al[23]	64 (38)	97	98	4
Gorczyca et al[22]	65 (100)	93	100	0
Layfield et al[19]	66 (100)	100	100	0
Valkov and Bojikin[13]	54 (94)	96	100	0
Obers and Phillips[20]	17 (100)	100	100	2

*NR: not reported

sectable tumors. As FNA has an exceedingly low complication rate compared to traditional tissue biopsy, it is much safer and may be repeated several times during a single biopsy session. We are unaware of a single instance in which malignant cells were implanted or disseminated in a child by FNA. Finally, procurement and interpretation of an aspiration biopsy specimen is less expensive than a tissue examination, especially when the pathologist is the aspirator as well as the interpreter.

Published series regarding pediatric FNA show high rates of sensitivity and specificity in distinguishing a benign process from a malignant neoplasm (Table 1.2). Results from these series, however, are not truly comparable because while some are FNA from all types of childhood masses, others represent only the malignant neoplasms at that institution, and some are from only one anatomic region. Nonetheless, Table 1.2 illustrates that several centers are practicing FNA in children, and obtaining results comparable to those reported in the adult literature. In many of these papers, the authors report being able to extend their interpretation beyond benign versus malignant to issue specific diagnoses that facilitated rapid treatment.

From a technical viewpoint, there is nothing unique about the procurement or preparation of cytologic specimens from children. It is not our intent to delve deeply into the details of preparation of specimens but a few general statements seem warranted. We rely on the complementariness of the Papanicolaou stain and a Romanowsky stain (eg, Wright-Giemsa or Diff-Quik) for almost all aspiration specimens and many body fluid specimens. This is especially true for CSF and any fluid from a patient with known or suspected lymphoreticular neoplasm. The Papanicolaou stain often permits a better evaluation of the classic nuclear features such as chromatin granularity and distribution. The advantage of Diff-Quik stain over the Papanicolaou stain is obvious for all benign and malignant lymphoreticular specimens.[28] This is especially true of aspiration biopsies of hyperplastic lymph nodes in which alcohol fixation reduces the apparent degree of polymorphism as the lymphocytes assume an artificially greater uniformity of size and appearance. Of course, the same can be said for the interpretation of CSF in children with acute leukemia. Another example involves aspiration biopsies of masses with background stroma. The neuropil background of neuroblastoma, for instance, often stains a brilliant magenta with Diff-Quik, whereas it stains pale green and is not always discernible with Papanicolaou stains.

In addition to the type of stain used, one might debate the merits of different types of fluid specimen preparation. Later chapters consider membrane filter and cytocentrifuge preparations, but a few brief statements may be appropriate here. Cells collected on filters are alcohol fixed and Papanicolaou stained. Most often, Diff-Quik or another Romanowsky stain is applied to cells in cytospin preparations. In a cell-for-cell comparison, cells will appear larger in the cytospin slides.

Importantly, direct smears and cytospin slides, but not filter preparations, often permit the direct application of ancillary diagnostic tests. Most commonly, immunocytochemistry is the modality of choice in this setting.[31] For ultrastructural examination, cells from exfoliative or aspiration specimens can be directly fixed in glutaraldehyde.[12,20,31] This cellular suspension can be centrifuged and the resultant pellet can be thin-sectioned for EM examination.

Published series regarding pediatric FNA show high rates of sensitivity and specificity in distinguishing a benign process from a malignant neoplasm

As stated earlier, we believe it is preferable for a pathologist to be present for aspiration biopsies.[1,14,21] Some believe that it is most desirable to have the pathologist perform the aspiration. By being on site, the cytopathologist may acquire additional valuable clinical and radiographic information to integrate with the morphology. In addition, by rendering an immediate diagnostic decision, the pathologist can selectively triage additionally procured cellular material for the most appropriate ancillary diagnostic tests.[31]

References

1. Frable WJ. Thin-needle aspiration biopsy. A personal experience with 469 cases. *Am J Clin Pathol* 65:168-182, 1976.

2. Bottles K, Miller TR, Cohen MB, Ljung B-M. Fine needle aspiration biopsy. Has its time come? *Am J Med* 81:525-531, 1986.

3. Hajdu SI, Ehya H, Frable WJ, Geisinger KR, Gompel CM, Kern WH, Löwhagen T, Oertel YC, Ramzy I, Rilke FO, Saigo PE, Suprun HZ, Yazdi HM. The value and limitations of aspiration cytology in the diagnosis of primary tumors. A symposium. *Acta Cytol* 33:741-790, 1989.

4. Helson L, Krochmal P, Hajdu SI. Diagnostic value of cytologic specimens obtained from children with cancer. *Ann Clin Lab Sci* 5:294-297, 1975.

5. Geisinger KR, Hajdu SI, Helson L. Exfoliative cytology of non-lymphoreticular neoplasms in children. *Acta Cytol* 28:16-28, 1984.

6. Buchino JJ. Cytopathology in Pediatrics. Karger Basel. 1991.

7. Jereb B, Us-Krasovec M, Jereb M. Thin needle biopsy of solid tumors in children. *Med Pediatr Oncol* 4:213-220, 1978.

8. Schaller RT, Schaller JF, Buschmann C, Kiviat N. The usefulness of percutaneous fine-needle aspiration biopsy in infants and children. *J Pediatr Surg* 18:398-405, 1983.

9. Baran GW, Haaga JR, Shurin SB, Alfidi RJ. CT-guided percutaneous biopsies in pediatric patients. *Pediatr Radiol* 14:161-164, 1984.

10. Taylor SR, Nunez C. Fine-needle aspiration biopsy in a pediatric population. Report of 64 consecutive cases. *Cancer* 54:1449-1453, 1984.

11. Diament MJ, Stanley P, Taylor S. Percutaneous fine needle biopsy in pediatrics. *Pediatr Radiol* 15:409-411, 1985.

12. Akhtar M, Ali MA, Sabbah R, Bakry M, Nash JE. Fine-needle aspiration biopsy diagnosis of round cell malignant tumors in childhood. *Cancer* 55:1805-1817, 1985.

13. Valkov I, Bojikin B. Fine-needle aspiration biopsy of abdominal and retroperitoneal tumors in infants and children. *Diagn Cytopathol* 3:129-133, 1987.

14. Wakely PE Jr, Kardos TF, Frable WJ. Application of fine needle aspiration biopsy to pediatrics. *Hum Pathol* 19:1383-1386, 1988.

15. Verdeguer A, Castel V, Torres V, Olague R, Ferris J, Esquembre C, et al. Fine-needle aspiration biopsy in children. Experience in 70 cases. *Med Pediatr Oncol* 16:98-100, 1988.

16. Rajwanshi A, Raok LN, Marwaha RK, Nijhawan VS, Gupta SK. Role of fine-needle aspiration cytology in childhood malignancies. *Diagn Cytopathol* 5:378-382, 1989.

17. Cohen MB, Bottles K, Ablin AR, Miller TR. The use of fine-needle aspiration biopsy in children. *West J Med* 150:665-667, 1989.

18. Shakoor KA. Fine needle aspiration cytology in advanced pediatric tumors. *Pediatr Pathol* 9:713-718, 1989.

19. Layfield LJ, Glasgow B, Ostrzega N, Reynolds CP. Fine-needle aspiration cytology and the diagnosis of neoplasms in the pediatric age group. *Diag Cytopathol* 7:451-461, 1991.

20. Obers V, Phillips JI. Fine needle aspiration of pediatric abdominal masses. Cytologic and Electron Microscopic Diagnosis. *Acta Cytol* 35:165-170, 1991.

21. Silverman JF, Gurley AM, Holbrook CT, Joshi VV. Pediatric fine-needle aspiration biopsy. *Am J Clin Pathol* 95:653-659, 1991.

22. Gorczyca W, Bedner E, Juszkiewicz P, Chosia M. Aspiration cytology in the diagnosis of malignant tumors in children. *Amer J Pediatr Hematol Oncol* 14:129-135, 1992.

23. Howell LP, Russell LA, Howard PH, Teplitz RL. The cytology of pediatric masses: a differential diagnostic approach. *Diag Cytopathol* 8:107-115, 1992.

24. McGahey BE, Moriarty AT, Nelson WA, Hull MT. Fine-needle aspiration biopsy of small round blue cell tumors of childhood. *Cancer* 69:1067-1073, 1992.

25. Wakely PE, Frable WJ, Kornstein MJ. Role of intraoperative cytopathology in pediatric surgical pathology. *Hum Pathol* 24:311-315, 1993.

26. Young JL Jr, Ries LG, Silverberg E, Horm JW, Miller RW. Cancer incidence, survival, and mortality for children younger than age 15 years. *Cancer* 58:598-602, 1986.

27. Miller RW. Frequency and environmental epidemiology of childhood cancer. In: Principles and Practice of Pediatric Oncology. PA Pizzo, DG Poplack, eds. JB Lippincott, Philadelphia, 1989, p 3-18.

28. Silverman JF, Frable WJ. The use of the Diff-Quik stain in the immediate interpretation of fine-needle aspiration biopsies. *Diagn Cytopathol* 6:366-369, 1990.

29. Dinges H-P, Wirnsberger G, Höfler H. Immunocytochemistry in cytology. Comparative evaluation of different techniques. *Anal Quan Cytol Histol* 11:22-32, 1989.

30. Osamura RY. Applications of immunocytochemistry to diagnostic cytopathology. *Diagn Cytopathol* 5:55-63, 1989.

31. Gurley AM, Silverman JF, Lassaletta MM, Wiley JE, Holbrook CT, Joshi VV. The utility of ancillary studies in pediatric FNA cytology. *Diagn Cytopathol* 8:137-146, 1992.

32. Dabbs DJ, Silverman JF. Selective use of electron microscopy in fine needle aspiration cytology. *Acta Cytol* 32:880-884, 1988.

33. Bloustein P, Silverberg SG. Rapid cytologic examination of surgical specimens. *Pathol Ann* 12:251-278, 1977.

34. Suen KC, Wood WS, Syed AA, Quenville NF, Clement PB. Role of imprint cytology in intraoperative diagnosis: value and limitations. *J Clin Pathol* 31:328-337, 1978.

35. Wilkerson JA, Bonin JM. Intraoperative cytology: An Adjunct to Frozen Sections. Igaku-Shoin, New York, 1987.

36. Nochomovitz L, Sidawy M, Jannotta F, Silverberg S, Schwartz A. Intraoperative Consultation: A Guide to Smears, Imprints, and Frozen Sections. American Society of Clinical Pathologists Press. Chicago, 1989.

CHAPTER TWO

Acute Leukemias

In the United States, the most common form of cancer in children is leukemia.[1,2] Annually, the various forms of leukemia account for 30% to 35% of all new pediatric malignancies. The overwhelming majority are acute leukemias, as less than 5% of all childhood leukemias are of the chronic form; chronic myelogenous leukemia is the most frequent of the latter.[2] This is in contrast to adults in whom the majority of all leukemias are chronic with chronic lymphocytic leukemias the most common. At least 75% of all of the acute leukemias in children have a lymphoid heritage (acute lymphoblastic leukemia, ALL). The remaining 20% are acute nonlymphocytic leukemias (ANLL).[3]

As both ALL and ANLL essentially involve the replacement of normal bone marrow by primitive neoplastic leukocytes, the early and major clinical features in both diseases are similar due to a marked disruption of the normal bone marrow functions.[2,3] The majority of children will have had symptoms and signs of their disease for no more than 2 months prior to diagnosis. Initial complaints are usually nonspecific, such as lethargy and anorexia. As more of the normal hematopoietic elements are overwhelmed, the clinical features directly reflect the degree of pancytopenia. Fever is usually secondary to granulocytopenia with infection. Bleeding in the form of petechiae, purpura and epistaxis are most commonly related to thrombocytopenia. Anemia presents with fatigue and pallor. In ALL, the majority of patients have pancytopenia, two-thirds have hepatosplenomegaly and 50% have lymphadenopathy at presentation.[2] Organomegaly is less frequent with ANLL.[3] Nearly one-fourth of children with ALL have bone and joint pain at the time of presentation. This is related to infiltrates of leukemic blasts in the bone and periosteum and to bleeding in the latter site.

Acute Lymphoblastic Leukemia

The incidence of ALL in patients less than 15 years of age in this country is 4 per 100,000.[2] It has a peak incidence at 4 years of age due predominantly to the "common ALL antigen" (CD10, CALLA) form. Childhood ALL is more common in males than in females, in part reflecting the greater proportion of T-cell ALL in boys, and in whites than in blacks, in part reflecting the greater frequency of the CALLA form in whites.

Genetics provide a major contribution to the development of ALL, as witnessed by the relationship between ALL and constitutional chromosomal abnormalities, the high incidence of ALL in identical twins and familial leukemias.[2] The best recognized association of ALL with a chromosomal syndrome is the greatly increased incidence of lymphoblastic leukemia in children with Down's syndrome (trisomy 21). An accelerated frequency of ALL occurs in association with increasing maternal age, as does Down's syndrome. In monozygotic twins, the concordance rate approaches 20% to 25%. The incidence of ALL is greater in families in which one or more members has had leukemia. All of these data support major genetic influences. Among environmental factors, exposure to ionizing radiation is the best established leukemogen.[1] It remains undecided whether or not such exposure in utero significantly increases the risk of subsequent leukemia.

As stated in the excellent review by Poplack, ALL in children is quite heterogenous from a number of viewpoints including morphology, immunophenotyping and cell genetics.[2] The cytomorphology is of greatest interest to cytologists. The French-American-British (FAB) classification of ALL is based on Wright-stained smears, is very widely

Table 2.1
Morphologic Features of Different Acute Lymphoblastic Leukemias[*]

Cellular Feature	L_1	L_2	L_3
Cell Size	Small, uniform	Variable	Large, uniform
Nuclear Contour	Round, smooth	Variable, may be very irregular with convolutions	Round, smooth
Nucleoli	Rare, inconspicuous	1 or more, small to prominent	1 to 5 prominent
Cytoplasm	Scanty, may have vacuoles	Moderate, may have vacuoles	Moderate, intensely basophilic, prominent vacuoles

[*]Based on data from references 4 and 8.

accepted and divides this leukemia into three forms (L_1, L_2 and L_3).[4] In children, 85% of all cases of ALL are L_1, which is characterized by relatively small, uniform lymphoblasts with high nuclear to cytoplasmic (N/C) ratios (Table 2.1). Nuclear contours are generally smooth and regular, and the chromatin is somewhat clumped but homogeneous; nucleoli are inconspicuous (Images 2.1 through 2.7). L_2 morphology is present in 14% of children and includes blasts of larger and more variable sizes. Nuclei are often irregularly shaped with prominent notches and clefts (Images 2.8 and 2.9). Complex irregularities of the nuclear envelope are commonplace. Although the chromatin is clumped, it is more heterogenous and variable than in L_1 cells. At least one nucleolus usually is readily apparent. N/C ratios are variable and generally lower than in L_1. The L_3 form of ALL corresponds to Burkitt's lymphoma, and thus is composed of uniform large blasts with moderate volumes of intensely basophilic and pyroninophilic cytoplasm with lipid-laden vacuoles. Nuclei are round and uniform, and have finely granular chromatin with multiple obvious nucleoli (Image 2.10).

The L_3 form comprises the B-cell variant of ALL which contributes to only about 1% of all childhood cases. The majority (80%) are considered to be of precursor B cell origin; within this group, approximately 80% are positive for CALLA."[5] The remaining 15% to 20% or so of children have a T-cell neoplasm. Although this is not the appropriate forum for an in-depth discussion of the immunologic typing of ALL, it is relevant to note certain distinguishing features of T-cell ALL. Typically, this form occurs in older children, especially males, who have a very high peripheral blood white cell count at the time of initial diagnosis. About 50% will also have a neoplastic mass in the mediastinum. These patients probably have a greater incidence of involvement of the central nervous system (CNS) by tumor cells. Both pre-B cell and T-cell ALL are positive for terminal deoxynucleotidyl transferase (Tdt), a nuclear antigen.[5]

In ALL, a large number of factors have prognostic implications.[2,6] The better established parameters include the initial peripheral white blood cell count, age at diagnosis, sex, race, FAB type, immunologic type, ploidy and organomegaly. Low cell counts, age between 2 and 10 years, females, whites, L_1 morphology, CALLA-positive pre-B cell phenotype, hyperdiploidy and the absence of hepatosplenomegaly are all associated with a better prognosis. Of these, the factors with the strongest prognostic weight are the initial peripheral blood white blood cell count and patient age.[2] Recently, Cerezo et al found the presence of large azurophilic granules in the cytoplasm of blasts (acute granular ALL) had a negative impact on patient outcome, independent of genetic lineage.[7] This feature was more often present in cells with L_2 morphology than those with the L_1 type. Very recently, Lilleyman and colleagues found a better prognosis for children whose L_1 or L_2 blasts had cytoplasmic vacuoles.[8] In a number of studies, patients with ALL have been stratified into different treatment programs on the basis of some of these risk factors. This tailoring of therapy to "fit" the individual patient is one of the latest in the recent encouraging improvements in the care of these children. As a group, 60% of all children with ALL are cured of their disease.[2]

The diagnosis of ALL is generally made by examination of a bone marrow aspirate and biopsy.[2] It is very rare for ALL to be diagnosed or

The diagnosis of ALL is generally made by examination of a bone marrow aspirate and biopsy

even suggested initially by either exfoliative or aspiration cytology.[9] However, extramedullary spread of ALL is very common and clinically important, as it often signals an impending bone marrow relapse before it becomes evident in either the peripheral blood or bone marrow. Furthermore, it may cause problems locally, at times as a mass lesion. Prior to the introduction of CNS prophylactic therapy (generally craniospinal radiation and intrathecal methotrexate), many patients had CNS relapses, as the CNS is probably the most important sanctuary for leukemic cells. CNS leukemia develops as a result of leukemic metastasis during periods of active hematologic disease; this may occur secondary to either hematogenous spread or extension from involved cranial bone marrow.[2,10,11] Diagnosis of leukemic involvement of the CNS requires the identification of blasts in exfoliative specimens of the cerebrospinal fluid (CSF); this is the area of greatest use of diagnostic cytology in ALL (Image 2.1). Surveillance lumbar punctures are thus an integral component of therapeutic protocols. Less than 1 in 20 children have positive CSF samples at the time of initial diagnosis.[2] Statistically, both T-cell ALL and the acute monocytic leukemias (M_4 and M_5) show a higher incidence of CNS infiltration. With current protocols, CNS involvement may be seen in up to 10% of patients and thus remains an important problem. CNS relapse may be symptomatic, generally with signs of elevated intracranial pressure, but more often is occult (asymptomatic). In either case, these children are at very high risk to develop a systemic (bone marrow) relapse as leukemic elements may seed extrameningeal sites. Unfortunately, this often proves refractory to therapy and thus is fatal.

Diagnosis of leukemic involvement of the CNS requires the identification of blasts in exfoliative specimens of the cerebrospinal fluid (CSF); this is the area of greatest use of diagnostic cytology in ALL

Acute Nonlymphocytic Leukemia

Nearly 20% of all pediatric leukemias are ANLL.[3] This percentage holds constant throughout childhood except for the newborn period when it is more common than ALL. In the United States, no sex or racial predispositions are recognized. Seven major subtypes of ANLL are now recognized by the FAB classification system (Images 2.11 through 2.16).[12-14] It is not the intent of this discussion to review these subtypes, but suffice it to say that it is based on the degree to which the neoplastic leukocytes resemble the various myeloid cell line components (myeloblasts, promyelocytes, monocytes, erythroblasts and megakaryoblasts) cytologically and cytochemically (Table 2.2). In patients younger than 2 years, the monocytic leukemias (M_5) are the most frequent, whereas in older children, myeloblastic and myelomonocytic (M_1, M_2, M_4) leukemias predominate. Each subtype is associated with different specific karyotypic abnormalities. The majority of cases of ANLL in children are hypodiploid. In a very low percentage of instances, blasts are Tdt-positive.

At the time of initial diagnosis, leukemic blasts are present in the CSF in 5% to 20% of ANLL patients.[3,15,16] Several investigations suggest that this early CNS disease may be associated with patient age less than 2 years, high peripheral white blood cell count and the M_4 and M_5 subtypes.[15,16] These three factors may also be associated with a

Table 2.2

Morphologic, Cytochemical and Immunocytochemical Features of
Different Acute Myelogenous Leukemias

Type	Diagnostic Features
Undifferentiated	Little maturation with few if any promyelocytes.
Myeloblastic (M_1)	> 3% myeloperoxidase (MPX) positive.
Myeloblastic with Maturation (M_2)	Over 50% of cell blasts plus promyelocytes and presence of more mature forms.
Promyelocytic (M_3)	Hypergranular blasts and promyelocytes. Some cells have monocytoid nuclei.
Myelomonocytic (M_4)	Both neutrophilic and monocytic lines involved with monocytic cells comprising > 20% and < 80%. Monocytic cells are nonspecific esterase (ANAE) positive. Neutrophilic cells are MPX positive.
Monocytic (M_5)	> 80% are of monocytic lineage. ANAE positive.
Erythroleukemic	Both neutrophilic and erythroid precursors present. Erythroid cells are often PAS positive and may be multinucleated.
Megakaryoblastic (M_7)	Positive for platelet peroxidase by immunoelectron microscopy, or immunocytochemical demonstration of von Willebrand Factor or glycoprotein IIb/IIIa.

Table 2.3

Acute Leukemia - Cytomorphology

Intercellular cohesion is not seen; leukemic elements occur as single, solitary cells. In aspiration smears, pseudocohesion may be seen.

Leukemic blasts are 2 to 3 times larger than mature lymphocytes with larger nuclei; very high N/C ratio.

Cytoplasm: Pap stain - scanty, cyanophilic, nonspecific.

Giemsa stain - more apparent, basophilic, may show diagnostic

features, eg, Auer rods, primary granules, lipid-positive vacuoles.

Nuclei: Pap stain - distinct nuclear membranes, finely granular chromatin.

Giemsa stain - fine to more coarsely reticulated chromatin.

Irregularities of nuclear membrane contours in ALL-L_2 & AML-M_4 & M_5.

Except in ALL-L_1, nucleoli are well developed.

poorer overall prognosis. Prior to the advent of CNS preventive therapy, up to 20% of patients had relapses within the CNS. Currently, CNS relapse occurs in less than 10%.

As stated above, the major arenas for diagnostic cytology in the acute leukemias is in the identification of the uncommon early involvement of the CNS and in monitoring for the more frequent relapse. Thus, many laboratories that deal with nongynecologic exfoliative specimens examine CSF for these purposes. The literature still debates the merits and disadvantages of different preparatory techniques. In the largest published study, Davey et al found Millipore filtration and cytocentrifugation to be equally sensitive in detecting involvement by acute leukemia and recommended that laboratories did not need to perform both procedures. They preferred cytocentrifuged CSF samples as the morphology found therein more closely resembled that in bone marrow aspirates.[17] In this study, the authors compared 300 CSF specimens from 17 children with acute leukemias (16 ALL; 1 ANLL). For all 300 fluids, both a filter preparation stained by the Papanicolaou technique and a cytospin preparation stained with Wright's stain were evaluated. In 91 cases, blasts were present in at least one of the two paired preparations. Both members of these pairs were positive for blasts in 77 pairs (85% agreement). Of the 14 pairs with discordant results, 7 pairs had positive filters and negative cytopsins, and 7 produced the opposite results. When all 300 pairs were considered, there was agreement in 95%. The major cause of a discrepancy within the pairs was inadequate staining or cellular preservation. When faced with a relatively scanty volume of CSF, we agree with Davey and her colleagues that a cytospin preparation is preferable.[17] We and others agree, however, with the companion editorial by Gondos, which favored employing both of these complementary modalities; although it increases cost, it also increases diagnostic sensitivity.[18,19]

In Papanicolaou-stained smears of CSF, leukemic blasts are usually easily identified (Table 2.3) although they are smaller than on the air-dried Wright-stained slides.[19-22] They are larger than normal lymphocytes with larger nuclei and have very high N/C ratios (Images 2.17 through 2.20). Very characteristically, their nuclear membranes are thick and distinctive and appear to blend focally with the cell membranes.[19-22] They may be irregular with clefts, protrusions and convolutions, especially in ALL; in ANLL, smoother outlines are more likely. Chromatin is usually finely granular and evenly distributed and nucleoli and/or chromocenters are often readily apparent. In ANLL, cells with greater volumes of cytoplasm may be present. In the M_4 and M_5 forms, nuclei may be more reniform and the N/C ratio may be considerably reduced (their cytomorphology in Wright-stained specimens is discussed above). In all specimen types, intercellular cohesion is lacking, thus true cellular aggregation is absent.

The important considerations in the differential diagnosis of acute leukemia in the CSF includes benign reactive pleocytosis, contamination of the CSF by blast-containing peripheral blood, and primitive primary brain tumors.[11,17,19-25] The reactive inflammatory cell infiltrates may be highly cellular and include immature-appearing mononuclear cells (Image 2.21). In the series reported by McIntosh and Ritchey, the No. 1 cause of pleocytosis in children with acute leukemia was an inflammatory reaction induced by prophylactic CNS therapy, that is, the arachnoiditis secondary to intrathecal chemotherapy or radiation.[23] Other causes of benign pleocytosis include infectious (especially viral) meningitis, immune reconstitution following therapy, and bleeding including that associated with traumatic lumbar puncture.[19,20,23,24] On a single cell-for-cell basis, it is our opinion that one may not be able to distinguish between benign and malignant cells in this setting. Of course, an appropriate clinical history is always important when examining the CSF, as for other cytologic specimens.

The major consideration in the differential diagnosis of benign pleocytosis is, of course, meningeal leukemia.[10,11] During the last several decades, the criteria for an absolute diagnosis of CNS leukemia have evolved as the clinical importance of this determination has grown. If,

The major consideration in the differential diagnosis of benign pleocytosis is, of course, meningeal leukemia

on the one hand, a patient has CNS leukemia, additional therapy is required, and to withhold it due to a false negative CSF diagnosis could prove fatal. However, therapy aimed at preventing or eradicating the CNS of malignant blasts is also not innocuous; thus, a false-positive diagnosis could prove harmful to the patient. For several decades, an outright diagnosis required both a hemocytometer count of 10 or more white blood cells per microliter and the presence of morphologically unequivocal blasts. McIntosh and Ritchey evaluated 15 children with malignant lymphoid tumors with CSF specimens that had fewer than 11 cells/μL with 1 or more unequivocal blasts.[23] Only 3 of these patients developed CNS leukemia. All 3 had between 5 and 10 cells/μL and 2 or more blasts in their fluids. Despite the presence of blasts, 4 other children did not progress to CNS disease during long follow-up periods. No child with either cell counts less than 5 or only 1 blast per specimen developed CNS leukemia. As a result, these authors cautioned that one should have a relatively conservative outlook with such specimens.[23] This concept is supported by Borowitz et al.[21] Davey et al, in contrast, believed that the CSF is involved whenever blasts are present, even if in low numbers, as long as peripheral blood contamination can be excluded.[17] That is, a CSF specimen should be considered positive for leukemia if unequivocal blasts are present, regardless of the cell count, since all specimens in their series with low counts (5 or fewer white cells/μL) were either immediately preceded or followed by a specimen demonstrating florid CNS involvement. Evans et al found that one-quarter of CSF samples with high white cell counts did not have blasts and that nearly one-third with a normal count did contain blasts.[24] Of those with blast cells in a normal count fluid, blasts ranged from 2% to 39%. Of those with high total counts but no blasts, only a small minority of patients suffered subsequent CNS relapses. These authors also did not find a good correlation between specimens with low cell counts and the numbers of cells on a cytospin preparation.[24] Generally, the CSF is now considered positive in patients with ALL when there are more than 5 white cells/mL and definite lymphoblasts are present.[6] Recently, Odom and colleagues published a detailed study in which they evaluated the clinical significance for children with ALL of CSF specimens with fewer than 6 white cells/mL in a hemocytometer chamber and 5% or more blasts in a cytospin preparation.[26] 58 children yielded 109 such specimens. The entire study included 332 children, 25 of whom developed CNS relapses. Of these 25, 22 had one or more abnormal low-count specimens, as described above. Approximately 60% of children in remission with one or more such CSF specimens developed relapses within the CNS. This was especially true in those children with two or more abnormal low count specimens. Interestingly, these findings appear not to carry the same weight in CSF specimens obtained at the time of initial diagnosis, but rather only in children in clinical remission.[26] This, of course, confirms the utility of surveillance lumbar punctures in this clinical setting. Aaronson et al described 112 specimens for 38 children with acute leukemia.[20] Cell counts were actually performed on the Papanicolaou-stained smears (and not in hemocytometer chambers). Their criteria for a positive CSF specimen included the presence of definite leukemic blasts and a predominance of blasts over other cell types. When 40% or more of cells were blasts, then the CSF was considered positive. Absolute blast counts were not significant, as high blast counts were found in some benign conditions; however, in these conditions, they comprised only 5% of the cells present. Furthermore, absolute blast counts did not correlate with either clinical symptomology or with the degree of meningeal infiltration seen at autopsy.

As suggested by others, comparison of current CSF specimens with prior positive CSF specimens and with the peripheral blood and marrow can be helpful.[21,22] When faced with only Papanicolaou-stained CSF smears, it may be preferable to be cautious when evaluating mixed cellular infiltrates. As stated above, it is preferable to have slides stained with both Wright and Papanicolaou stains.[18,19] In very infrequent instances, however, the tumor cells in the CSF may have distinctly different cytologic morphology from those present in the marrow.[27] In difficult cases, one may resort to staining for Tdt.[28,29] This *nuclear* antigen is positive in the overwhelming majority of cases of pediatric ALL and should be negative in benign reactive cells within the CSF. Flow cytometry for ploidy and immunostaining for surface antigens have also been proposed to overcome this problem. No more than approximately 3% of all cells in normal CSF are CALLA-positive.[30-32] However, Tdt is the most specific and perhaps the most sensitive of the three as a marker for leukemic cells.[11,29] Another useful step is "tincture of time." In equivocal cases, repeat lumbar puncture after a period may very well answer the question.[21-23]

The single most common problem in daily practice is the potential contamination of CSF by blast-containing peripheral blood in the course of a bloody tap.[17,19,21-23,33] This seems most likely to occur before remission has been induced (Image 2.22). The question, of course, is whether or not the blasts are due to true infiltrates by leukemic cells in the meninges or are simply carried over as part of the peripheral blood. Only a very small volume of peripheral blood is necessary to "contaminate significantly" the CSF with white cells.[33] At times, comparison of the CSF with the peripheral blood smear may be helpful. If the blasts comprise a much greater proportion of the total cellular population in the CSF than in the peripheral blood, it is probable that CNS disease is present. Davey et al have claimed that it is easier to recognize peripheral blood contamination in a Wright-stained cytospin preparation compared to a Papanicolaou-stained membrane filter.[17] This is due, at least in part, to the lysis of erythrocytes by ethanol.[33] We may need, however, to resort to actual cell counts of the white and red blood cells within the CSF and blood. Insertion of these figures into a formula will then give a corrected total white cell count for the CSF specimen. The formula that we utilize is that supplied by Kjeldsberg and Knight.[34] It consists of:

$$W = WBC_f - \frac{WBC_b - RBC_f}{RBC_b}$$

where: W = CSF white cell count before the addition of blood
WBC_f = total CSF white cell count
WBC_b = white cell count in blood
RBC_f = red cell count in CSF
RBC_b = red cell count in blood

The CSF may also be directly contaminated by bone marrow when the spinal needle inadvertently enters the vertebral marrow during a lumbar puncture (Image 2.23). Craver and Carson have utilized the presence of intermediate stage normoblasts to identify such contamination.[35]

Medulloblastoma and related primitive tumors are made up of small malignant cells that may resemble leukemic blasts (Image 2.24). [20,22,25] Aaronson and colleagues claimed that the chromatin in these primitive neuroectodermal tumor cells is more homogenous and hyperchromatic and the nucleoli are more prominent than in leukemic blasts.[20] More importantly, these neoplastic elements have a proclivity for intercellular cohesion, including the formation of rosettes (Image 2.25).[20,25] Such aggregation does not occur with the leukemias.

Rosenthal calls attention to the additional problems that may be encountered in the evaluation of CSF in children receiving intrathecal chemotherapy.[22] The degenerative changes in nuclei can be impressive. Progressively, the chromatin will form larger aggregates, the nucleus may become totally pyknotic and eventually lyse (Images 2.26 and 2.27). She recommends study of the nuclear membranes, which may be disrupted as a telltale sign that they are degenerative. Degenerative changes, however, were not considered to be well developed by Aaronson and colleagues.[20] In their series, positive CSF specimens abruptly converted to negative with therapy without intermediate or transitional morphologic stages.

As stated above, chronic leukemias are quite unusual in children. Furthermore, in contrast to adults in whom chronic lymphocytic leukemia is most frequent, the most common type in the pediatric population is chronic granulocytic leukemia (CGL). It is decidedly rare for the CSF to contain malignant elements in CGL or its blast crises.[36]

Many of these guidelines hold for the evaluation of other exfoliative specimens as well. It is not rare at all to be called upon to look for leukemic cells in serous effusions, especially in our experience, pleural fluids. In this situation as well, both Romanowsky and Papanicolaou-stained specimens are preferable. Quite infrequently, we have seen leukemic blasts in urine and bronchial specimens. The latter were usually obtained from children with pulmonary infiltrates with a suspicion of infection; the presence of malignant elements is usually a surprise to the pediatrician.

Usually, ancillary diagnostic tests are unnecessary in exfoliative cytologic specimens. They may have a greater role to play in the diagnosis of fine needle aspiration (FNA) material. As discussed earlier, evaluation of Tdt will help to confirm the vast majority of cases of ALL.[28,29] Leukemic blasts and lymphomatous elements will react with leukocyte common antigen (CD45), whereas other small cell tumors of childhood will not.[37] Blasts are negative for desmin, neuron-specific enolase and cytokeratin. Electron microscopy is generally not diagnostically helpful (or at least essential) in the leukemias.

It is relatively uncommon for the acute leukemias to form mass lesions (including lymphadenopathy), although it certainly does occur, especially as an unexpected relapse. Several groups have reported using FNA to examine testicular enlargement in boys with ALL.[38-40] We have no personal experience with this situation, but FNA appears to be more sensitive than the more conventional wedge biopsy. In positive gonads, leukemic elements dominate the cytologic picture with only a few Sertoli cells present.[38-40]

In FNA smears, leukemic cells individually resemble those seen in exfoliative specimens, except their N/C ratio may be slightly lower and they may have more irregular cellular contours (Images 2.28 through 2.31). True intercellular cohesion is absent, although tumor cells may appear "aggregated." Certainly, organoid structures and differentiation are not present. Lymphoglandular bodies may be diffusely scattered about the smear background.

Although they will be discussed in much greater detail in subsequent sections of this book, the malignant lymphomas should be mentioned here as well. Tumor cells in the non-Hodgkin's lymphomas may be morphologically indistinguishable from or may very closely resemble leukemic blasts. It is very uncommon for any of the childhood lymphomas to involve the CNS at the time of initial presentation. Frequency is increased when the bone marrow is positive at diagnosis and with the large cell type of lymphoma. Yet, when lymphomatous elements are present within the CSF early in the course, this is a bad prognostic indicator. CSF cytology is part of the initial diagnostic workup of children with non-Hodgkin's lymphomas (Images 2.32 through 2.34). According to Magrath, spread to the CNS, however, will occur in a large proportion of patients if CNS prophylactic therapy is not provided.[41] Helson's extensive review included 37 children with non-Hodgkin's malignant lymphomas who provided a total of 321 CSF specimens.[42] Of these, 16 (5%) were positive for malignant cells. The study by McIntosh and Ritchey included 25 children with non-Hodgkin's lymphomas, only one of whom had tumor cells in the CSF and suffered a relapse. As discussed by Jones et al, primary CNS lymphomas are exceedingly uncommon in pediatric patients.[43] Just as rare is CNS involvement in Hodgkin's disease at any point in the clinical course. A cytologic examination of the CSF is generally not included in the evaluation of children with Hodgkin's disease,[44] and in Helson's study, the CSF was not examined cytologically in any of the 27 children with Hodgkin's disease. We have not seen neoplastic Reed-Sternberg cells in the CSF of a child.

Image 2.1

The CSF may be hypercellular ("over-run" with lymphoblasts) in ALL, both at the time of initial diagnosis and at relapse. In such cases, the diagnosis of malignancy is obvious. When cytospin preparations such as this one are so crowded with cells, they may give the impression of aggregation of tumor cells. This pseudocohesion needs to be distinguished from true intercellular cohesion. (Romanowsky).

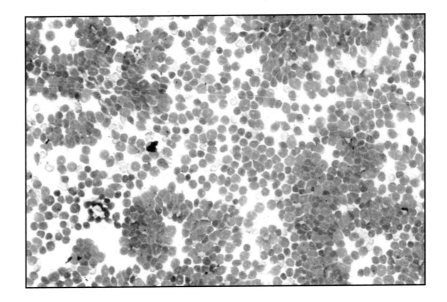

Image 2.2

The tumor cells in acute leukemia and other lymphoreticular malignancies occur in fluids as a single cell suspension due to the lack of intercellular cohesion. Even at low magnifications, the malignant lymphoblasts appear larger than normal lymphocytes; the prominent heterogeneity of a reactive process is absent. (Romanowsky).

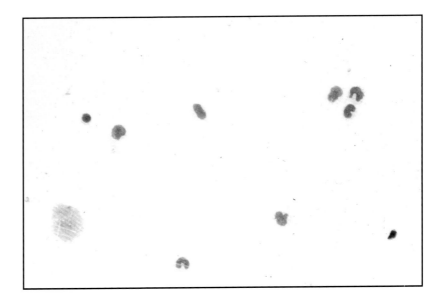

Image 2.3

In ALL-L$_1$, cytoplasm is barely perceptible in many blasts. Occasional cells may have cytoplasmic vacuoles, as present in a few of these neoplastic elements. Chromatin is clumped, but nucleoli are evident in a few nuclei. (Romanowsky).

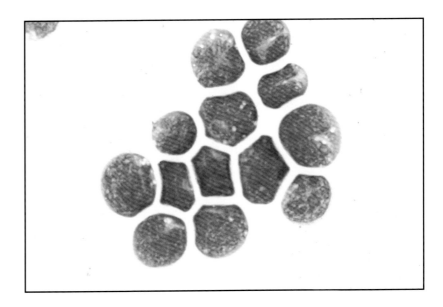

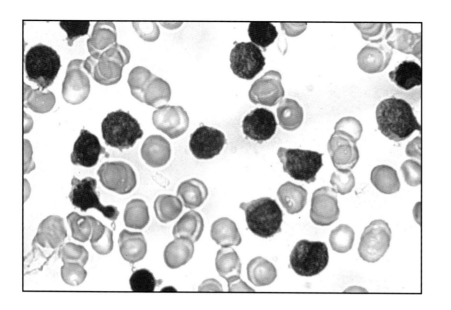

Image 2.4
In the L₁ form of ALL the lymphoblasts are small and uniform. They have a single round nucleus with relatively smooth contours. Chromatin is clumped and nucleoli are generally small and inconspicuous. N/C are high with only a thin rim of basophilic cytoplasm visible in a few cells. (Romanowsky).

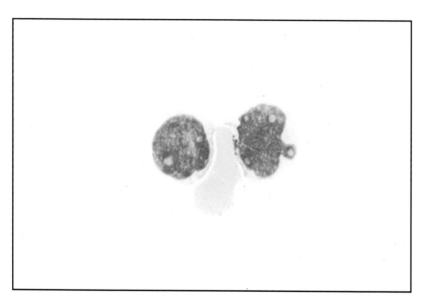

Image 2.5
Although uncommon, a characteristic appearance of malignant lymphoblasts in ALL and some lymphomas is the outward protrusion of the nuclear envelope as seen in the cell on the right. Chromatin is finely reticulated and evenly dispersed in both nuclei, which have small nucleoli (ALL-L₁). (Romanowsky).

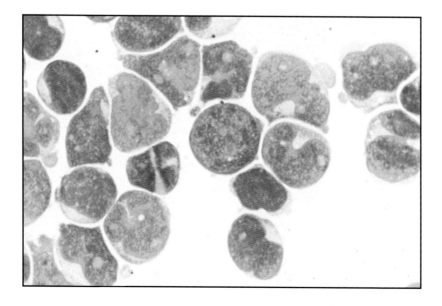

Image 2.6
Compared to touch preparations, greater irregularities in nuclear outlines may be evident with cytospin preparations, as seen in this example of ALL-L₁. (Romanowsky).

Image 2.7
This is an example of recurrent ALL-L₁ in a 5-year-old boy. Nucleoli are visible and are more apparent than prior to chemotherapy. Note the persistence of high N/C ratio and chromatin clumping and the mitotic figure. (Romanowsky).

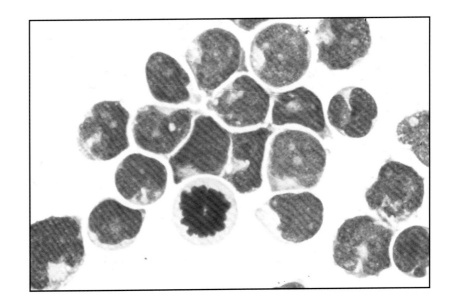

Image 2.8
In ALL-L₂, some of the lymphoblasts are larger than in ALL-L₁, with a spectrum of cellular sizes. (Romanowsky).

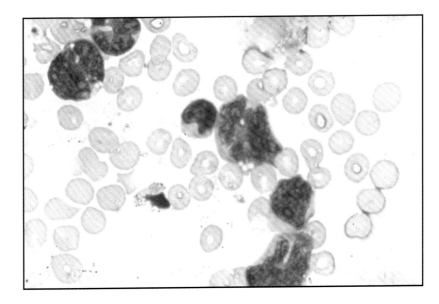

Image 2.9
In ALL-L₂, irregularities of the nuclear outlines are expected and they may be quite complex. They may include multiple small notches due to convolutions and deep indentations of the nuclear membranes. Cytoplasmic vacuoles may be apparent. (Romanowsky).

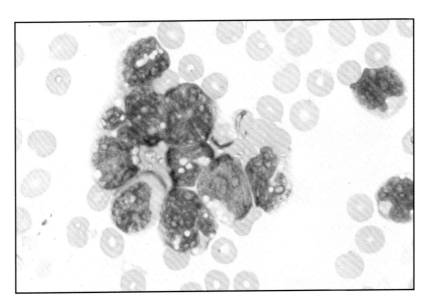

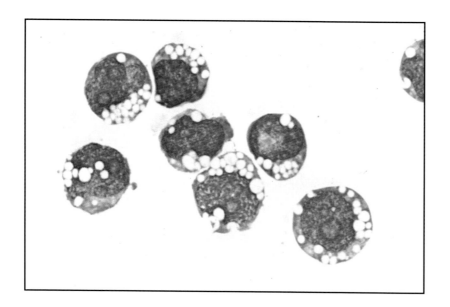

Image 2.10
In the uncommon L$_3$ form of ALL, the lymphoblasts are larger and relatively uniform. Compared with the L$_1$ variant, nuclei are larger, have a more open chromatin pattern, and multiple obvious nucleoli. Nuclear contours are generally round and smooth. Cytoplasm is usually readily apparent, deeply basophilic, and often highly vacuolated. (Romanowsky).

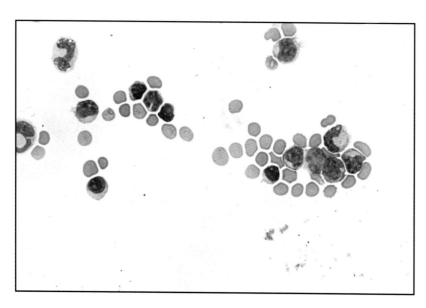

Image 2.11
This CSF specimen is positive for acute myeloblastic leukemia (AML). A greater degree of heterogeneity is seen among the malignant cells that is typical of ALL. Note the absence of fully mature granulocytes. (Romanowsky).

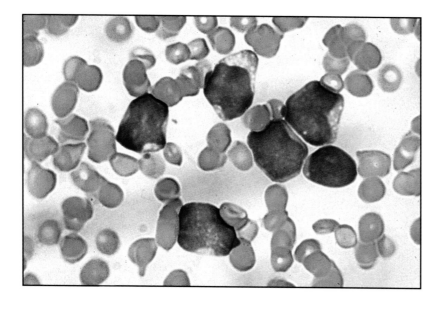

Image 2.12
In AML-M$_1$, the myeloblasts have a very high N/C ratio and show no evidence of differentiation. Their chromatin is finely reticulated and uniformly distributed throughout the round nuclei. One or more well-defined nucleoli may be seen. (Romanowsky).

Image 2.13
In AML-M$_2$, some of the malignant cells may resemble promyelocytes and metamyelocytes, although cytoplasmic granularity often is poorly developed. (Romanowsky).

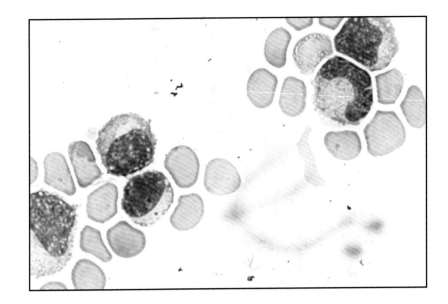

Image 2.14
This is an example of recurrent AML presenting in the CSF. Secondary granulocytic granules appear to be present in the cytoplasm of several malignant cells. (Romanowsky).

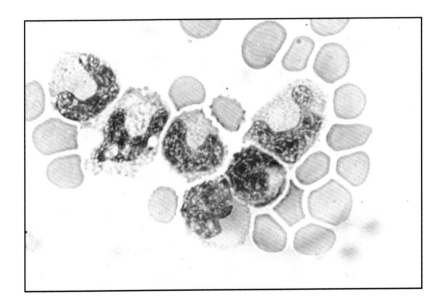

Image 2.15
This is an example of AML-M$_3$ (from an adult patient). The neoplastic cells have abundant cytoplasm that contains numerous small primary granules (microgranular variant). Only very rarely do these cells present in the CSF. (Romanowsky).

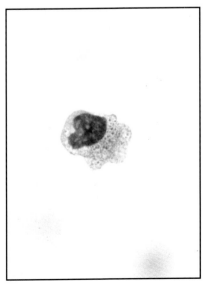
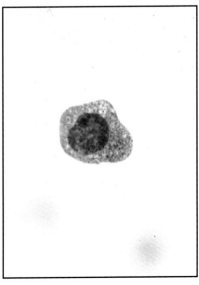

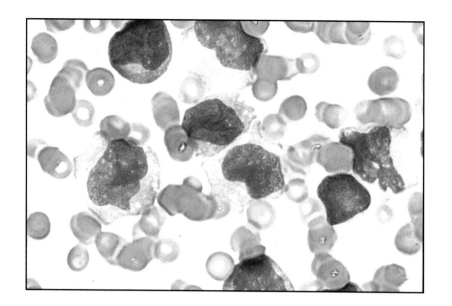

Image 2.16
In AML-M₅, greater volumes of cytoplasm may be present. It has a characteristic slate-gray hue and may contain multiple minute vacuoles. Nuclear contour is varied from round to quite irregular. Typically, some will be reniform. Chromatin is finely reticulated and nucleoli may be seen. (Romanowsky).

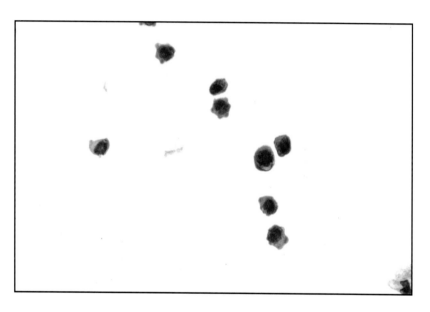

Image 2.17
Leukemic myeloblasts from a child with AML-M₂ present as a single cell suspension in this CSF prepared by the Papanicolaou method. Compared to the Romanowsky-stain preparations, the tumor cells are smaller. Yet, their malignant nature is obvious due to their large hyperchromatic nuclei and high N/C ratio. Although these malignant cells are not highly uniform, they do not exhibit the heterogenicity typical of a benign reactive pleocytosis. (Papanicolaou).

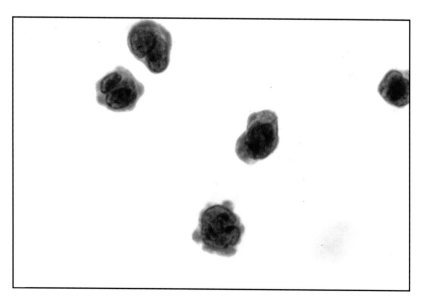

Image 2.18
Distinct thick nuclear membranes are present in these leukemic myeloblasts (M₂) due to peripheral chromatin condensation. The chromatin is finely granular and rather evenly distributed throughout the nuclei, which are quite variable in outline. Nucleoli are apparent. Somewhat great volumes of cytoplasm than expected in ALL are evident. (Papanicolaou).

Image 2.19
This is the same CSF specimen as in Image 2.18. Again, note the distinct nuclear membranes, the uniformly distributed chromatin, and the small nucleoli. (Papanicolaou).

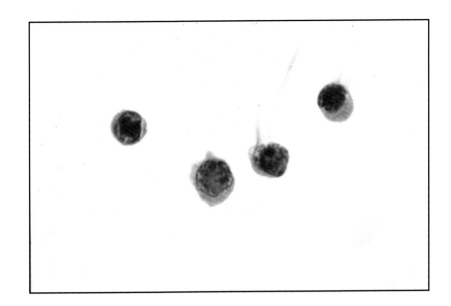

Image 2.20
A composite of CSF specimens from three children with ALL with involvement of the meninges. Note the relative uniformity of the leukemic blasts with their single round nucleus, distinct nuclear membranes, and finely granular chromatin. (Papanicolaou).

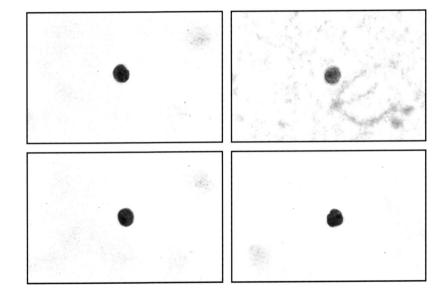

Image 2.21
Benign pleocytosis in a child treated for ALL. Although the CSF is cellular, malignant blasts are absent. Instead, there is an admixture of numerous monocytoid forms and a few granulocytes. Nuclei have condensed chromatin. Cytoplasm is moderately abundant and the N/C ratio is low. (Romanowsky).

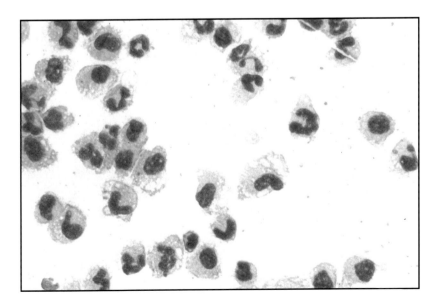

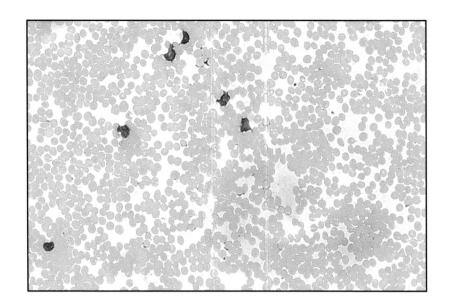

Image 2.22
Contamination of the CSF with peripheral blood due to a traumatic lumbar puncture. This specimen was obtained from a 4-year-old girl at the time of her initial diagnosis. Blasts were circulating in the blood, creating a potential false-positive CSF specimen. There are numerous erythrocytes present. (Romanowsky).

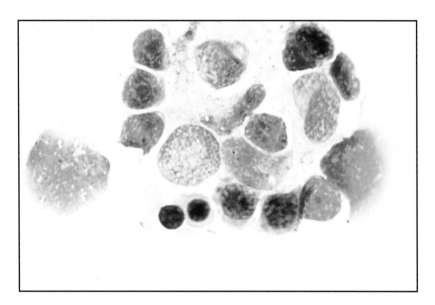

Image 2.23
Large primitive noncohesive cells are present in this CSF specimen due to contamination by vertebral bone marrow. Various stages of normoblasts are seen. (Romanowsky). (Courtesy of Dr R Craver).

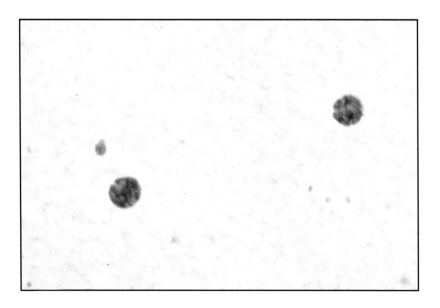

Image 2.24
CSF from a child with recurrent medulloblastoma. The specimen is dominated by individually dispersed malignant cells, each with a single round nucleus and a very high N/C ratio. It may be very difficult to distinguish from leukemic elements. (Papanicolaou).

Image 2.25
CSF from another child with medulloblastoma. True intercellular cohesion including molding is evident among the malignant cells. (Papanicolaou).

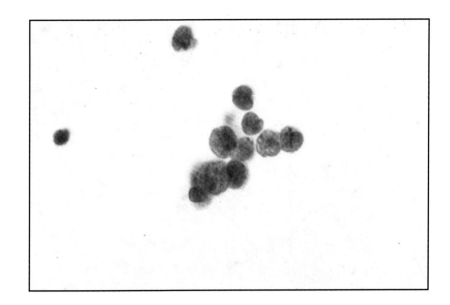

Image 2.26
CSF from a child with partially treated Burkitt's lymphoma. In this blast, relatively early degenerative changes include condensation of chromatin and focal disruption of the nuclear envelope. (Romanowsky).

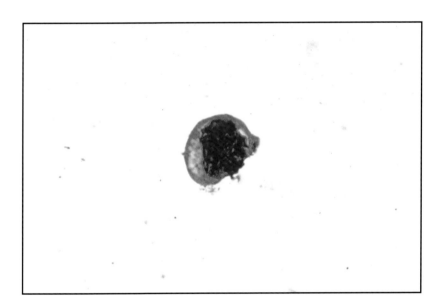

Image 2.27
CSF from a child with a partially treated Burkitt's lymphoma (see Image 2.25). The chromatin forms an almost homogenous mass without any detectable structure. Marked irregularities of the nuclear membrane are unexpected in Burkitt's lymphoma and probably reflect irreversible cell damage secondary to chemotherapy. Its cytoplasm has lost some of its basophilia and its vacuoles. (Romanowsky).

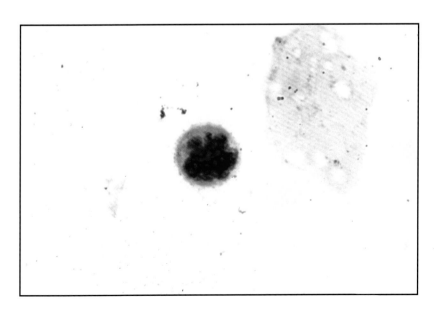

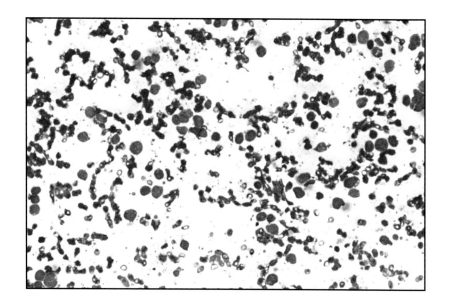

Image 2.28
Smear of a parotid FNA in an 8-year-old boy with ALL-L$_1$ in apparent remission. The smear contains numerous isolated tumor cells with very high N/C ratio. Even at low magnification, their uniformity is apparent. Lymphoglandular bodies are evident in the background. (Romanowsky).

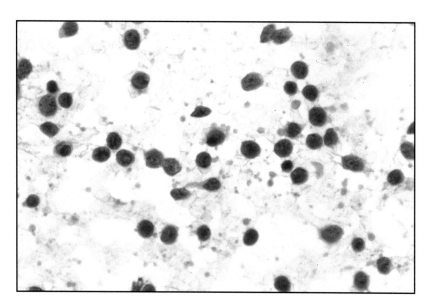

Image 2.29
This is the Papanicolaou-stained smear from the specimen shown in Image 2.28. Note again the uniformity of the blasts and the lymphoglandular bodies.

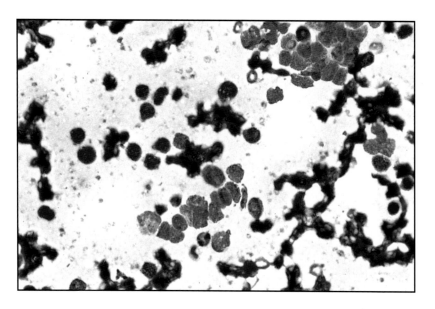

Image 2.30
Smear of a parotid FNA specimen (see Image 2.28). Pseudocohesion is evident among the leukemic elements. This aggregation may occur in aspirates, but will not be seen in exfoliative specimens. Note the presence of isolated malignant cells and lymphoglandular bodies. (Romanowsky).

Image 2.31
The same specimen as in Image 2.28. Individual blasts have round nuclei with finely reticulated chromatin and inconspicuous nucleoli. (Romanowsky).

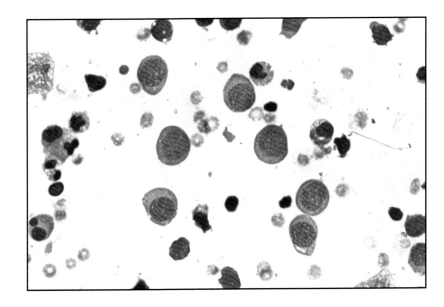

Image 2.32
CSF in a patient in whom the meninges were involved by lymphoblastic lymphoma. Presenting as a single cell suspension, the lymphomatous blasts have thick and somewhat irregular nuclear membranes, fine chromatin, generally inconspicuous nucleoli and high N/C ratio. (Papanicolaou).

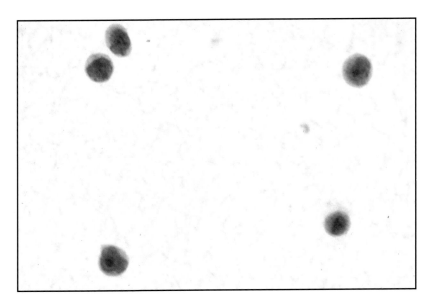

Image 2.33
Lymphoblastic lymphoma is usually a T-cell tumor and often the malignant cells have complex twisted nuclei. They have very fine, even chromatin and lack nucleoli. (Romanowsky).

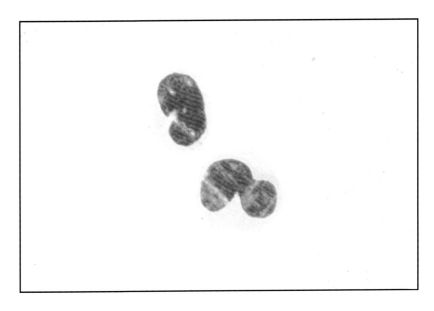

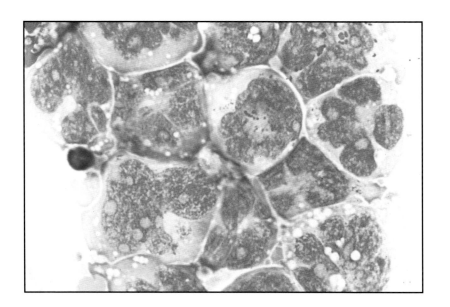

Image 2.34
In large cell lymphoma, malignant cells larger than those in either lymphoblastic or Burkitt's lymphomas will be present. In this CSF specimen, deep nuclear indentations and other complex irregularities are evident, as are well developed and often multiple nucleoli. Cytoplasm is also readily apparent. (Romanowsky).

References

1. Miller RW. Frequency and environmental epidemiology of childhood cancer. In: Principles and Practice of Pediatric Oncology. PA Pizzo, DG Poplack, eds. JB Lippincott, Philadelphia, 1989.

2. Poplack DG. Acute lymphoblastic leukemia. In: Principles and Practice of Pediatric Oncology. PA Pizzo, DG Poplack, eds. JB Lippincott, Philadelphia, 1989.

3. Grier HE, Weinstein HJ. Acute nonlymphocytic leukemia. In: Principles and Practice of Pediatric Oncology. PA Pizzo, DG Poplack, eds. JB Lippincott, Philadelphia, 1989.

4. Bennett JM, Catovsky MD, Daniel MT, Flandrin G, Galton DAG, Gralnick HR, Sultan C. Proposals for the classification of the acute leukemias. French-American-British Cooperative Group. *Br J Haematol* 33:451, 1976.

5. Cabrera ME. Immunologic classification of acute lymphoblastic leukemia. *Am J Ped Hematol Oncol* 12:283-291, 1990.

6. Mastrangelo R, Poplack D, Bleyer A, Riccardi R, Sather H, D'Angio G. Report and recommendations of the Rome workshop concerning poor-prognosis acute lymphoblastic leukemia in children: biologic basis for staging, stratification, and treatment. *Med Pediatr Oncol* 14:191-194, 1986.

7. Cerezo L, Shuster JJ, Pullen J, Brock B, Borowitz MJ, Falletta JM, Crist WM, Head DR. Laboratory correlates and prognostic significance of granular acute lymphoblastic leukemia in children. A Pediatric Oncology Group Study. *Am J Clin Pathol* 95:526-531, 1991.

8. Lilleyman JS, Hann IM, Stevens RF, Richards SM, Eden OB, Chessells JM, Baily CC. Cytomorphology of childhood lymphoblastic leukemia: a prospective study of 2000 patients. *Br J Haematol* 81:52-57, 1992.

9. Ganick DJ, Sondel PM, Gilbert EF, Borcherding W. Leukemia presenting as central nervous disease without bone marrow involvement. *Med Ped Oncol* 11:229-232, 1983.

10. Bleyer WA. Biology and pathogenesis of CNS leukemia. *Am J Ped Hematol Oncol* 11:57-63, 1989.

11. Lauer SJ, Kirchner PA, Camitta BM. Identification of leukemic cells in the cerebrospinal fluid from children with acute lymphoblastic leukemia: advances and dilemmas. *Am J Ped Hematol Oncol* 11:64-73, 1989.

12. Bennett JM, Catovsky MD, Daniel MT, Flandrin G, Galton DAG, Gralnick HR, Sultan C. Proposed revised criteria for the classification of acute myeloid leukemia. A report of the French-American-British Cooperative Group. *Ann Intern Med* 103:620-625, 1985.

13. Bennett JM, Catovsky MD, Daniel MT, Flandrin G, Galton DAG, Gralnick HR, Sultan C. Criteria for the diagnosis of acute leukemia of megakaryocyte lineage (M_7). A report of the French-American-British Cooperative Group. *Ann Intern Med* 103:460-462, 1985.

14. Windebank KP, Tefferi A, Smithson WA, Li C-Y, Solberg LA Jr, Priest JR, Elliot SC, de Alarcon PA, Weinblatt ME, Burgert EO Jr. Acute megakaryocytic leukemia (M_7) in children. *Mayo Clin Proc* 64:1339-1351, 1989.

15. Pui C-H, Dahl GV, Kalwinsky DK, Look AT, Mirro J, Dodge RK, Simone JV. Central nervous system leukemia in children with acute nonlymphoblastic leukemia. *Blood* 66:1062-1067, 1985.

16. Grier HE, Gelber RD, Camitta BM, Delorey MJ, Link MP, Price KN, Leavitt PR, Weinstein HJ. Prognostic factors in childhood acute myelogenous leukemia. *J Clin Oncol* 5:1026-1032, 1985.

17. Davey DD, Foucar K, Giller R. Millipore filter vs. cytocentrifuge for detection of childhood central nervous system leukemia. *Arch Pathol Lab Med* 110:705-708, 1986.

18. Gondos B. Millipore filter vs. cytocentrifuge for evaluation of cerebrospinal fluid. *Arch Pathol Lab Med* 110:687-688, 1986.

19. Bigner SH, Johnson WW. The cytopathology of cerebrospinal fluid. I. Nonneoplastic conditions, lymphoma and leukemia. *Acta Cytol* 25:335-353, 1981.

20. Aaronson AG, Hajdu SI, Melamed MR. Spinal fluid cytology during chemotherapy of leukemia of the central nervous system in children. *Am J Clin Pathol* 63:528-537, 1975.

21. Borowitz M, Bigner SH, Johnston WW. Diagnostic problems in the cytologic evaluation of cerebrospinal fluid for lymphoma and leukemia. *Acta Cytol* 25:665-674, 1981.

22. Rosenthal DL. Cytology of the Central Nervous System. K Karger, Basel, 1984.

23. McIntosh S, Ritchey AK. Diagnostic problems in cerebrospinal fluid of children with lymphoid malignancies. *Am J Ped Hematol Oncol* 8:28-31, 1986.

24. Evans DIK, O'Rourke C, Morris Jones P. The cerebrospinal fluid in acute leukaemia of childhood: studies with the cytocentrifuge. *J Clin Pathol* 27:226-230, 1974.

25. Geisinger KR, Hajdu SI, Helson L. Exfoliative cytology of non-lymphoreticular neoplasms in children. *Acta Cytol* 28:16-28, 1984.

26. Odom LF, Wilson H, Cullen J, Bank J, Blake M, Jamieson B. Significance of blasts in low-cell-count cerebrospinal fluid specimens from children with acute lymphoblastic leukemia. *Cancer* 66:1748-1754, 1990.

27. Hanada T, Ono I, Moriyama N, Koike K. Cytoplasmic granules in leukaemic cells of the cerebrospinal fluid in a child with non-granular acute lymphocytic leukemia. *Eur J Ped* 150:839-840, 1991.

28. Casper JT, Lauer SJ, Kirchner PA, Gottschall JT, Camitta BM. Evaluation of cerebrospinal fluid mononuclear cells obtained from children with acute lymphocytic leukemia: advantages of combining cytomorphology and terminal deoxynucleotidyl transferase. *Am J Clin Pathol* 80:666-670, 1983.

29. Hooijkaas H, Hählen K, Adriaansen HJ, Dekker I, van Zanen GE, van Dongen JJM. Terminal deoxynucleotidyl transferase (Tdt)-positive cells in cerebrospinal fluid and development of overt CNS leukemia: a 5-year follow-up study in 113 children with a Tdt-positive leukemia of non-Hodgkins' lymphoma. *Blood* 74:416-422, 1989.

30. Redner A, Melamed MR, Andreeff M. Detection of central nervous system relapse in acute leukemia by multi parameter flow cytometry of DNA, RNA, and CALLA. *Ann NY Acad Sci* 468:241-255, 1986.

31. Homans AC, Forman EN, Barker BE. Use of monoclonal antibodies to identify cerebrospinal fluid lymphoblasts in children with acute lymphoblastic leukemia. *Blood* 66:1321-1325, 1985.

32. Homans AC, Barker BE, Forman EN, Cornell CJ, Dickerman JD, Truman JT. Immunophenotypic characteristics of cerebrospinal fluid cells in children with acute lymphoblastic leukemia at diagnosis. *Blood* 76:1807-1811, 1990.

33. Rohlfing MB, Barton TK, Bigner SH, Johnston WW. Contamination of cerebrospinal fluid specimens with hematogenous blasts in patients with leukemia. *Acta Cytol* 25:611-615, 1981

34. Kjeldsberg CR, Knight JA. Body Fluids. Laboratory Examination of Amniotic Cerebrospinal, Seminal, Serous, and Synovial Fluids. American Society of Clinical Pathologists Press, Chicago, 1982.

35. Craver RD, Carson TH. Hematopoietic elements in cerebrospinal fluid in children. *Am J Clin Pathol* 95:532-535, 1991.

36. Altman AJ. Chronic leukemias of childhood. In: Principles and Practice of Pediatric Oncology. PA Pizzo, DG Poplack, eds. JB Lippincott, Philadelphia, 1989, p383-396.

37. Zelter PM, Bodey B, Marlin A, Kemshead J. Immunophenotype profile of childhood medulloblastomas and supratentorial primitive neuroectodermal tumors using 16 monoclonal antibodies. *Cancer* 66:273-283, 1990.

38. Rupp M, Hafix MA, Hoover L, Sun CC. Fine needle aspiration in the evaluation of testicular leukemic infiltration. *Acta Cytol* 31:57-58, 1987.

39. Layfield LJ, Hilborne LH, Ljung B-M, Feig S, Ehrlich RM. Use of fine needle aspiration cytology for the diagnosis of testicular relapse in patients with acute lymphoblastic leukemia. *J Urol* 139:1020-1022, 1988.

40. Akhtar M, Ali MA, Burgess A, Aur RJA. Fine-needle aspiration biopsy (FNAB) diagnosis of testicular involvement in acute lymphoblastic leukemia in children. *Diagn Cytopathol* 7:504-507, 1991.

41. Magrath IT. Malignant non-Hodgkin's lymphomas. In: Principles and Practice of Pediatric Oncology. PA Pizzo, DG Poplack, eds. JB Lippincott, Philadelphia, 1989, p415-455.

42. Helson L, Krochmal P, Hajdu SI. Diagnostic value of cytologic specimens obtained from children with cancer. *Ann Clin Lab Sci* 5:294-297, 1975.

43. Jones GR, Mason WH, Fishman LS, DeClerck YA. Primary central nervous system lymphoma without intracranial mass in a child. Diagnosis by documentation of monoclonality. *Cancer* 56:2804-2808, 1985.

44. Leventhal BG, Donaldson SS. Hodgkin's Disease. In: Principles and Practice of Pediatric Oncology. PA Pizzo, DG Poplack, eds. JB Lippincott, Philadelphia, 1989, p457-476.

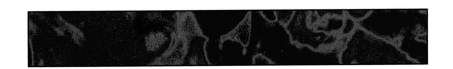

CHAPTER THREE

Cerebrospinal Fluid and the Central Nervous System

In children, cerebrospinal fluid (CSF) is the most commonly and widely examined cytologic specimen type, attesting to its conspicuous clinical importance.[1,2] The utmost value of the cytologic diagnosis and monitoring of CSF for meningeal infiltration by leukemic and lymphomatous elements has already been discussed. Infections resulting in meningitis are relatively common in the pediatric population and in this situation, the cytologic evaluation of the CSF may provide very early data upon which to direct and support appropriate therapy. Primary brain tumors are the most frequent solid neoplasms in children. Compared with adults, central nervous system (CNS) neoplasms are much more likely to disseminate via the CSF pathways; this also bolsters the role of CSF cytology in searching for tumor cells both at the time of initial diagnosis and during antineoplastic treatments. Although probably not as common as in adults, nonlymphoreticular, non-CNS tumors may metastasize to the subarachnoid space.[1-3]

Cerebrospinal fluid is constantly manufactured by the choroid plexus, a modified form of ependyma, predominantly within the lateral ventricles, but also in the third and fourth ventricles. This fluid flows through the ventricular system into the subarachnoid space, the cavity between the arachnoid and the pia mater which encases the brain and spinal cord. CSF provides nourishment and mechanical protection for these structures. Within the subarachnoid space, CSF flows down about the cord and upward over the brain. Most CSF is reabsorbed superiorly within the arachnoid villi. In hydrocephalus, the flow of CSF is significantly hindered, eventuating in variable dilatation of the ventricles.

Most often, CSF is obtained via a lumbar spinal tap in which a needle enters the subarachnoid space below the spinal cord. Fluid occasionally is obtained directly by aspirating a ventricle. Infrequently, we have seen exfoliative cytologic specimens from children derived either from an Ommaya reservoir shunt (which is used for chemotherapy administration) or from a direct intraoperative brain washing. In the last three specimen types, one can expect to see minute fragments of glial and neuronal elements (Images 3.1 through 3.3). In the latter cell type, the presence of prominent nucleoli should not be mistaken for a feature of neoplastic cells.[4]

The morphologic evaluation of CSF may appear to be straightforward relative to many other types of cytologic specimens. However, cytologic interpretations may provide diagnostically crucial information upon which important therapeutic decisions are based, and thus a systematic approach is required. As reviewed by Bigner, adequate clinical data must accompany the fluid specimen to the laboratory.[4] This fact must be impressed upon all clinicians who submit CNS specimens for study as clinicopathologic correlations are essential in order to arrive at the most meaningful interpretation. It is also important for all practitioners to recognize the importance of a timely, rapid delivery of CSF to the laboratory; if this is not feasible, then the fluid needs immediate refrigeration. Patient age and sex are, of course, required, for the incidence and location of different primary brain tumor changes with age throughout the pediatric population. It is important to know whether or not the patient has a clinical picture suggestive or diagnostic of meningitis as infiltrates of the meninges by malignant cells may clinically mimic nonneoplastic inflammatory states. The pathologist also should be informed about the presence of signs and symptoms relating to an intracranial mass lesion and any prior history of neoplasm, whether primary within the CNS or elsewhere. Clinicians should also relate whether or not the fluid was derived from a lumbar puncture or a less common site. What may be totally acceptable morphologically in a ventricular sample may be most unusual in a lumbar spinal fluid.

Cytologic interpretations may provide diagnostically crucial information upon which therapeutic decisions are based, and thus a systematic approach is required

CSF Preparation

The initial step with most CSF specimens is an enumeration of the cells present. This is generally performed manually with a counting chamber. The absolute number of cells in cytologic smears depends upon the starting volume of fluid. The two most widely accepted methods for processing CSF for morphologic examination are membrane filtration and cytocentrifugation.[5] In the former, CSF is drawn through a thin membrane by a vacuum, fixed in ethanol, and stained by the Papanicolaou method. The filter is then affixed to a glass slide. With the latter method, the material is concentrated by mild centrifugation of fluid onto slides. The cells are air-dried and generally stained with one of the Romanowsky stains. As mentioned in the leukemia chapter, debate has centered on the advantages and disadvantages of these two approaches.[4,5] Membrane filtration permits greater recovery of cells and superior cellular preservation, but requires more time and expertise in preparation. The cytocentrifuge method can be performed with a smaller volume of CSF, and is an easier and a more rapid process. Whereas membrane filters are essentially restricted to the Papanicolaou stain, a large number of stains can be used with cytocentrifuge specimens.[1,2] Furthermore, these slides are amenable to immunocytochemical and in situ hybridization procedures.[4] The luxury of doing both procedures is optimal. If not possible, however, then cytocentrifugation is preferred whenever a leukemia or lymphoma is known or suspected, and when special stains are expected to be necessary. In the evaluation of primary brain tumors, we prefer the Papanicolaou method.

Normal CSF

The normal range of inflammatory cells in lumbar CSF varies with age

In contrast to adults, the normal range of inflammatory cells in lumbar CSF varies with age. With puberty, the adult levels of 0 to 5 mononuclear leukocytes per microliter is reached.[6,7] In children up to 1 year of age, counts of up to 30 wbc/μL are acceptable, although the majority of normal patients in this group will have much lower counts. Values tend to be especially high in neonates. Declining numbers of leukocytes are expected as children progress from infancy to puberty.[6] The vast majority of cells in nonneonates are lymphocytes, although monocytes may also be seen. This may not be the case for neonates, as both Dalens and Pappu and their coworkers have reported that the macrophage (histocyte) is the predominant cellular element in newborns.[8,9] It is classically taught that polymorphonuclear leukocytes are not normally present in uncontaminated CSF. However, several authors have claimed that very infrequent neutrophils may be seen in otherwise unremarkable specimens from children without any apparent CNS disorder.[2,7-10] Bonadio claimed that up to approximately one-third of the white blood cells may be neutrophils, and that this may be considered clinically unimportant in CSF specimens that have a normal total cell count.[10] This conclusion was based on his study of 106 children older than 1 month of age with culture and Gram stained-negative fluids. From their evaluation of 371 patients, Portnoy and Olson argue, on the other hand, that a lower threshold is preferable in order to avoid misdiagnoses (false-negative interpretations) in children with meningitis.[7]

The cells lining the ventricular surface may also be considered normal constituents of the CSF. Although they are recognized only very infrequently in lumbar spinal fluids, these elements are normally present in ventricular fluid specimens and may be quite numerous (Image 3.4). Whether derived from the ependymal or the choroid plexus, they are morphologically indistinguishable from each other. Histologically, these elements form a simple columnar epithelium composed of cells with a small basally oriented nucleus and a low N/C ratio. This appearance is recapitulated after they exfoliate in aggregates from the surface. Typically, they are seen as clusters of cuboidal cells with indistinct borders and small, uniform and polarized nuclei with smooth, round contours.[1,2,11]   These clusters appear quite cohesive and may contain more than 50 cells. Nucleoli are inconspicuous and the N/C ratio is distinctly low. Individual ependymal and choroidal cells also may be visualized on occasion; such isolated cells have a proclivity to "round up" which may make their specific recognition more difficult. Wilkins and Odom found these epithelial cells to occur most often and to be present in greatest numbers in hydrocephalic infants.[11]   Although Dalens et al stated that aggregates of choroidal and ependymal cells are a consistent finding in neonates, Pappu et al claimed that ependymal cells are not seen in this group.[8,9]   These cells can generally be recognized as benign, but as will be discussed later, they need to be distinguished from certain low-grade neoplasms, namely, well-differentiated ependymomas and choroid plexus papillomas.

Under normal conditions, erythrocytes should be very scarce in CSF. When blood does enter the subarachnoid space, either spontaneously or following a "traumatic tap," then they may be present in such numbers that other cellular elements are obscured. It is easier to recognize red blood cells in cytocentrifuge slides, as alcohol and possibly the filter itself lyse erythrocytes in membrane filter preparations (Image 3.5).

Subarachnoid Hemorrhage

Hemorrhage into the subarachnoid space may occur at any age in the pediatric population, but it is probably most common and clinically important in the neonatal period. Most often, this bleeding occurs within the first few days of life in premature infants. Although exact etiology and pathogenesis remain unknown, hemorrhage most frequently originates in the germinal matrix beneath the ependymal lining of the lateral ventricles (intraventricular hemorrhage). This matrix consists of small primitive or undifferentiated cells. Similarly, but less frequently, hemorrhage arises in the external granular layer of the cerebellum. Early in the course of the bleed, fully intact erythrocytes overwhelm the cytologic picture of the CSF.

Following a pathologic bleed, phagocytosis of intact red blood cells by macrophages (erythrophagocytosis) may occur (Images 3.6 through 3.13).[4]   Hemosiderin-laden macrophages (siderophages) may also be seen; the latter may be seen in the CSF of neonates for several weeks following intrapartum intracranial hemorrhage.[8]   However, siderophages and erythrophages may be seen in CSF obtained some time after a preceding traumatic tap and thus cannot be used as absolute evidence of a pathologic bleed.[4,12]

Most often, bleeding occurs within the first few days of life in premature infants

CSF Contaminants

Probably the most frequent cellular contaminant of CSF is squamous epithelium derived from the skin during the needle puncture.

Although nucleated squamous cells are possible, usually keratinized enucleated elements are seen. Generally, they are not a cause of diagnostic confusion as they are easy to recognize and there is, for all practical purposes no other CNS source. However, through the courtesy of Dr R Craver, we have seen an example of squamous cell contamination via rupture of a dermoid cyst (Images 3.14 and 3.15). Other less common but diagnostically more challenging contaminants include immature hematopoietic precursor cells (Image 3.16) and primitive neuroepithelial elements (Images 3.17 through 3.20).[13,14] In both of these, cells with immature chromatin patterns, round contours, and very high N/C ratio are present within the CSF. Craver and Carson published a study of 5 infants, none of whom were older than 2 months, in whom hematopoietic elements were found in lumbar CSF specimens.[13] In all 5 patients, both myeloid and erythroid precursor cells were present within the fluid. These authors used the presence of basophilic or polychromatophilic normoblasts as the major criterion for contamination of the CSF by bone marrow due to unintentional penetration of the vertebral body during the performance of the spinal tap. They did not find megakaryocytes in the specimens. Three additional older children all of whom had been treated for acute lymphoblastic leukemia were also reported. The presence of primitive hematopoietic elements would be quite disconcerting in this latter situation.[13] Fischer and colleagues described the presence of immature cells resembling hematopoietic blasts in the CSF from 4 infants.[14] All 4 had hydrocephalus due to intraventricular hemorrhage, which was associated with prematurity in 3. In contrast to the immature hematopoietic elements described by Craver and Carson, these blast-like elements occurred as cohesive cellular aggregates in the CSF.[13,14] Fisher et al described the cells as having round to oval nuclei with finely granular, uniformly distributed chromatin and small nucleoli set within basophilic cytoplasm which ranged from slight to moderate in volume.[14] It is important to recognize that these cells demonstrated intercellular cohesion (Images 3.17 and 3.18). Such relationships would not be expected in hematopoietic elements whether benign or malignant. By immunocytochemistry, these cells were decorated with neuron specific enolase but were non-reactive with a panel of antileukocyte antibodies. These authors postulated that these cellular aggregates, which they termed primitive cell clusters, were probably derived from the germinal matrix cells, which may be found beneath the ependyma of premature infants.[14] In addition to leukemic blasts, these elements need to be distinguished from medulloblastoma cells; the latter were described as being typically larger than these germinal matrix cells. Fisher et al point out two other important factors which may be useful in the differential diagnosis.[14] These primitive cell clusters were not present in the first lumbar puncture obtained in the children, but appeared after the hydrocephalus was diagnosed. A morphologic clue was the universal presence of hemosiderin-containing macrophages. These, of course, may have been secondary to the preceding hemorrhage.

Takeda et al described a 5-month-old infant with contamination by notochord material.[15] The CSF in this child had aggregates of large cellular elements that contained abundant frothy cytoplasm with relatively indistinct intercellular borders. The nuclei were described as round to oval, hyperchromatic and having coarse clumps of chromatin. It was believed that these cells were derived from the notochord of the nucleus pulposus, again due to the inadvertent puncture of a vertebral body (Images 3.21 and 3.22).

Infectious Meningitis

A clinically important and relatively common syndrome in children that directly affects the CSF is meningitis.[16] Often, this inflammatory process is secondary to infection of the meninges by bacteria. The specific causative organism is, at least, in part, related to patient age. In the first 2 months of life, Gram-negative bacilli (enteric pathogens) and the group B streptococci are the major causative agents, although *Listeria* appears to be increasing in frequency. It has been traditionally taught that the most common cause of bacterial meningitis in children older than 2 months is *Haemophilus influenzae*, type b, followed by *Neisseria meningitides* and *Streptococcus pneumoniae*. However, the development and widespread use of a successful vaccine against *H influenzae* has already dramatically reduced the absolute incidence of infections by this organism.[17,18] The clinical spectrum of disease produced by bacterial meningitis is highly variable among patients.[16] Fever is generally present and may be associated with nausea, vomiting, photophobia, and nuchal rigidity, although some infants may manifest only irritability. Unfortunately, seizures occur in at least one-quarter of all infected children. As bacterial meningitis may have sequelae that include significant neurologic damage and even death, these infections are considered almost a medical emergency.

In most instances, spinal tap to acquire CSF for diagnostic purposes is almost always indicated when bacterial meningitis is suspected. The examination of the CSF should occur very promptly and include a total cell count as well as a morphologic examination. Usually, the latter includes a Romanowsky-stained smear of the cytocentrifuged sediment and an additional Gram-stained slide. Generally, therapy may be initiated based on the findings in the above tests. The importance of the rapidity of examination is related partly to the fact that the leukocytes in the CSF will start to disintegrate within 2 hours of collection.

Typically, the total white blood cell count is significantly elevated with bacterial meningitis. The predominant component is the neutrophilic leukocyte (Images 3.23 through 3.26). Usually more than one hundred and at times thousands of white blood cells/mL are present in the CSF (pleocytosis) with greater than 90% comprising neutrophils. However, as cited by Bonadio, children may suffer bacterial meningitis without a pleocytosis or with an initial cellular predominance of lymphocytes.[10]

Bonadio and Smith recently described 101 children who had acute bacterial meningitis secondary to *H influenzae*, type b.[19] These authors compared the morphologic findings in the CSF at the time of diagnosis with those found 48 to 72 hours after antibiotic therapy. Only one of the children in the entire series had a positive CSF bacterial culture on

Spinal tap to acquire CSF for diagnostic purposes is almost always indicated when bacterial meningitis is suspected

the subsequent examination. Although there was a significant decrease in the total number of inflammatory cells in the CSF, pleocytosis persisted in all of the children. Most of these pediatric patients demonstrated a decline in the proportion of neutrophils, and in 14% there was a conversion to a lymphocyte predominance. The overwhelming majority (98%) evolved from a positive to a negative Gram-stain on the CSF sediment (Images 3.27 through 3.29).

Bonadio and colleagues also investigated the differentiation of traumatic tap from the cytomorphologic findings of bacterial meningitis in children.[20] They evaluated the cellular findings in infected children with a traumatic lumbar puncture (defined by them as >1000 rbc/μL). This is an important subject as traumatic puncture is frequent in children, comprising 20% of all specimens in Bonadio's experience. Utilizing a simple mathematical formula to correct for the contamination of peripheral blood, they found that all children with bacterial meningitis had a ratio of observed leukocyte count to predicted leukocyte count of at least 1. Furthermore, 93% of the patients had a ratio greater than 10. By contrast, only 3% of the children without meningitis but with a traumatic tap had a ratio greater than 10; 63 of the patients had a ratio less than 1. Using this mathematical ratio they found a diagnostic sensitivity of 93% and a diagnostic specificity of 95%. Other helpful clues in separating children with and without bacterial meningitis was the Gram-stain, which was negative in all children without meningitis, and a neutrophilic predominance, present in only 11% of those without infection. They concluded that it was exceedingly uncommon for children over 1 month of age to have the CSF abnormalities that are typically associated with bacterial meningitis to be obscured by contamination with peripheral blood.[20]

Aseptic meningitis may be defined as inflammation of the meninges in the absence of evidence of a bacterial pathogen in the CSF as detected by usual laboratory techniques, namely, culture and Gram stain. Most often, a viral infection, especially Echovirus, is responsible, but the list of etiologic factors is quite impressive. Typically, older children and adolescents suffer from fever, headache and meningismus, with an associated pleocytosis. Fortunately, most cases follow a benign course and resolve spontaneously.

The cytologic picture of aseptic meningitis is variable, depending in part on the underlying cause, the immune status of the patient, and the point of time in the clinical course at which the CSF is sampled. Classically, a mononuclear cell infiltrate in the CSF is expected (Images 3.30 through 3.36). Recently, Amir et al evaluated 98 children with aseptic meningitis, presumably viral in origin, with differential cell counts.[21] The neutrophil was the predominant cell within the CSF during the first 24 hours of symptoms in most patients, but declined in numbers so as to comprise only a minority of all white cells enumerated after 24 hours. Lymphocytes predominated thereafter. Using the Wright-Giemsa stain, Baker and Lenane reported the presence of atypical lymphocytes as the best discriminator between bacterial and viral meningitis.[22] When defined as a large lymphoid cell with basophilic cytoplasm, coarse chromatin and prominent nucleoli, this cell was a highly specific (although somewhat insensitive) cytomarker of viral meningitis (Image 3.37). When faced with large immunoblast-like

Most often, a viral infection, especially Echovirus, is responsible, but the list of etiologic factors is quite impressive

cells in patients without a history of malignant lymphoma, a conservative "watch and see" approach has been suggested by Bigner.[4] On the other hand, in patients with known lymphoma and a similar cytologic CSF picture, she recommends immunotyping for monoclonality. Woodruff found such disconcerting lymphoid cells in the CSF of some infants without evidence of infection.[12]   Rarely, eosinophils may be prominent in examples of chronic meningitis.[23] *Cryptococcus neoformans* is one nonbacterial agent that may be specifically identified morphologically in cases of meningitis.[1,4]   These fungi appear as round structures with variable diameters, narrow-neck budding, and a refractile capsule (Images 3.38 through 3.41).[1,24]

In addition to hemorrhagic situations, histiocytes may be the predominant nucleated cell within the CSF in a number of other circumstances.[2,25]   Certainly, they may be numerous or even dominate infectious and noninfectious examples of pleocytosis (Images 3.42 and 3.43). In most of these cases, their benign reactive appearance is readily appreciated by their pale, fine chromatin granules, smooth nuclear contours and low N/C ratio; additionally, their relatively abundant cytoplasm may be vacuolated or contain unrecognizable phagocytized debris. Rosenthal has extensively discussed the conditions in which atypical and malignant-appearing histiocytes may appear in the CSF.[2] Among those conditions that may affect children are inborn errors of metabolism (storage disorders) and the Histiocytosis X syndromes (Images 3.44 through 3.46).[25] Wolfson has detailed the cytologic findings in the very rare cerebral histiocytosis.[26]

One of the major therapeutic innovations for patients with hydrocephalus is the surgical placement of a systemic shunt.[27,28]   Most often, this carries CSF from the ventricular system to the peritoneal cavity, but other sites, for example, cardiac atrium, receive this excess fluid. Unfortunately, problems may develop due to the presence of the shunt. Shunts, for example, may become infected, leading to ventriculitis.[29] Serial morphologic examinations of the fluid from the shunt in patients with ventriculitis demonstrate a pattern of changes similar to those seen in lumbar CSF in meningitis (Image 3.47). Early in the course, neutrophils may predominate, but they are replaced later by lymphocytes and macrophages, especially the latter. In turn, infection may lead to obstruction of the shunt by inflammatory debris or scar tissue. Other causes of obstruction include plugs of tumor cells and foreign body inflammatory giant cells (Images 3.48 through 3.50). The latter are probably related to the host response to the foreign material of the shunt itself. As discussed by Bigner et al, these reactive elements should not lead to an erroneous interpretation of granulomatous infection, sarcoid or tumor.[27]   The host response to the shunt may also include eosinophilic leukocytes (Image 3.51).[30,31]

Bigner et al also reviewed the possibility that reactive and neoplastic cells indigenous to the CNS may travel through the shunt and appear in unusual sites, mostly the peritoneal cavity.[27] Tumor cells of glial, embryonal and germ cell types have all been rarely described as producing shunt-related metastases and ascites. Benign choroid plexus cells may also follow this pathway. We have seen an example of ascites in a child with a choroid plexus papilloma.[32]   However, cytologic examination of the peritoneal fluid failed to reveal neoplastic cells.

One of the major therapeutic innovations for patients with hydrocephalus is the surgical placement of a systemic shunt

Perhaps the effusion was related to the greatly increased production of CSF by the tumor, which was the cause of the hydrocephalus.

CNS Neoplasms

As a group, primary neoplasms of the CNS are the most common type of solid tumor in children[33]; only the leukemias are more frequent. This is in contrast to adults in whom CNS malignancies account for less than 2% of all cancers. Furthermore, both the histologic types and anatomic distribution of pediatric CNS neoplasms are quite different from those in adults. For example, in children, the majority are infratentorial and often midline, whereas in adults, laterally situated supratentorial tumors predominate. Both meningiomas and oligodendrogliomas occur relatively frequently in adults but are quite rare in children. Conversely, medulloblastomas and midline germ cell tumors occur much more often in the pediatric population. Even within this younger group, these patterns may vary with age. For readers desiring much greater detail about this complex topic, the encyclopedic review by Heideman and colleagues is highly recommended.[33]

A consequence of these age-related differences in sites of origin and types of CNS tumors is that neoplastic cells are identified within the CSF relatively more commonly in children than in adults. Neoplasms which are especially likely to shed into the CSF are the primitive neuroectodermal tumors (including medulloblastoma), ependymomas, germ cell tumors, high-grade gliomas and choroid plexus tumors.

It is important to know the incidence rates for leptomeningeal dissemination of the different CNS tumors. Packer et al have provided the single largest study that addresses this question in children.[34] They reviewed the CSF cytology and myelography in 314 pediatric patients with primary brain tumors. Overall, 19% showed leptomeningeal spread; in half of these (mostly primitive neuroectodermal tumors), such dissemination occurred before diagnosis. As documented in their investigation, spread was seen in 50% of the primitive neuroectodermal tumors (PNETs), 32% of anaplastic astrocytomas, 20% of ependymomas, 14% of germ cell tumors, no more than 5% of low-grade noncerebellar astrocytomas, and none of the low-grade cerebellar astrocytomas.

Before describing these individual neoplasms in greater detail it is important to discuss briefly the mechanisms that have been proposed to account for tumor cell entry into the CSF and the production of craniospinal metastasis.[34-40] Of course, proximity of the primary neoplasm to the ependymal or leptomeningeal lining is important. Thus, ependymomas and choroid plexus tumors have an advantage to spread in the CSF as they generally grow as intraventricular masses. Other neoplasms, especially midline germ cell tumors and medulloblastomas, also often develop very closely to the lining surfaces. Tumor-specific biologic aggressiveness is also probably important. High-grade astrocytomas with cellular pleomorphism, hyperchromasia and brisk mitotic activity, for example, are more likely to exfoliate into the CSF and remain viable than a benign or low-grade astrocytoma. Reaction of

Neoplastic cells are identified within the CSF relatively more commonly in children than in adults

the meninges to the presence of tumor may affect shedding of cells. For example, cerebellar astrocytomas typically induce a well-developed desmoplastic response, which may act as a barrier to dissemination.[33,35-37] Individual differences in tumor cells' ability to adhere to surfaces, both normal and abnormal, eg, denuded ependyma, may very well play a role.[37,40] Finally, the iatrogenic roles of surgery and shunts need to be considered.

Medulloblastoma

Medulloblastomas are the prototypic PNET of the CNS. They account for 10% to 20% of all CNS tumors of childhood and nearly half of the posterior fossa neoplasms.[33] Their incidence peaks at 5 years of age, and they are more common in boys. Most arise within the cerebellar vermis. Grossly, they are usually friable and soft; this may aid in their dissemination into the CSF.[40] As with other PNETs, they are cellular neoplasms, composed of sheets of small malignant cells with a high N/C ratio and a proclivity for molding. Homer-Wright rosettes and perivascular pseudorosettes may be seen. Within their solitary hyperchromatic nucleus, nucleoli are poorly visualized, but mitotic figures are common. Pleomorphism with giant cells is not seen. 5 year survival rates may now significantly exceed 50%.[41-44]

Deutsch recently reported the results of staging by CSF cytology and myelography in 52 children with medulloblastoma.[41] 46% had evidence of dissemination beyond the posterior fossa at the time of initial diagnosis; this was especially likely in children under 5 years. Only 4 patients had a preoperative lumbar CSF cytology examination; 3 were positive and in 2 of these, there was no other evidence of subarachnoid spread. In 23, preoperative lateral ventricular fluid cytology was evaluated; in the 4 with positive preparations there were other signs of dissemination. Of the 14 children with spinal cord involvement (stage M3) at the time of diagnosis, 11 had positive cytology. 11 of 41 patients with postoperative lumbar spinal cytology had tumor cells present. Some authorities believe that the evaluation of CSF in the early (up to 2 weeks) postoperative period does not have much clinical value, as tumor cells may have been dislodged during surgery.[42,43] Flannery et al reported CSF cytology to be positive in 10% of their series of 31 children.[43] Morphologic examination was performed approximately 1 month after surgery and thus "false-positive" contamination was avoided.

PNETs occur in other sites in the CNS.[33,45] In the pineal gland, for example, they are referred to as pineoblastomas. The very rare cerebral neuroblastomas usually occur as hemispheric masses. Finally, retinoblastoma is also considered within this nosologic category. Subtle histologic differences may be encountered among these entities, all considered to be PNETs. However, it needs to be emphasized that on the basis of their cytomorphologic features in exfoliative specimens, they are indistinguishable from one another. Thus, in their evaluation, the cytologist needs to integrate all clinical and especially radiographic data. In the presence of nonlymphoreticular small malignant cells and a predominant fourth ventricle (cerebellar) mass lesion, the diagnosis is medulloblastoma until proven otherwise. If, on the other hand, radiographic scans reveal a mass in the region of the pineal gland, then

On the basis of their cytomorphologic features in exfoliative specimens, PNETs are indistinguishable from one another

tumor cells with the same exact light microscopic appearance are consistent with a pineoblastoma.[1,46]

Cytologic specimens of the CSF are often quite cellular in patients with medulloblastoma and perhaps less so with the other PNETs (Image 3.52). Intraoperative wash and shunt drainage specimens may be cellular, regardless of the primary site. In any case, they consist of a uniform population of small obviously malignant cells with very high N/C ratio (Table 3.1). Nuclei are round to angulated with finely granular, evenly distributed chromatin particles. One or two small nucleoli may be evident as may mitotic figures. Degenerative changes are common, especially just following therapy (usually surgical resection and postoperative radiotherapy); even in specimens from untreated patients, karyorrhexis is frequently observed. Only a thin rim of nondescript basophilic cytoplasm surrounds the nuclei of solitary cells, but it is often much more obvious within cellular clusters, such as tetrads or pseudorosettes (Images 3.53 through 3.56). In pseudorosettes, a ring of obviously malignant nuclei surrounds central cytoplasm. Nuclear molding is also characteristic. At times, histologic examination demonstrates divergent lines of differentiation, eg, skeletal muscle (medullomyoblastomas) or neuronal features within the tumor.[44] We have never seen evidence of such differentiation in exfoliative cytologic preparations nor have such cases been documented in the cytologic literature.

Table 3.1
Medulloblastoma

Smears are variably cellular and consist of uniform populations of small tumor cells with high N/C ratios.

Nuclei: round; hyperchromatic with even, finely granular chromatin; 1 or 2 small nucleoli; molding may be seen; degenerative changes common.

Cytoplasm: scanty in single cells; more obvious in aggregates, especially in pseudorosettes.

Astrocytomas

As a group, the astrocytomas are the most frequent primary CNS tumor in children, as well as in adults, but they are less often encountered in exfoliative cytopathology specimens. The anatomic distribution and histologic appearances of astrocytomas in children are at variance with those in adults.[33,39] For example, only 1/3 of all childhood astrocytomas are supratentorial which is the preferred site in older individuals. Astrocytomas in the cerebellum and brain stem each account for 10% to 20% of all pediatric CNS tumors, whereas these sites are infrequently involved in adults. The incidence curve for supratentorial astrocytomas in the pediatric population is bimodal with the first peak occurring in children between 2 to 4 years of age and the second in adolescents.[33] Boys are more often affected than girls. Clinically, patients suffer from increased intracranial pressure with headaches, nausea, vomiting, seizures and localized neurologic deficits.

The histologic features, both architectural and cytologic, of astrocytomas are highly heterogenous.[1,2] The low-grade end of the spectrum may be very difficult to distinguish from benign reactive gliosis. They may be composed of uniform-appearing mononucleated astrocytes with stellate or fibrillar contours and pale cytoplasm. The nuclei are smooth and round, have finely granular chromatin, and small relatively inconspicuous nucleoli. Glioblastoma multiforme forms the other end of the spectrum. Marked pleomorphism includes the presence of bizarre tumor giant cells with multiple, hyperchromatic and irregular nuclei. High levels of cellularity, foci of necrosis with a peripheral palisade of tumor cells, and endothelial proliferation are histologic hallmarks.

Clinically evident spread of astrocytomas is relatively uncommon.[34-36,38-40] Most of these occur within the craniospinal axis and only rarely extraneurally. The reported incidence rates for CSF dissemination are quite variable and depend on a number of factors including the histologic grade and location of the tumor, and the method of study (CSF cytology versus myelography versus autopsy). In one very large study, for example, involving over 1000 high-grade supratentorial tumors, nearly 7% of the patients developed metastases postoperatively.[47] However, in this investigation, in which positive CSF cytology alone was not considered adequate to document metastasis, the vast majority of patients were adults. In the previously mentioned study by Packer et al, 1/3 of the anaplastic astrocytomas showed leptomeningeal spread, with a much greater proclivity for infratentorial tumors to disseminate.[34] None of the low-grade cerebellar neoplasms and only 2% of similar noncerebellar tumors metastasized; in this review of children with brain tumors either positive CSF cytology or myelography were considered sufficient to demonstrate such spread.[34] On the other hand, some excellent review publications do not even discuss metastases.[39] As a generalization, the higher the grade of the astrocytoma, the more likely it is to produce cerebrospinal spread and to yield positive cytologic specimens.

In our experience and that of others, CSF cytology examination in children with low-grade tumors is almost always negative.[1,2] Neoplastic elements are uncommonly seen in fluid specimens and when present may be difficult to recognize as tumor cells (Table 3.2). Even when positive, the specimens are generally sparsely cellular and consist of rather small dispersed cells.[1-3,48,49] As the individual cells exfoliate, they tend to develop round contours in fluid, although a minority may maintain blunt cytoplasmic tails or projections or appear elongated (Images 3.57 through 3.62). Cytoplasm is pale and cyanophilic, and characteristically has indistinct borders. As expected from their histology, nuclei are round and smooth with uniformly dispersed finely granular chromatin and possibly a small nucleolus.

Literature review documents a relatively scanty number of published case reports and small studies of children with low-grade astrocy-

The higher the grade of the astrocytoma, the more likely it is to produce cerebrospinal spread and to yield positive cytologic specimens

Table 3.2
Low-Grade Astrocytomas

Usually sparsely cellular, consisting of dispersed rather small cells

Nuclei: smooth and round; pale, finely granular chromatin; small nucleolus

Cytoplasm: in exfoliated specimens, pale, cyanophilic; indistinct borders; tails or projections in a few; in aspirates more apparent but variable; often one or more long or blunt processes; Rosenthal fibers

Background: in aspiration smears, fibrillar; blood vessels "coated" with tumor cells

---

tomas with spinoaxial metastasis and a relatively poor clinical course. Even then, cytologic examination of fluid specimens is either negative or not even mentioned in the publication.[36,38,50,51] McLaughlin's series of 5 patients with juvenile piloid astrocytomas included an 8-year-old boy with subarachnoid space spread and "medulloblast-like" cells in the CSF.[52] However, histologically these neoplasms showed foci of nuclear pleomorphism or oligodendrogliomatous differentiation.

High-grade gliomas include malignant astrocytomas and glioblastomas. As with the low-grade tumors, it is unusual to find neoplastic cells in lumbar CSF, although this phenomenon does occur somewhat more frequently with the more poorly differentiated astrocytomas. Accordingly, published cytologic reports are also scanty. In contrast, intraoperative wash specimens are often very cellular in patients with these tumors. The largest single published study devoted to children that we are aware of is that of Kandt and colleagues.[53] Leptomeningeal dissemination was documented antemortem in 6 of 13 (46%) children with grade III or IV astrocytomas. The mean age for these 6 patients was 8 years, and most were supratentorial in location. Overall, 5 of these 6 had a cytologic examination of lumbar CSF; tumor cells were present in 3, including 1 patient at the time of initial diagnosis. Necrotic debris was seen in an additional child. Eade and Urich reported a series of five young patients with metastasizing gliomas but only 1 could be considered pediatric.[35] In 1 patient (the 21-year-old subject), "atypical cells" were present within the CSF. These authors stated that although a larger proportion of childhood gliomas occur closer to the

Table 3.3
Glioblastoma

Marked pleomorphism.

Small cells predominate with variably hyperchromatic and irregular nuclei and high N/C ratio and indistinct cellular borders.

Tumor giant cells with 1 or more large, bizarre nuclei with prominent nucleoli or degenerative changes.

Degeneration and necrosis prominent.

In aspirates, syncytial-appearing endothelial proliferations.

---

ventricular surfaces than in adults, spread within the CSF is rare. Much more recently, Grant et al reported positive cytologic findings in 11 individuals with malignant gliomas, 2 of whom were teenagers.[54] This represented at least 4% of all of their astrocytoma patients.

In fact, only rarely are the cytomorphologic features detailed or illustrated.[1,2,49,53] Pleomorphism is variable but generally marked (Table 3.3). According to Rosenthal, the most typical attribute of these high-grade neoplasms is the remarkable variability from cell to cell (Images 3.63 through 3.66).[2] As expected from their histopathology, there can be bizarre, monstrous tumor giant cells. Their nuclei may be quite large and irregular in contour with hyperchromatic chromatin that varies from finely or coarsely granular to homogenous and dense; macronucleoli may be present but also are variable. Although less "eye-catching," smaller malignant cells usually predominate. These are most often round or oval, but infrequently stellate or elongated shapes may also be seen. These more irregular cellular contours are generally confined to wash specimens which are rapidly fixed. Most cells have a solitary hyperchromatic nucleus that ranges from round and smooth to highly irregular in shape. For the most part, N/C ratios are high. Cytoplasm usually stains cyanophilic and is nonspecific in appearance. Cellular borders are characteristically indistinct (Image 3.66). Degenerative changes are common and a necrotic diathesis may be prominent in washes of glioblastoma multiforme (Image 3.67).

Ependymoma

Up to 10% of all pediatric brain tumors are ependymomas.[33] Although ependymomas are the most common primary tumor of the spinal cord in adults, they are rare in this site in children. In children, they originate most often in the fourth ventricle. They clinically may resemble medulloblastomas and present with nonspecific features of increased intracranial pressure. When they occur as supratentorial masses, they present with localized cerebral defects similar to high-grade astrocytomas.[33] Grossly, their typical appearance is that of a rather well delineated firm mass. Microscopically, a wide range of differentiation may be seen, although the majority are well differentiated. However, both malignant ependymomas and ependymoblastomas exist; in the latter, the cells may resemble the elements in PNETs. The characteristic histologic feature is the true rosette, in which columnar tumor cells are polarized about a central lumen. Papillary formations and perivascular pseudorosettes are other components. Most often, the neoplastic cells appear well differentiated or even benign, with low N/C ratio and small bland nuclei. 5-year survival rates approximate 33%.

Due in large part to their frequent location within the ventricular system, leptomeningeal dissemination is not uncommon, even for tumors with banal histologic appearances. Rosenthal states that these tumors shed more cells into the CSF than any other primary neoplasm.[2] According to Packer et al, 20% produce antemortem evidence of spread, but, as stated by Bigner, documented examples of ependymoma cells in the CSF are very sparse.[4,34] On a cell-for-cell basis, tumor cells from well-differentiated ependymomas may be mor-

Both malignant ependymomas and ependymoblastomas exist; in the latter, the cells may resemble the elements in PNETs

phologically indistinguishable from normal ependymal elements (Table 3.4). They have a single small round nucleus that is displaced to one end of the cell.[1,2,49] However, spontaneously exfoliated ependymal cells do so as solitary elements, whereas their neoplastic counterparts shed into the CSF in small cohesive aggregates, including rosettes (Image 3.68). We have seen an example of an ependymoma in which long tapering cellular processes were recognizable in the cell block (Image 3.69). Bigner and Johnston illustrated the cells of an anaplastic (malignant) ependymoma in CSF which had the features of a PNET (Image 3.70).[1]

Table 3.4
Well Differentiated Ependymomas

Cohesive 3 dimensional aggregates, some with papillary configurations.
Columnar to cuboidal tumor cells with well defined borders.
Single round nucleus, generally polarized; variable finely to coarsely granular chromatin.
Low N/C ratio.

Choroid Plexus Neoplasms

Tumors of the choroid plexus also are directly exposed to the flow of CSF. Both papillomas and adenocarcinomas occur predominantly in children.[33] They arise most frequently within the lateral ventricles and in the first few years of life. Hydrocephalus is the rule and is related to the production of excess amounts of CSF by the neoplastic cells and/or to obstruction to the flow of CSF. Whereas most children with choroid plexus papillomas can expect a long-term survival, the vast majority with carcinomas will die of the disease.[33,55-57] However, recently Packer et al reported a series of children with choroid plexus carcinomas in whom there was a 45% progression-free remission at 4 years from the time of diagnosis, and they demonstrated that prognosis was associated with the degree of resection of tumor.[57] Histologically, the benign tumors have a distinctly papillary growth pattern and are basically indistinguishable from normal choroid plexus. A single layer of columnar or cuboidal cells with low N/C ratio line fibrovascular cores. Carcinomas, in contrast, are composed of obviously malignant cells which still retain a papillary architecture, at least focally.

As might be expected from the histopathology of choroid plexus papillomas, it may be very difficult or impossible in cytologic preparations to distinguish papilloma cells from cells of the normal plexus or ependyma.[1,2,4,55] As stated by Bigner, this can be especially difficult in direct ventricular samples.[4]   Buchino and Mason have detailed the cytomorphologic features of a 9-month-old boy.[55]   In addition to single tumor cells, there were numerous cohesive papillary clusters (Image 3.71).   Cuboidal cells had round regular nuclei with finely granular, uniformly distributed chromatin and relatively large volumes of cytoplasm.   Both mitotic figures and nuclear molding were distinctly absent.   Our experiences have been the same; although nuclei may overlap one another in large aggregates, nuclear molding is not seen (Table 3.5). The cells have a distinct epithelial quality in which cellular borders may be well visualized.   Small but obvious nucleoli may also be present.

We have seen an interesting example of a 1-year-old girl who presented with the clinical signs and symptoms of acute meningitis (Image 3.72).   Following a course of antibiotics, a lumbar CSF specimen was obtained.   There was an intense mixed inflammatory infiltrate.   Scattered throughout this infiltrate were a number of cohesive benign epithelial aggregates with features consistent with choroid plexus papilloma.   The diagnostic report suggested this neoplasm and was subsequently proven at surgery.

In addition to normal choroidal elements, Buchino and Mason offered the following differential diagnosis: papillary ependymomas and PNET.[55]   In the former, multiple cell layers may line stromal cores often with nuclear molding.   However, papillary configurations, in our experience, are not always evident, and as noted above, there may be crowded nuclei within 3-dimensional cellular balls.   The features of PNETs, including hyperchromatic angulated nuclei with fine to coarse chromatin granules and mitotic figures, very high N/C ratio and molding, are not evident within the papillomas.   Although papilloma cells may be seen in fluid specimens with some frequency, it remains unknown what their clinical significance is, if any.

In a series of 11 children with choroid plexus carcinomas, two had positive postoperative CSF specimens, but no other evidence of spread.[57]   A cytomorphologic description was not provided.   Kim et al detailed the cellular features of an anaplastic plexus carcinoma from a 13-month-old boy.[56]   Tumor cells occurred singly and in variably cohesive aggregates.   The cells were rather small, round in contour and had a high N/C ratio.   An important attribute was their pleomorphic nuclei with prominent irregularities in the nuclear envelope.   Kim et al stated that the striking nuclear changes helped to distinguish these tumor cells from those of a PNET, which have smoother contours.[56]

Although nuclei may overlap one another in large aggregates, nuclear molding is not seen

Table 3.5
Choroid Plexus Papilloma

Cohesive cellular aggregates; in aspirates, papillary and monolayer arrangements.

Cuboidal tumor cells with distinct borders.

Single round nucleus with fine chromatin and a small nucleolus.

Relatively low N/C ratio.

Pineal Neoplasms

A small but significant proportion of pediatric brain tumors arise in the region of the pineal gland. These neoplasms actually comprise a heterogenous array of biologically and morphologically diverse proliferations. Most series state that the majority are germ cell tumors with germinomas leading the way.[30,58,59] However, Packer et al found a relatively equal distribution of germ cells tumors, gliomas and parenchymal pineal tumors.[60] In any case, because of this diversity, a morphologic diagnosis is required as the clinical presentation is generally the same, regardless of the tumor's histology. This clinical picture is dominated by symptoms and signs of increased intracranial pressure and hydrocephalus. Some authors, but not others, have found the use of biochemical markers in the CSF, eg, α-fetoprotein and human chorionic gonadotropin helpful in the differential diagnosis.[60-62]

Table 3.6
Germinoma

Fluids consist of uniform large mononucleated cells dispersed as solitary elements. Aspirates are cellular and consist of similar tumor cells, either single or in small loosely cohesive aggregates at times mixed with lymphocytes.

Nuclei: large vesicular, smooth with prominent nucleoli.

Cytoplasm: Scanty to moderate; delicate, at times appears vacuolate; distinct cell borders.

Tigroid background in aspirates.

Due in part to their location near the anterior aspect of the third ventricle, tumor cells theoretically have ready access to the CSF pathways.[63] However, it appears as if only a minority of patients will manifest neoplastic elements in their CSF.[58,60] For example, in one large series, none of the children with germ cell tumors had a positive cytology specimen at the time of diagnosis, and only 2 of 8 with parenchymal neoplasms were positive; in both, their diagnosis was pineoblastoma.[60] 3 children with gliomas had negative ventricular fluid examinations. Similarly, CSF cytologies for the germ cell tumors were uniformally negative in another large series.[58] 2 of 7 patients (both with pineoblastomas) had positive cytologic specimens in a third series.[64]

Germ Cell Tumors

When germinomas do exfoliate into ventricular or spinal fluid, they have a characteristic appearance (Table 3.6). The malignant cells stand out as large mononucleated cells with a very prominent nucleolus.[1,2,65-67] Nuclear membranes are distinct and chromatin is vesicular (Image 3.73). Most often, a solitary large nucleolus is evident, but they may be multiple. Cytoplasm is scanty and usually dense and cyanophilic. In fluids, the cells are usually dispersed as solitary elements, but small loosely cohesive flat arrays may be seen. Several authors have described an accompanying infiltrate of small lymphocytes. We are unaware of the documented use of immunocytochemistry on CSF specimens for germ cell tumors. As measured biochemically, serum and CSF α-fetoprotein should be negative, but chorionic gonadotropin may be elevated in pure germinomas if syncytiotrophoblasts are present. Both yolk sac tumors and embryonal carcinomas present as high-grade adenocarcinomatous elements, both singly and in 3-dimensional aggregates.[64] Eccentric large smooth nuclei with nucleoli and high N/C ratio are apparent in the exfoliated cells; their cytoplasm may be vacuolated or clear. From a routine light microscopic evaluation, their appearances would be indistinguishable from one another and from metastatic adenocarcinoma. Some tumor cells should be decorated with cytokeratin and α-fetoprotein and possibly with chorionic gonadotrophin by immunocytochemistry. We know of no report of the cytologic features of a primary choriocarcinoma in CSF. One might anticipate an admixture of large mono- and multinucleated cells. Cytoplasm would be bubbly or clear in the former and denser in the latter. Nuclei would be obviously malignant and show degenerative changes. A positive chorionic gonadotrophin staining reaction would also be expected. Teratomas, both mature and immature, may arise in the pineal region. Thus, almost any cell type could theoretically appear in the CSF, but this phenomenon is quite unusual. Most often, primitive neuroblastic cells would exfoliate and would be indistinguishable from pure PNET in routine smears. Kamiyama et al reported a case of immature teratoma of the spinal cord in a 14-year-old boy which yielded clusters of glandular cells, individual squamous, and skeletal muscle fibers in a postoperative CSF specimen; although neuroblasts were present in the primary neoplasm, they were not recognized cytologically.[68] Germ cell tumors need to be diagnosed very accurately as they are often responsive to nonsurgical therapies and thus are not excised.

Germ cell tumors need to be diagnosed very accurately as they are often responsive to nonsurgical therapies and thus are not excised

Pineal Parenchymal Tumors

Pineal parenchymal tumors include pineoblastoma and pineocytoma. The former is more common, especially in children. Pineoblastoma is a member of the PNET family and accordingly, histologically it is composed of small mononucleated tumor cells with a hyperchromatic nucleus and a very high N/C ratio. Chromatin is finely granular and small nucleoli may be apparent; the neoplastic elements grow in broad sheets, which may be punctuated by small pseudorosettes. As their name implies, pineocytomas are more mature with an incomplete lobular pattern of small tumor cells. They are more sparsely cellular than in pineoblastoma. Their characteristic feature is the large rosette which is ovoid to irregular and consists of abundant fibrillated neural cellular processes. Grossly, parenchymal infiltration is seen with pineoblastoma but not with pineocytoma.

As pineoblastomas are PNETs, they are morphologically indistinguishable from medulloblastomas in exfoliative specimens (Table 3.1). Small hyperchromatic cells with very high N/C ratio are seen molded together in chains, sheets and rosettes, as well as dispersed individually (Image 3.74).[1-3,46] Similar to others, our personal experiences have been rather limited. On an individual case basis, it is probably impossible to differentiate pineocytoma from pineoblastoma in CSF.[46] However, greater degrees of nuclear molding and mitotic activity would favor the latter neoplasm.

Retinoblastoma

Another member of the PNET family, retinoblastoma, needs to be mentioned separately.[69] First, investigations of this tumor have provided a wealth of information concerning the genetics of neoplasms in man. Although fascinating, it is certainly beyond the scope of this text to discuss the contributions and insights gained by such studies. It is the one known instance in which a recognized prezygotic chromosomal defect consistently predisposes to a specific neoplasm. Both sporadic and familial forms exist with a high incidence of bilateral involvement in the latter. Furthermore, this malignant tumor is quite curable. Diagnosis is usually based on the combination of ophthalmoscopic and radiologic findings without a preoperative tissue examination. Histologically, necrosis is often a prominent feature. Although not always present, characteristic features include Flexner-Wintersteiner rosettes and fleurettes. The former are cellular aggregates centered about true lumens; the latter are radially arranged tumor cells.

Such well-developed structures are unexpected in cytologic examinations of the CSF.[3,70,71] Small cells with the features of other PNETs are seen in smears (Image 3.75). Greenberg and Goldberg reported 3 children with positive CSF specimens despite negative brain scans and the absence of suggestive clinical features.[70] Some but not all authors recommend that a CSF cytologic examination be incorporated into the work-up.[69,71]

Metastatic Neoplasms

If primary brain tumors and lymphoreticular neoplasms are excluded from consideration, it is very uncommon for the CSF from children to contain metastatic tumor cells. Yet, essentially all forms of malignancy may metastasize to the meninges and thus exfoliate cells into the CSF.[3,72] Overall, in our experience, the two major nonlymphoreticular cancers to result in positive metastatic fluid specimens are neuroblastoma and rhabdomyosarcomas.[3] Cytomorphologically, neuroblastoma cells would fully resemble those of medulloblastoma and other PNETs (Image 3.76).[73] We are unaware of any routine means to separate these tumor types in exfoliative specimens. Furthermore, immunocytochemistry and electron microscopy would also probably be noncontributory. Fortunately, from a diagnostic viewpoint, it is very unlikely that a patient with a primary extracranial neuroblastoma will present initially with neurologic manifestations and positive CSF cytology specimens.[73] Primary cerebral neuroblastomas are exceedingly rare and present clinically with signs of mass lesions, rather than meningeal irritation.

Children with rhabdomyosarcoma and positive CSF specimens usually have a primary neoplasm in the head and neck region.[3] Their close proximity to the subarachnoid space and their local invasiveness probably account for this phenomenon. Tomei et al have described 2 children with rare primary intracranial rhabdomyosarcomas.[74] In both patients, leptomeningeal spread was documented and in 1, malignant cells were noted within the CSF. In cytologic preparations, both isolated and aggregated neoplastic cells may be seen and are usually obvious.[3] Cellular size is more variable than with other small cell tumors (Image 3.77). Nuclei are hyperchromatic with fine, even chromatin and often visible nucleoli. Irregularities of nuclear contours are more consistently present than with neuroblastoma. Although most cells have a single, somewhat eccentrically placed nucleus, binucleated cells certainly may be found. Frequently, cytoplasm is more voluminous than in other small cell tumors. We have not seen an example of rhabdomyosarcoma in which cross-striations were evident in an exfoliated cytologic preparation.

Although exceedingly uncommon, other cancers may appear in CSF specimens.[3,70,75] In most circumstances, the primary neoplasm will have been diagnostically established earlier.

It is very unlikely that a patient with a primary extracranial neuroblastoma will present initially with neurologic manifestations and positive CSF cytology specimens

Stereotactic Biopsy and FNA

A morphologic diagnosis of intracranial neoplasms is necessary for determining the optimal form of therapy and the prognosis for children with primary CNS tumors. With deep-seated mass lesions, however, the risk of severe neurologic complications secondary to a biopsy procedure has frequently deterred a histologic interpretation. Accordingly, neurosurgeons have frequently based their working diagnosis on a combination of clinical and radiologic findings. Prime examples of this include brain stem gliomas and tumors of the pineal gland.[76] Recent advances in radiologic imaging techniques and smaller needles have allowed neurosurgeons to obtain tissue from deep intracranial lesions with significantly less morbidity than that associated with an open craniotomy. The addition of stereotactic monitoring has further aided in the accurate placement of the biopsy needle.[77-85] Most published studies recording either radiologic- and/or stereotactic-directed biopsies have used a histologic examination of a thin tissue core and/or a cytologic evaluation of crush smears performed on a portion of that core biopsy specimen. Less frequently, the use of FNA biopsies of intracranial masses has been reported. Although many published series do not provide the exact ages of the patients included in their investigation, it appears that FNA is used very sparingly in children with primary intracranial lesions. In fact, reports dedicated to or concentrating on the use of stereotactic biopsies (with or without cytologic crush preparations) in the pediatric population are very limited[74]; we are unaware of a large published series of FNA smears of CNS lesions in children.

The actual operative procedure for obtaining stereotactic biopsy specimens has been eloquently detailed and illustrated by Chandrasoma and Apuzzo in their excellent monograph.[84] Briefly, any of several different stereotactic apparatuses may be used to interface with the CT scan to provide the exact target coordinates. This accuracy permits needle sampling of both the center and the periphery of small mass lesions. The biopsy itself is performed through a small burr hole in the skull. In adults, this generally can be performed using only local anesthesia. However, as stated by Schmitt et al, light anesthesia is probably preferable in children.[77] This technique is also discussed briefly in our chapter dealing with radiologic imaging.

When the stereotactic equipment is used to obtain a tissue core or multiple minute fragments of CNS tissue, an initial step is to prepare a smear from these samples. A small portion of each tissue fragment is placed directly on a glass slide. A second slide is used to prepare the smear. In general, we use the same technique as we use in the preparation of smears for aspiration cytology. The long axes of the two slides are parallel to each other and pressure is applied to squash the fragments of tissue and the slides are then drawn apart in a longitudinal fashion. As detailed by Chandrasoma, the amount of pressure required in order to make such specimens varies with the firmness of the tissue samples.[84] In most centers in the United States, the slides are fixed immediately in 95% ethanol and stained with hematoxylin and eosin. Others prefer rapid Papanicolaou stains on these smears. When a fine needle is used to obtain an aspiration specimen, smears are prepared in the same manner as they are for aspiration biopsies in any other body site. Both air-dried Romanowsky and alcohol-fixed Papanicolaou stains may be used. Romanowsky is also used by some workers in crush preparations.[82]

The major indications for the use of stereotactic biopsies with crush smears and/or FNA biopsies of the CNS include obtaining material for morphologic diagnosis of mass lesions involving relatively inaccessible sites. The latter include the deep cerebrum including basal ganglia and the hypothalamus, the suprasellar area, the region surrounding the third ventricle, the pineal gland, and the lower brain stem. The stereotactic approach results in only a minimum of injury to normal brain tissue. Diffuse lesions such as infections and storage disorders comprise another indication. Patients considered inoperable due to poor general health may be evaluated by stereotactic biopsy when a craniotomy would be considered probably out of the question. The technique is applicable to very young infants as well.[77]

Patients considered inoperable due to poor general health may be evaluated by stereotactic biopsy when a craniotomy would be considered probably out of the question

Cytomorphology

Although the neurosurgeon tries to avoid sampling normal brain tissue, its inclusion in a stereotactically obtained specimen is unavoidable in certain circumstances. In smears of normal CNS tissue, nuclei of astrocytes will be most numerous. They are characterized by a round or slightly ovoid configuration with very finely granular, pale-stained chromatin and inconspicuous or inapparent nucleoli. In general, cytoplasm is not visible. One may also visualize the nuclei of oligodendrocytes. The latter will be slightly smaller and more perfectly round than those of the astrocytes. Furthermore, the chromatin is more darkly stained, although it is uniformly distributed throughout the nucleus. A perinuclear halo may be apparent, but in general cytoplasm is inconspicuous. These nuclei are set within an eosinophilic fibrillary background which corresponds to the neuropil. Delicate capillaries may be seen but are infrequent. In certain parts of the brain, neurons may also be sampled. These cells and their nuclei are larger than those of normal glia. They are characterized by a round, vesicular nucleus with a prominent, even large nucleolus, all set eccentrically within polygonal eosinophilic cytoplasm.

As one might expect, the differential diagnosis of normal brain tissue may include reactive gliosis and even low-grade astrocytomas. In general, both gliosis and low-grade neoplasms will be hypercellular relative to normal brain (Image 3.78). In fact, the differential diagnosis between benign gliosis and low-grade astrocytomas may be much more difficult. This distinction may be almost impossible according to some authorities.[82,83,85] Other authors offer diagnostic clues to this differential situation.[82,84] In gliosis, cytoplasm may be more apparent among the reactive astrocytes appearing as denser, more eosinophilic cell bodies often with evident cellular processes.[80,82,83,84] Cytoplasm may also be much more apparent in the neoplastic elements of low-grade astrocytomas (Image 3.79). However, this is a less uniform phenomenon than in reactive gliosis. In low-grade astrocytomas, Rosenthal fibers may be recognized in smears.[80,86] Nuclei may or may not be larger and/or more pleomorphic than in a nonneoplastic setting (Table 3.2). Their chromatin also may or may not be more darkly stained. According to Chandrasoma, the smear background will be much more fibrillar in the low-grade astrocytomas (Image 3.80).[84] Blood vessels may be more prominent as the neoplastic astrocytes may be surrounded by a collar of increased numbers of astrocytes. A diagnostic aid is to correlate the cytomorphology with the radiologic appearance of the lesion. Reactive gliosis surrounding a nonneoplastic mass such as an abscess generally produces a ring-enhancing pattern, as do malignant astrocytomas. Well-differentiated astrocytomas are generally not ring-enhancing lesions.

High-grade astrocytomas include anaplastic astrocytoma and glioblastoma. Smears from these neoplasms will be definitely hypercellular and contain obviously malignant astrocytic elements (Image 3.81). The latter are characterized by larger and more variably sized and shaped hyperchromatic nuclei (Table 3.3). Chromatin may be coarsely granular, but generally retains a uniform distribution within the enlarged nuclei. At times, nucleoli may also be quite prominent.

A diagnostic aid is to correlate the cytomorphology with the radiologic appearance of the lesion

Another characteristic feature is proliferation of endothelial cells within the capillaries (Image 3.82).[80,82-85] In smears, this is seen as syncytial arrangements of the endothelial cells either in a parallel longitudinal manner or 3-dimensional irregular ball-like arrays. The endothelial nuclei generally remain elongated or plump and oval. They may appear quite dark due to the prominent overlapping of nuclei. Margination of neoplastic astrocytes along these vascular walls with an apparent intermingling with the endothelial cells is also recognized in some specimens. As with the low-grade astrocytomas, tumor cell cytoplasm may be much more apparent and even present bizarre configurations with blunt or elongated processes. Necrosis is required for a diagnosis of glioblastoma (Images 3.83 through 3.85). In smears, this occurs most often as irregular masses of granular debris without evident nuclei. As stated by Chandrasoma, it is more easily recognized as such when it occurs as the outlines of dead anucleated cells (ghosts).[84]

Although not specifically restricted to the pediatric population, the subependymal giant cell astrocytoma is a very uncommon, benign neoplasm that probably occurs only in patients with tuberous sclerosis complex.[87] Usually, these tumors occur along the wall of the lateral ventricles of patients with other features of tuberous sclerosis. The cytologic appearance of these neoplasms have been recorded only very infrequently.[78,87] These specimens have been described as being cellular and consisting of aggregates of large cells with variable contours. Cell borders may be smooth or disrupted by thick cellular processes producing a characteristic polarized appearance. These cells have moderate to abundant eosinophilic cytoplasm. At times, it presents as a very elongated or spindled contour (strap cells). Tumor cells with more than one nucleus are characteristic. Chromatin is generally benign in appearance with a finely granular uniform distribution. Mitotic activity is sparse and neither necrosis nor endothelial proliferation has been recorded. The differential diagnosis of this neoplasm is detailed by Altermatt and Scheithauer.[87]

Smears of ependymomas are generally cellular and often contain large, cohesive fragments of tumor cells (Table 3.4). The latter are characterized by round or slightly oval uniform nuclei with finely granular chromatin that is evenly distributed (Image 3.86). Nucleoli may or may not be apparent. The cell outline in ependymomas are characteristically well defined, demonstrating columnar or cuboidal configurations. These neoplastic cells may be distributed in monolayer sheets or occasionally in papillary or pseudopapillary structures.[78,83-85] Rosettes may be seen in smears of ependymomas.

These epithelial qualities are also easily recognized in tumors of the choroid plexus.[83,84] Definite papillary arrangements of the neoplastic cells will be seen in papillomas (Image 3.87). These 3 dimensional aggregates are composed of uniform neoplastic cells with round, pale staining nuclei and variable amounts of cytoplasm, although columnar contours are infrequent. Intercellular borders are readily appreciated (Table 3.5). These bland neoplastic cells may also be seen in monolayer arrangements (Image 3.88). Although Chandrasoma warns that the diagnosis of choroid plexus carcinoma should not be made on the basis of smears alone, Nguyen et al claimed that the cells are obviously malignant and demonstrated an epithelial quality in the crush prepara-

Although not specifically restricted to the pediatric population, the subependymal giant cell astrocytoma is a very uncommon, benign neoplasm that probably occurs only in patients with tuberous sclerosis complex

tions.[83,84] Their series includes two choroid plexus carcinomas; the intraoperative cytodiagnosis on the basis of the crush preparation was "cancer cells present" in both patients.[83]

Medulloblastomas present in smears as a typical small cell cancer composed of relatively dense populations of obviously malignant cells (Image 3.89). The latter are characterized by a single, hyperchromatic nucleus with coarsely granular and at times irregularly distributed chromatin (Table 3.1). The nuclear contours range from round to irregular and angulated. Nuclear to cytoplasmic ratios are characteristically very high with only a thin rim of apparent cytoplasm present. Within other aggregates, pseudorosettes may be seen, although they are uncommon (Image 3.90). More frequently, the neoplastic cells are aggregated into nondescript arrangements in which nuclear molding is readily apparent (Image 3.91). Necrosis may also be frequently seen, as are mitotic figures. As discussed earlier in this chapter, a number of different types of neoplasms may occur in and about the region of the pineal gland. Smears of pineoblastomas would be indistinguishable from those of medulloblastoma and other primitive neuroectodermal tumors. As described by Chandrasoma, smears from pineocytomas contain numerous regular neoplastic cells which are characterized as small and round.[84] Typically, they appear as round nuclei with finely granular chromatin, small nucleoli, and devoid of cytoplasm. By far, the most frequent malignant germ cell tumor to occur in this region is the germinoma (Table 3.6). In smears, the large neoplastic cells usually occur as solitary cells, or at most, in small loosely cohesive aggregates.[82,84] They are characterized by a solitary large round vesicular nucleus that houses one or more prominent nucleoli. The cell body may at times be seen as a scanty rim of pale-staining, at times vacuolated cytoplasm. This delicate cytoplasm is fragile, creating the characteristic tigroid background in smears stained with Diff-Quik. In addition, the smears will often contain numerous small mature-appearing lymphocytes. Granulomatous inflammation may also be seen in these tumors and be represented in the smears. Chandrasoma details the diagnostic difficulties that may be produced by this inflammatory infiltrate.[84]

Two benign neoplasms that occur in and about the region of the pituitary gland with a relatively high frequency in children are the adenoma and the craniopharyngioma. Both crush and aspiration smears of pituitary adenomas provide a characteristic picture.[79,80,84] These specimens will be cellular and composed of cells, each having a perfectly smooth round or oval nucleus with finely granular chromatin and occasionally a prominent nucleolus (Image 3.92). Characteristically, there may be considerable variation in nuclear size. However, this pleomorphism of size should not lead to a diagnosis of malignancy if one recognizes the uniformity of the smooth nuclear contours and correlates this with the clinical picture and the location of the stereotactic needle. Cytoplasm may be stripped away from the cells or be preserved as dense and polygonal in contour. With Diff-Quik–stained smears, the neoplastic cells may have a characteristic plasmacytoid appearance. The cells will occur both scattered individually and in loosely cohesive aggregates without any distinctive organoid arrangement.[79] Although some authors warn against the needle biopsy of a craniopharyngioma due to potential leakage of cyst contents, other authors have described

A number of different types of neoplasms may occur in and about the region of the pineal gland

well the appearance of this neoplasm in smears.[67,77-79,84] In order to make the diagnosis, one needs to recognize squamous epithelial cells without prominent cytologic atypia in these smears. Most often, the tumor cells are present in large, irregular cohesive aggregates. Liwnicz and colleagues state that the finding of squamous epithelial cells is also not diagnostic of craniopharyngioma.[78] Degenerative changes may also be frequent. In addition, one may find numerous histiocytes and inflammatory cells within the smears. In Diff-Quik–stained aspiration cells, cholesterol crystals may also be recognized by their "negative-staining" image. As warned by Chandrasoma, these crystals and histiocytes are not specific for craniopharyngioma.[84] These last points emphasize the constant need to correlate cytomorphologic features of CNS tumors with the clinical information and the exact site from which the biopsy specimen was procured. One nonneoplastic mass lesion seen with some frequency in stereotactically obtained specimens is the abscess. As one might expect, these smears will feature intact and degenerated neutrophils on a background of fibrinous proteinaceous debris (Image 3.93). Other cellular elements may include histiocytes, but neurons or glia will occur only rarely. Most often, microbial organisms will not be seen in the smears, but bacteria may be recognizable with the Diff-Quik–stained preparations. At times, fungi may also be seen in the smears (Images 3.94 and 3.95).

Accuracy of Stereotactic Specimens

As most reported series probably involve mostly or exclusively adult patients, the data may not be totally applicable to the pediatric population. Accuracy is best analyzed by comparing the results of the intraoperative diagnosis either by crush smears or aspiration smears with the final histologic diagnosis rendered on paraffin-embedded tissue sections. Review of the literature for crush preparations demonstrates an accuracy ranging from 77% to 95%.[77,80,82-85] Most series report an accuracy of at least 90%. Only the report of Schmitt and colleagues was restricted to children.[77] Although it is difficult to be totally certain from their manuscript, it appears that they had an accuracy of 90%. Fewer reports are dedicated to the accuracy of stereotactically-obtained FNA biopsy specimens.[78,79,88] None of these papers concentrated on this technique in children. Accuracy of reported series ranges from 87% to 92%. Silverman et al have calculated the diagnostic specificity, sensitivity and efficiency of FNA of CNS lesions, utilizing reported data.[88] Their calculations found a diagnostic sensitivity of 92%, specificity of 100% and an efficiency of 89%.

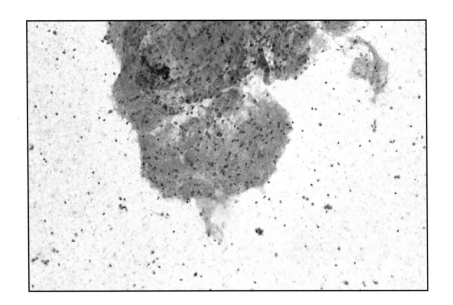

Image 3.1
Intraoperative brain wash specimen includes a relatively large fragment of glial tissue with a normal-appearing cellular density. It would be very difficult to distinguish this from a fragment of gliotic brain or a low-grade astrocytoma, and thus clinical history is crucial. Many small isolated cells are also present. (Papanicolaou).

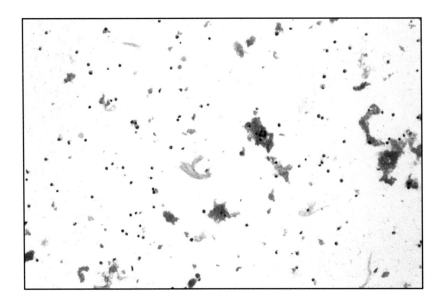

Image 3.2
Most intraoperative brain wash specimens contain only very small fragments of brain tissue with few if any visible nuclei. Most cells are usually dispersed singly and include many red and white blood cells. (Papanicolaou).

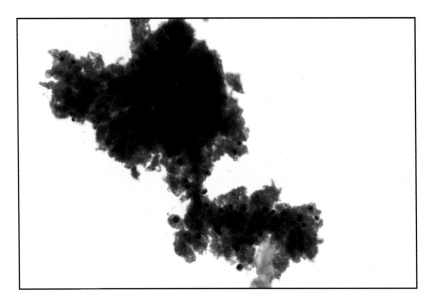

Image 3.3
Large 3-dimensional cellular masses may be seen in otherwise unremarkable specimens, as in this shunt fluid. Observation of the cells at the edges of such fragments permits visualization of the small, uniform and evenly spread benign elements, which are usually glial in nature. (Papanicolaou).

Image 3.4
This is a small round cluster of normal choroidal–ependymal cells in a child previously treated for acute leukemia. The nuclei are small and uniform and have smooth contours; cellular borders are indistinct. (Papanicolaou).

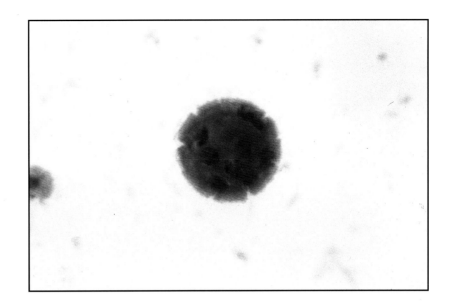

Image 3.5
CSF specimen from a child with sickle cell anemia. The peripheral blood was probably a contaminant. Note that many of the erythrocytes are deformed. (Romanowsky). (Courtesy of Dr R Craver).

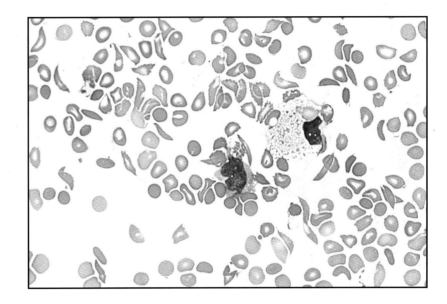

Image 3.6
The cytoplasm of individual and loosely aggregated histiocytes contain intact erythrocytes, some of which look like "ghost red cells," (erythrophagocytosis). Indentation of the phagocyte's nucleus by the intact red cells is a common feature. (Romanowsky). (Courtesy of Dr R Craver).

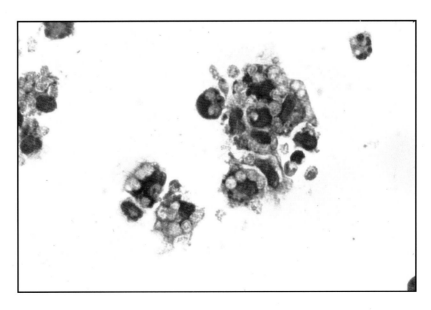

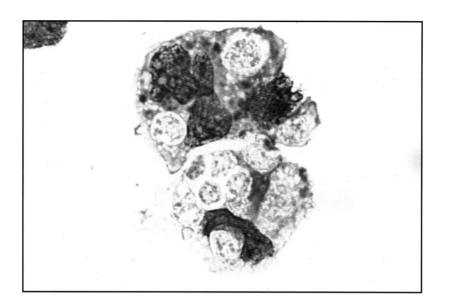

Image 3.7
The cytoplasm of the histiocytes is distended by erythrocytes in various stages of degeneration. The nature of these inclusions is obvious and usually correlates well with the clinical history. Nuclei may be disarmingly atypical but in this setting should not create a diagnostic problem. (Romanowsky). (Courtesy of Dr R Craver).

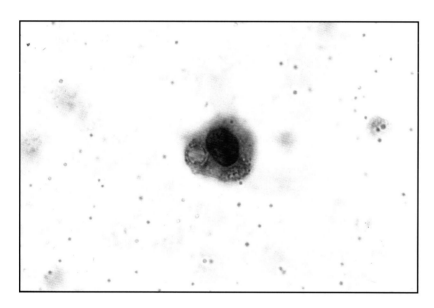

Image 3.8
With the Papanicolaou stain, the phagocyte's fine nuclear chromatin and the low N/C ratio are readily appreciated. Note the minute fragments of the erythrocytes in the background; these should not be mistaken for microbial organisms, eg, yeast.

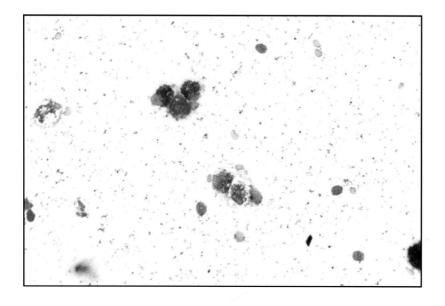

Image 3.9
Although red cell fragments are more commonly seen in filter preparations, (as in Image 3.8), they may also be present in cytospins. Lack of budding and variable size and shape allow distinction of fragments from *Candida* and other fungi. Other evidence of hemorrhage is also helpful. (Romanowsky). (Courtesy of Dr R Craver).

Image 3.10
This siderophage contains hemo-siderin. With the Romanowsky stains, this pigment takes on a dark blue to black coloration. (Courtesy of Dr R Craver).

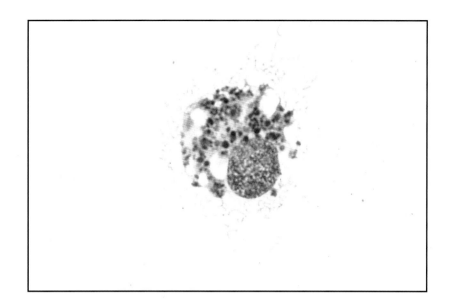

Image 3.11
The nucleus of the histiocytes may be displaced to the very edge of the cell or even obscured by the hemosiderin pigment granules. Note also the intact and fragmented erythrocytes. (Romanowsky).

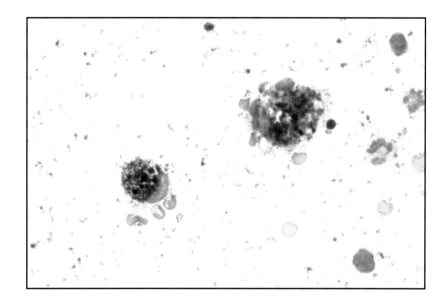

Image 3.12
With the Papanicolaou stain, hemo-siderin granules appear brown or green and may be more refractile.

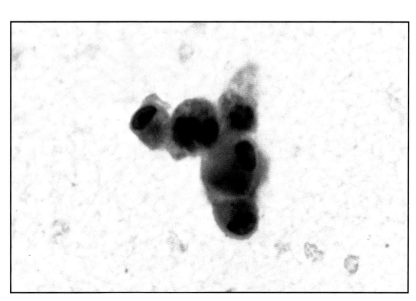

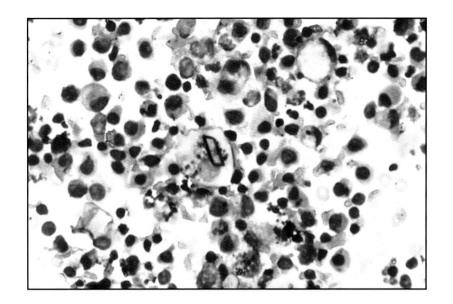

Image 3.13
Crystals of hematoidin may be seen in the cytoplasm of phagocytes. They are bright yellow and have sharp edges. (Romanowsky). (Courtesy of Dr R Craver).

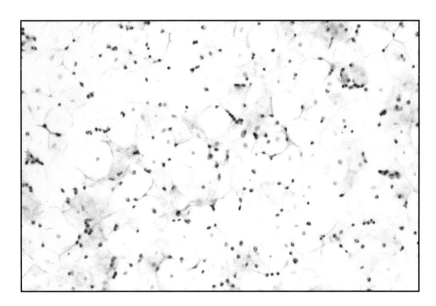

Image 3.14
CSF specimen from a child with a ruptured primary CNS dermoid is dominated by sheets of squamous epithelial cells. Neutrophils are also present. (Romanowsky). (Courtesy of Dr R Craver).

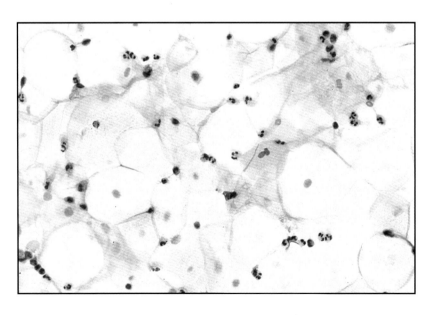

Image 3.15
This is a higher magnification of Image 3.14. It shows benign squames, each with a single small round nucleus set within abundant cytoplasm. The cells have polygonal contours and distinct borders. Morphologically, this would be impossible to distinguish from contamination of the CSF specimen by skin during a lumbar puncture. (Romanowsky). (Courtesy of Dr R Craver).

Image 3.16
Inadvertent bone marrow contamination of CSF in an infant. A cluster of normoblasts encircle a large histiocyte. (Romanowsky). (Courtesy of Dr R Craver).

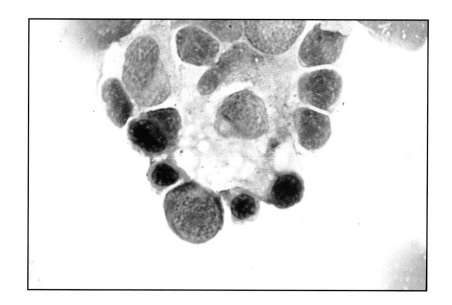

Image 3.17
Primitive cell clusters present in a rosette-like cohesive aggregate in CSF. The chromatin is finely reticulated and nucleoli are small but obvious. Nuclear contours are indented or notched. N/C ratio is high. (Romanowsky). (Courtesy of Dr J Goeken).

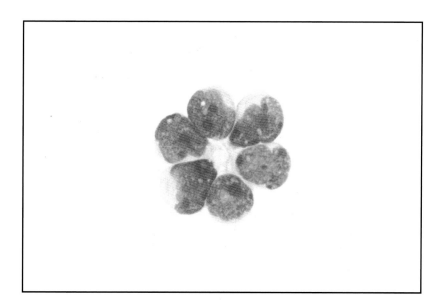

Image 3.18
With the Papanicolaou stain, the chromatin in the germinal matrix cells is finely granular and evenly distributed throughout the nuclei which are not truly hyperchromatic. Thin rims of cyanophilic cytoplasm surround the nuclei. Compare the size of these neural elements with that of the mononuclear cells, probably small lymphocytes.

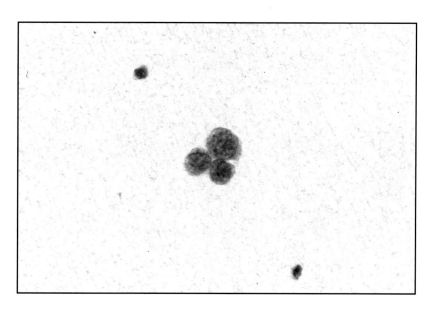

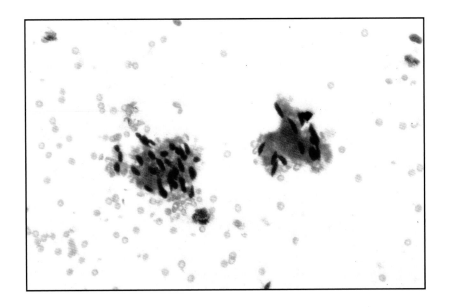

Image 3.19
Germinal matrix cells may exfoliate attached to small volumes of neuropil. In this setting, the differential diagnosis possibly includes glioma and medulloblastoma, but not leukemia. The clinical history is very important. Note the erythrocytes. (Romanowsky). (Courtesy of Dr R Craver).

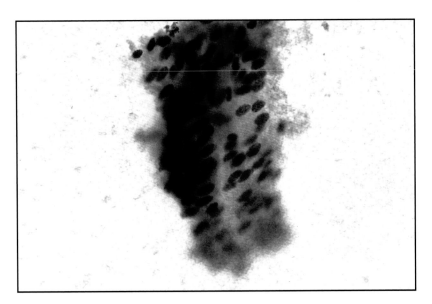

Image 3.20
Occasionally, the nuclei of the germinal matrix elements are aligned in parallel rows, a helpful hint of their true nature. (Papanicolaou).

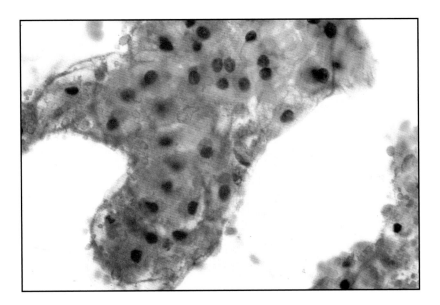

Image 3.21
CSF specimen contaminated with fragments of notochord due to sampling of a vertebral body. With the Papanicolaou stain, the notochordal nuclei are seen to be small, round, and have evenly dispersed fine chromatin granules; nucleoli are not evident. Cell borders are not well developed, but N/C ratio appears to be low.

Image 3.22
CSF specimen contaminated with notochord fragments (see Image 3.21). With the Diff-Quik stain, the meta-chromatic nature of the matrix is evident and permits easy recognition of the notochordal nature of the specimen. No primary brain tumor would resemble this appearance.

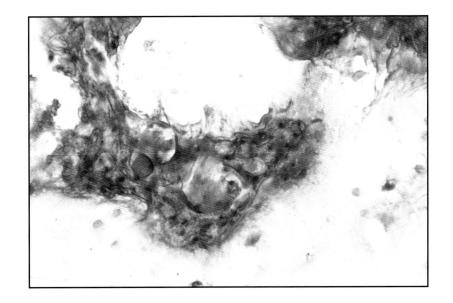

Image 3.23
In acute meningitis, one typically sees a pure "culture" of neutrophilic leukocytes. In this example, fibrin, debris and bacterial organisms are absent. (Romanowsky).

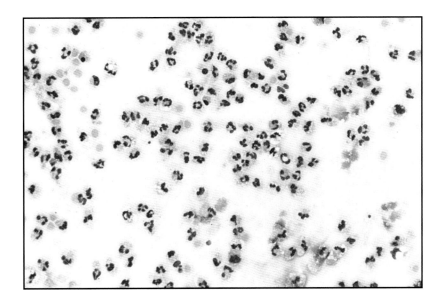

Image 3.24
CSF specimen contains numerous neutrophils admixed with fibrinous exudate. The segmented leukocytes often appear in loosely cohesive clumps. (Papanicolaou).

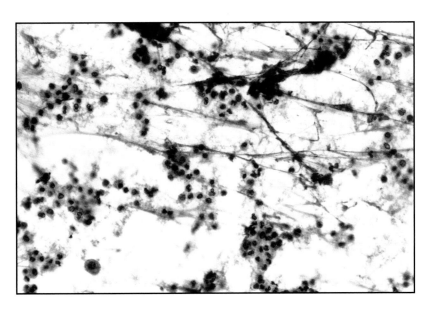

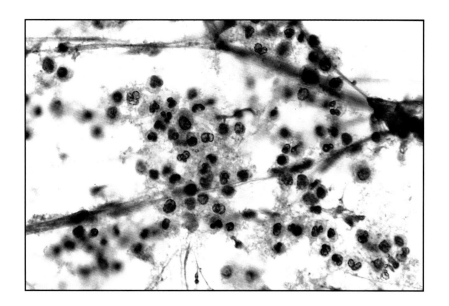

Image 3.25
Although neutrophils dominate the cytologic picture, mononuclear elements, both macrophages and lymphocytes, will comprise a minor cellular component. Note the fibrin strands. (Papanicolaou).

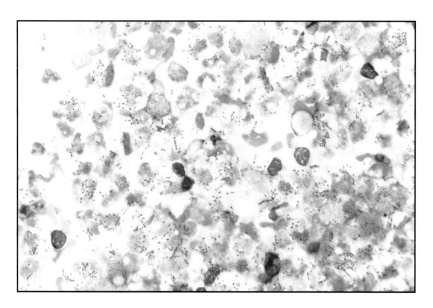

Image 3.26
CSF specimen is from a child with acute meningitis clinically; it contains numerous streptococci, both intra- and extracellularly. The Diff-Quik stain may allow recognition of many bacterial organisms that are not readily visualized with the Papanicolaou stain.

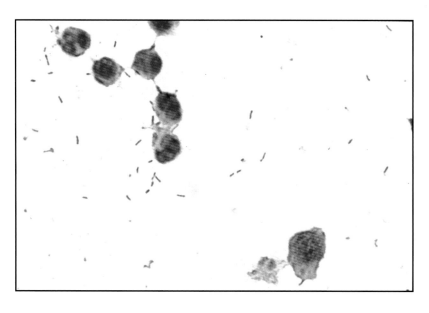

Image 3.27
In CSF, bacteria are better identified with a Gram-stain. This is an example of *Haemophilus influenzae* in which numerous short Gram-negative rods are present extracellularly. A few organisms are closely associated with neutrophils. (Courtesy of Dr B Wasilauskas).

Image 3.28
Streptococcus pneumoniae are typically seen as pairs of Gram-positive round cocci (doublets) within the cytoplasm of phagocytes. Often, they appear within small vacuoles. (Courtesy of Dr B Wasilauskas).

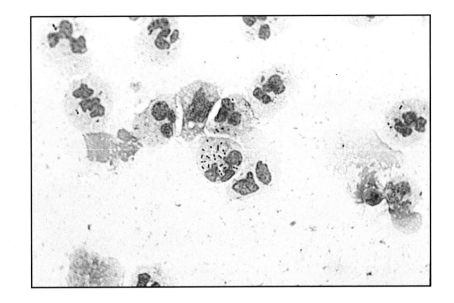

Image 3.29
Inflammatory cells are not seen in this Gram-stained CSF from a 2-year-old child with a clinical picture of acute meningitis due to a *Salmonella* infection. Note the plump Gram-negative rods. (Courtesy of Dr B Wasilauskas).

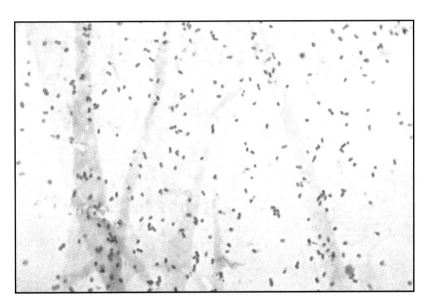

Image 3.30
The scanning lens view in chronic meningitis usually contains obviously increased numbers of small mononuclear cells diffusely distributed over the slide. Note the absence of the protein exudate typical of bacterial meningitis. (Papanicolaou).

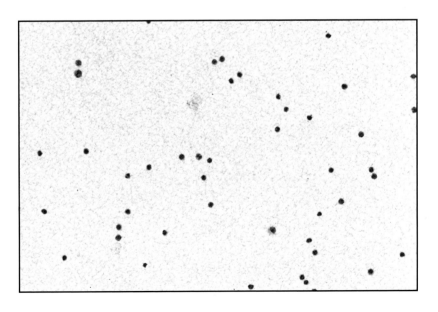

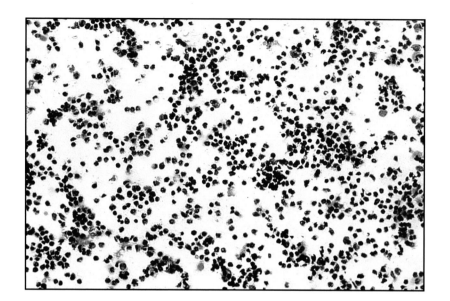

Image 3.31
Mononuclear cells may be so densely packed in CSF specimens, especially those prepared by cytocentrifugation, that they may appear to form cellular aggregates (pseudocohesion). (Romanowsky). (Courtesy of Dr R Craver).

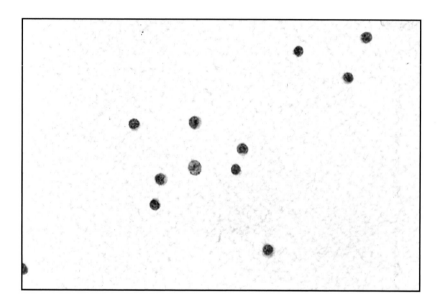

Image 3.32
In this example of viral meningitis, the lymphocytes occur as a single cell suspension and are rather uniform. Each has a single smooth round nucleus and a very high N/C ratio without nucleoli. (Papanicolaou).

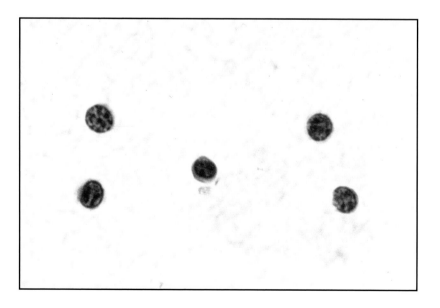

Image 3.33
Viral meningitis (higher magnification of Image 3.32) exhibits the coarse chromatin and smooth nuclear contours expected in most examples of chronic meningitis. This should not create a diagnostic difficulty. (Papanicolaou).

Image 3.34
Blast-like elements may appear in the CSF in cases of benign chronic meningitis. The cells are larger than mature lymphocytes and have a more open chromatin pattern and a nucleolus. This spectrum of appearances is a marker of a benign process. (Papanicolaou).

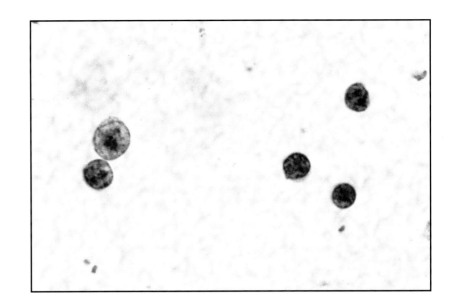

Image 3.35
CSF specimen from a child with herpes meningitis. Although small mature-appearing lymphocytes are present, many are larger and have a plasmacytoid appearance with an eccentric round nucleus, basophilic cytoplasm, and a perinuclear hof. (Romanowsky). (Courtesy of Dr R Craver).

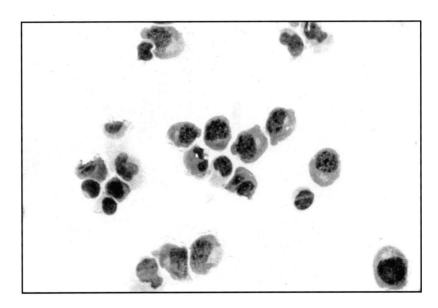

Image 3.36
CSF specimen shows herpes meningitis (see Image 3.35). A well-developed spectrum of lymphocytes is present with a range of sizes and appearances, which is consistent with a benign reactive process. Note the mitotic figure. (Romanowsky). (Courtesy of Dr R Craver).

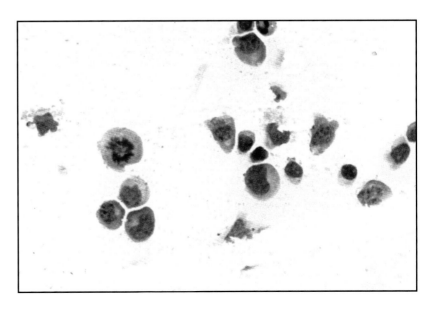

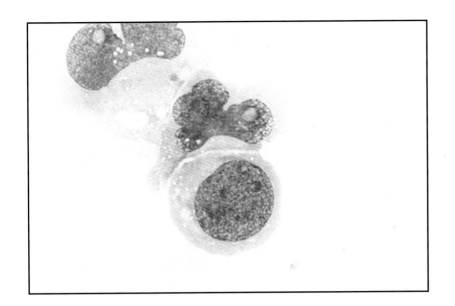

Image 3.37
Large primitive blast-like cells and other atypical mononuclear elements are present in the CSF of an infant with possible viral meningitis. There was no evidence of cancer. (Romanowsky).

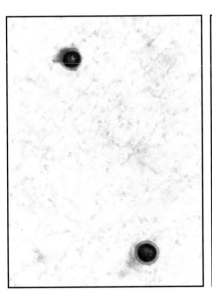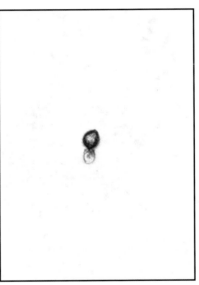

Image 3.38
CSF specimen from a child with ALL and cryptococcal meningitis. Two organisms are present at left. They are round with a stippled structure and a thick capsule. Narrow neck budding of *Cryptococcus* is seen on the right. Note the absence of inflammatory cells. (Papanicolaou).

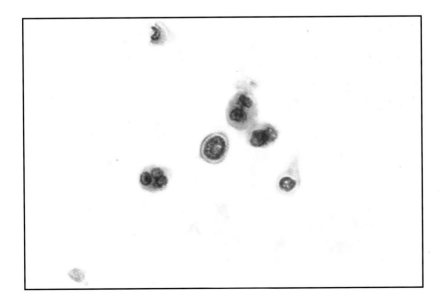

Image 3.39
Cryptococcus in the CSF of a child with AIDS. The organism, including its capsule, approximates the size of the inflammatory cells. (Papanicolaou).

Image 3.40
A methenamine-silver–stained cyto-spin preparation of CSF. Cryptococcal organisms characteristically show variability in size. A few cells demonstrate budding. (Gomori methenamine silver).

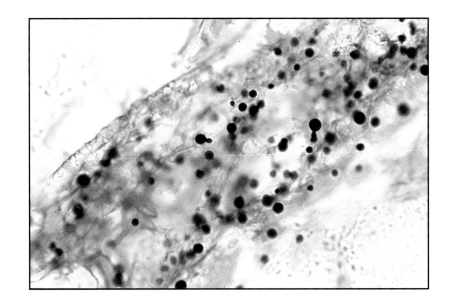

Image 3.41
A methenamine-silver–stained cytospin preparation of CSF (see Image 3.40). Budding yeast forms are clear, as are the outlines of thick capsules. (Gomori methenamine silver)

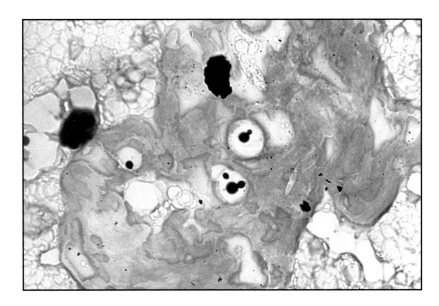

Image 3.42
CSF specimen from a child with *Candida* meningitis. The cytoplasm of this mononuclear phagocyte contains numerous phagocytized yeast cells. Pseudohyphae (not shown) are also present extracellularly. (Romanowsky). (Courtesy of Dr R Craver).

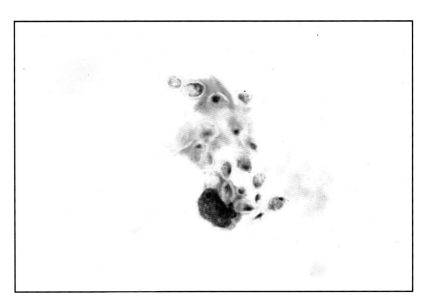

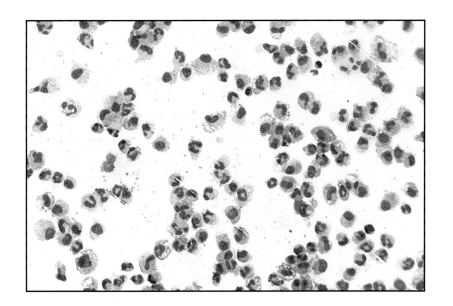

Image 3.43
This is an example of pleocytosis from a child adequately treated for ALL. This postchemotherapy CSF is dominated by benign histiocytes. They have eccentric, oval or bean-shaped nuclei, and low N/C ratio. Cytoplasm is granular to somewhat foamy. (Romanowsky).

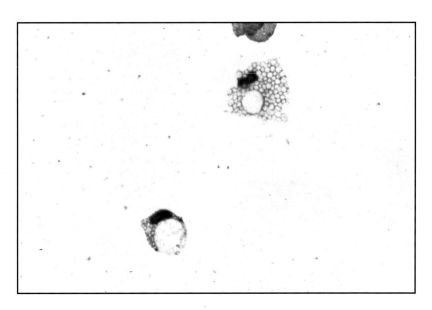

Image 3.44
CSF specimen is from a 3-month-old child with gangliosidosis (Tay-Sachs disease). The cytologic picture is dominated by individually dispersed histiocytes. Their cytoplasm is distended by abnormally accumulated ganglioside. One cell forms the classic signet-ring appearance. (Romanowsky). (Courtesy of Dr R Craver).

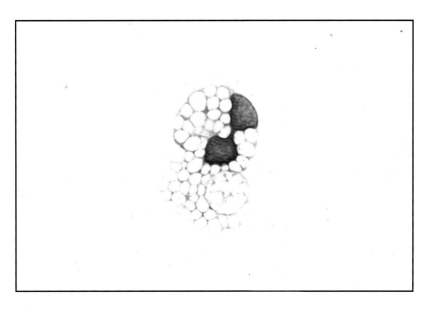

Image 3.45
CSF specimen from a child with gangliosidosis (see Image 3.44). The cytoplasm of this histiocyte is packed with small uniform lysosomal vacuoles. The N/C ratio is low and the nucleus appears deformed. (Romanowsky).

Image 3.46
CSF specimen from a child with gangliosidosis (see Image 3.44). Variable vacuoles occupy the cytoplasm of this histiocyte. Note the benign nature of the nucleus. This should not be mistaken for signet-ring carcinoma, which is exceedingly rare in young children. (Romanowsky).

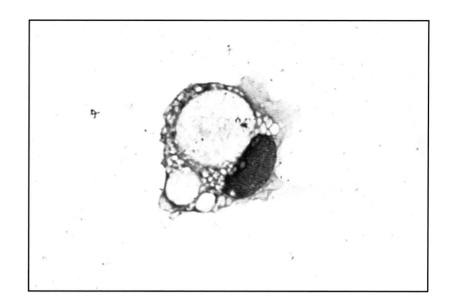

Image 3.47
In this example of ventriculitis, the cytologic picture of this shunt fluid specimen is dominated by intact and degenerated neutrophils. It correlated well with the clinical impression of acute bacterial ventriculitis. (Romanowsky).

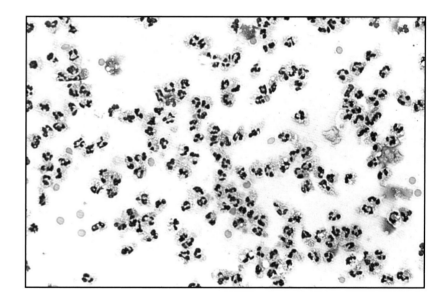

Image 3.48
CSF specimen was obtained during a shunt revision procedure. In addition to erythrocytes and a few lymphocytes, many of the cells are histiocytic elements probably related to the presence of a foreign body (the shunt). Most are mononucleated but others have multiple nuclei including one with a wreath-like arrangement. (Romanowsky). (Courtesy of Dr R Craver).

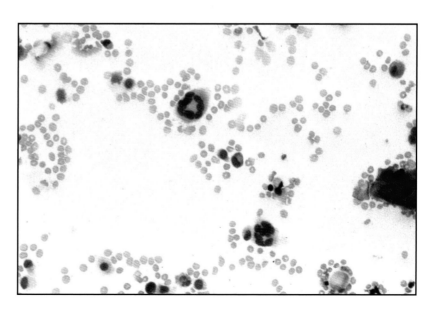

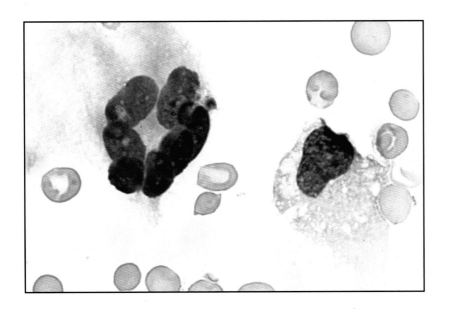

Image 3.49
CSF specimen obtained during shunt revision procedure (see Image 3.48). This multinucleated histiocyte has overlapped nuclei arranged in a circular manner like a wreath. Each nucleus has a smooth oval contour, dense chromatin and a small nucleolus; they are strikingly uniform. Adjacent is a foamy macrophage with a similar nucleus. (Romanowsky).

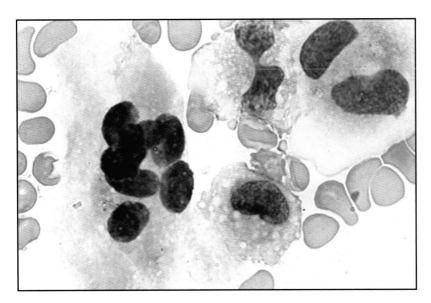

Image 3.50
CSF specimen obtained during shunt revision procedure (see Image 3.48). Although the sizes and shapes of these reactive elements are quite variable, their nuclei are all very uniform and they all have a low N/C ratio. (Romanowsky).

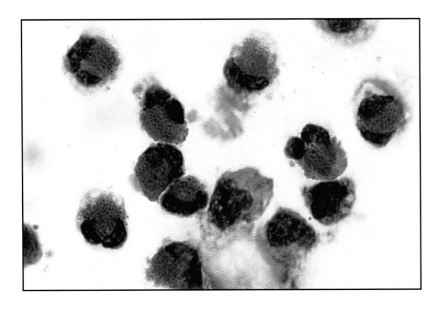

Image 3.51
Shunt fluid from a child with hydrocephalus is overrun by eosinophilic leukocytes admixed with lymphocytes and macrophages. Note the bilobed nuclei of the eosinophils. (Romanowsky). (Case courtesy of Dr R Craver).

Image 3.52

Medulloblastoma frequently presents in CSF as rather large masses, often 3-dimensional, with a patternless or sheet-like arrangement. The malignant cells are homogenous, each having a single round hyperchromatic nucleus and a very high N/C ratio. Note the molding. (Papanicolaou).

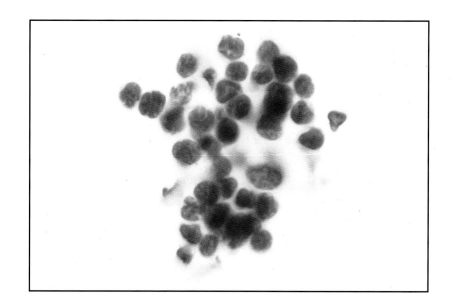

Image 3.53

In this rosette of medulloblastoma cells, a peripheral ring of uniform obviously malignant nuclei surround central cyanophilic cytoplasm. Their chromatin is finely granular and evenly distributed. Nucleoli are almost imperceptible. Note the isolated cell with the characteristic blunt tail of cytoplasm. The other individual tumor cell is pyknotic. (Papanicolaou).

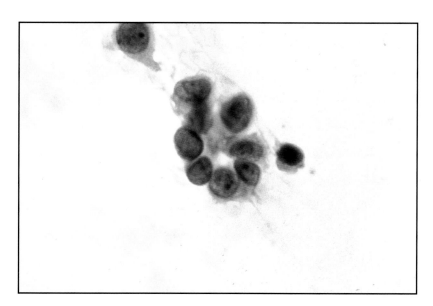

Image 3.54

This tetrad of medulloblastoma cells is composed of four uniform medulloblasts, all with a very high N/C ratio. (Papanicolaou).

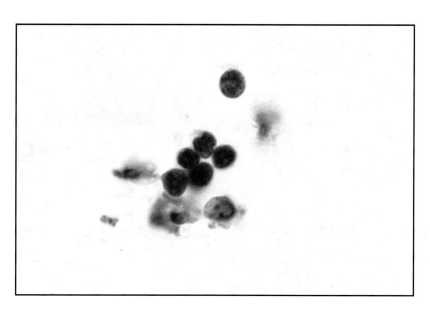

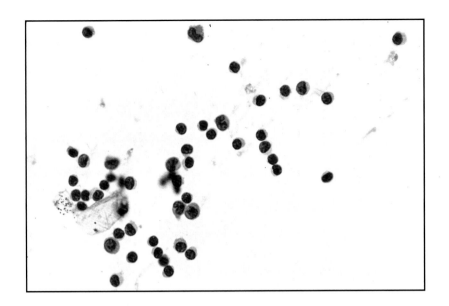

Image 3.55
CSF specimen is from a 4-year-old boy treated for medulloblastoma. Although the specimen is cellular, tumor cells are absent. Lymphocytes comprise the major component of this reactive pleocytosis. They are small and do not demonstrate true intercellular cohesion. (Papanicolaou).

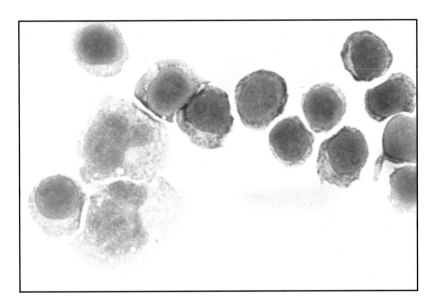

Image 3.56
CSF specimen is from a 4-year-old boy treated for medulloblastoma (see Image 3.55). Chromatin is more finely reticular in lymphocytes than in tumor cells. The lymphocytes have small but evident nucleoli. The larger histiocytes have more irregularly shaped nuclei and larger volumes of pale cytoplasm. (Romanowsky).

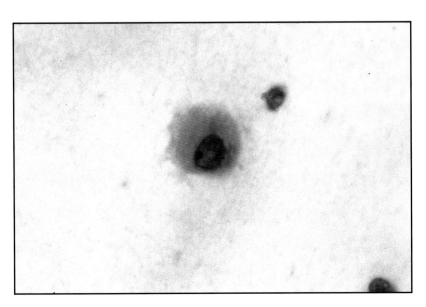

Image 3.57
Ventricular fluid specimen from a 10-year-old child with a low-grade astrocytoma. Cellularity is very scanty but includes solitary tumor cells. Each cell has a single round to oval nucleus with smooth contours, finely granular chromatin and a small nucleolus. The cell bodies stain a faint bluish-green and blend into the smear background. (Papanicolaou).

Image 3.58
Only a small minority of the tumor cells will display the characteristic bipolar cytoplasmic tails. N/C ratio is low and the nuclei have bland features. (Papanicolaou).

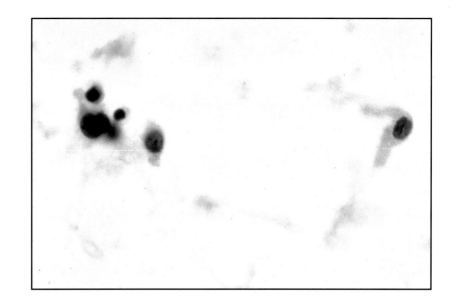

Image 3.59
Exfoliated tumor cell from a low-grade astrocytoma. The eccentric nucleus has pale staining, very finely granular chromatin and a small nucleolus. The peripheral cell border is fuzzy or indistinct. (Papanicolaou).

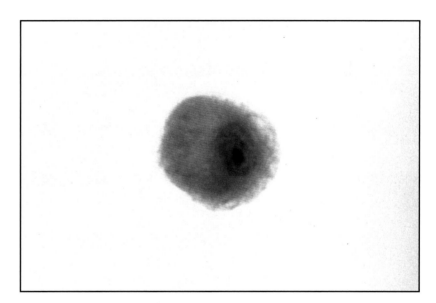

Image 3.60
Specimen from a 12-year-old with a recurrent astrocytoma. The eccentric nucleus is bland in appearance and cytoplasm is abundant and dense. Cell borders are not well defined. Note the size of the tumor cells compared to the adjacent neutrophil. (Romanowsky).

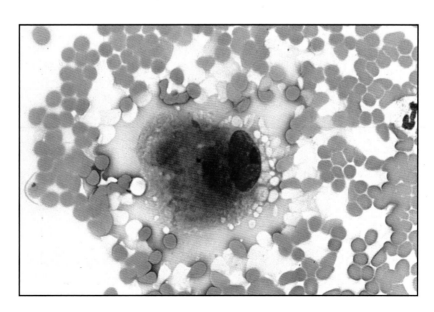

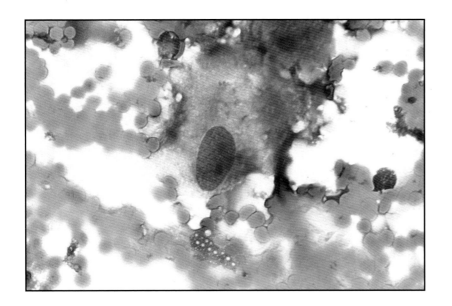

Image 3.61
This astrocytoma cell's nucleus almost appears in a different plane from its cytoplasm. The nuclear membrane is smooth and regular, as is expected in low-grade tumors. (Romanowsky).

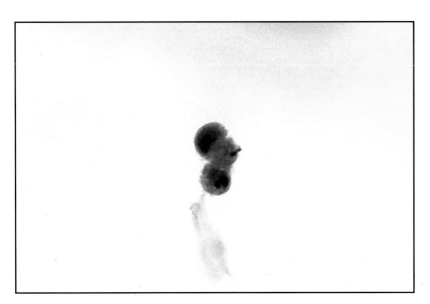

Image 3.62
Cellular aggregates are usually composed of a low number of neoplastic cells. Their cytoplasm is dense and cyanophilic with indistinct margins. (Papanicolaou).

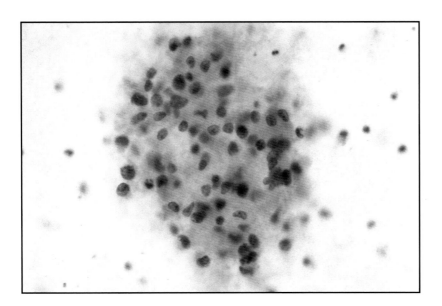

Image 3.63
Anaplastic astrocytomas, as in this CSF specimen from a young child, may be much more cellular than those seen in low-grade counterparts. This fragment of tumor shows a high density of hyperchromatic nuclei. It is difficult to judge N/C ratio. (Papanicolaou).

Image 3.64
CSF specimen from an 8-year-old boy with an anaplastic astrocytoma. Histologically, the tumor has areas composed of small malignant cells. This is the cytologic counterpart. Although their nuclei closely resemble those of a PNET, their cytoplasm appears more plentiful. (Papanicolaou).

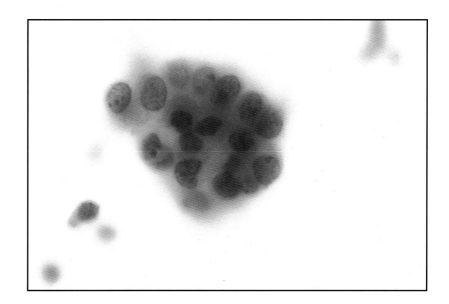

Image 3.65
In cytologic specimens from glioblastomas, the malignant nature of the tumor giant cells is obvious. They have one or more large often irregularly shaped nuclei. Chromatin is hyperchromatic or almost pyknotic in appearance and nucleoli may be well developed. (Papanicolaou).

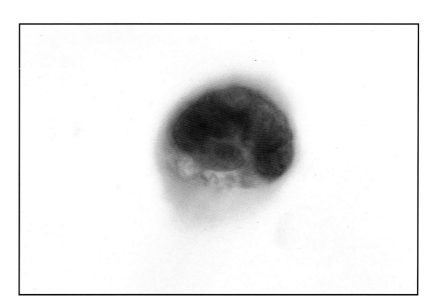

Image 3.66
In cytologic specimens, smaller tumor cells usually predominate. Most are round or oval, but a few may have elongated or stellate contours. Cytoplasm is cyanophilic and cell borders are rather indistinct. (Papanicolaou).

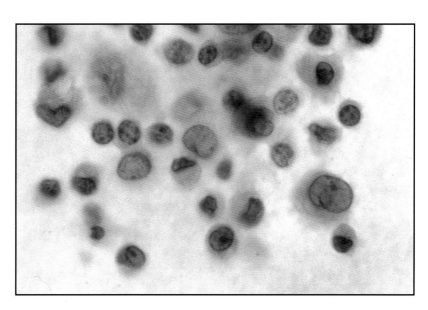

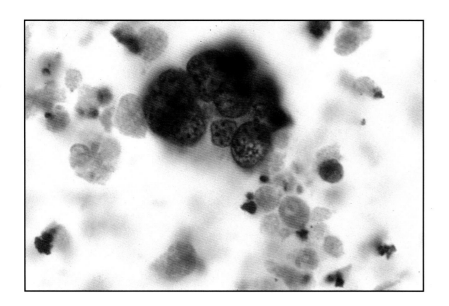

Image 3.67
As seen in this brain wash specimen, degenerative changes and necrotic debris are frequent in glioblastoma. (Papanicolaou).

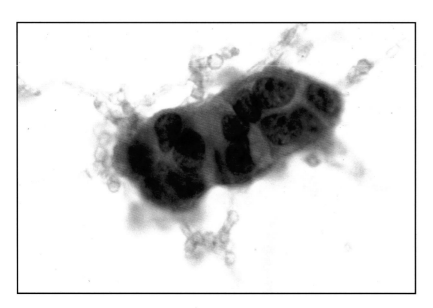

Image 3.68
Ependymoma cells in CSF of a 1-year-old child are present in a 3-dimensional aggregate with a smooth external contour. Many of the neoplastic elements have a columnar contour and contain a single polarized nucleus. The latter have finely granular chromatin and a single small nucleolus. (Papanicolaou).

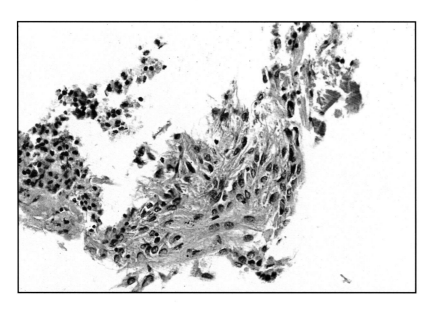

Image 3.69
Cell block preparation from the specimen shown in Image 3.68. Long tapering cellular processes are evident in some of the tumor cells. N/C ratio is low. (H & E).

Image 3.70
Poorly differentiated ependymal tumor in an 8-year-old boy. True lumen-containing rosettes are present. The malignant cells resemble those of a medulloblastoma. (Papanicolaou).

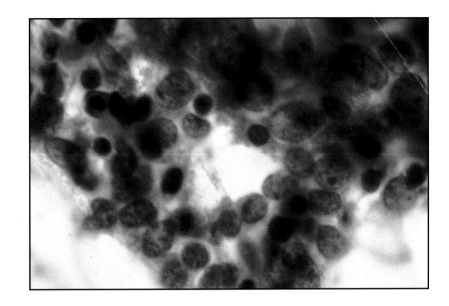

Image 3.71
Cells from a choroid plexus papilloma are present in this CSF from a 1-year-old child. This 3-dimensional papillary aggregate is composed of small uniform cells with an epithelial quality. They have a single small round nucleus with benign-appearing features. (Papanicolaou).

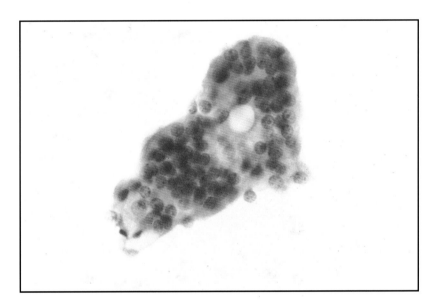

Image 3.72
CSF specimen from a 1-year-old girl who presented with a picture of acute meningitis. Scattered throughout a mixed inflammatory reaction are small cohesive clusters. These cells have an epithelial quality with defined cellular borders and polygonal contours. The small nuclei have a benign appearance. Subsequently, a choroid plexus papilloma was resected. (Papanicolaou). (Courtesy of Dr S Woodhouse).

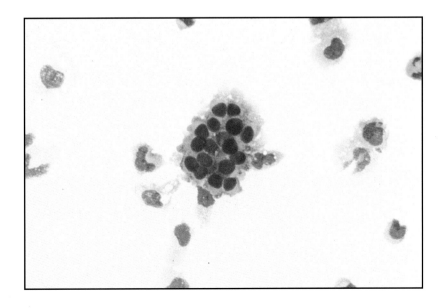

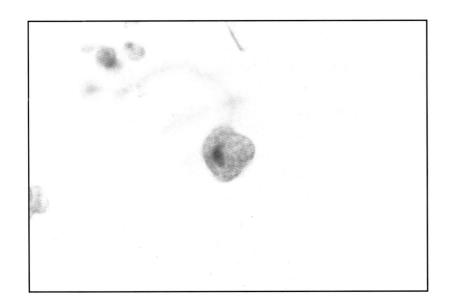

Image 3.73
CSF specimen contains very low numbers of individually dispersed germinoma cells. This nucleus is large and relatively vesicular with very finely granular, pale chromatin and a large nucleolus. Cytoplasm is not visible. A lymphocytic infiltrate is absent. (Papanicolaou).

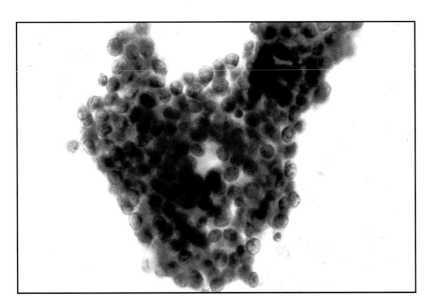

Image 3.74
Intraoperative wash specimen contains a large aggregate of pineoblastoma cells. They are indistinguishable from those of medulloblastoma in that they each have a single round, hyperchromatic nucleus and a very high N/C ratio. Rosette formation is present. (Papanicolaou).

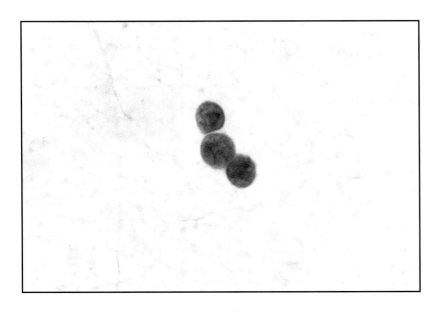

Image 3.75
Short chain of retinoblastoma cells is present in this CSF in a child with a known primary neoplasm. They manifest the features of other PNETs. (Papanicolaou).

Image 3.76

Rosette of metastatic neuroblastoma cells is morphologically indistinguishable from that of medulloblastoma. The uniform tumor cells each have a single round hyperchromatic nucleus with fine, even chromatin. They surround central cytoplasm. (Papanicolaou).

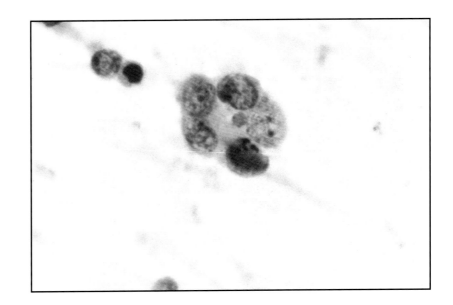

Image 3.77

CSF specimen is positive for metastatic rhabdomyosarcoma. This small cohesive cluster includes cells with eccentrically placed solitary nuclei. The latter have irregularly contoured membranes with folds and notches. Cytoplasm is moderate in volume and dense; striations are not visible. (Papanicolaou).

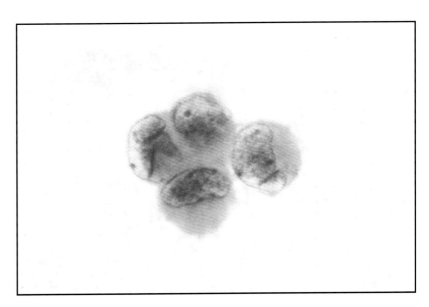

Image 3.78

Crush preparation of a stereotactically obtained biopsy of a low-grade astrocytoma. The cellularity is increased compared to that of normal brain tissue. The smear contains relatively uniform neoplastic astrocytes which are characterized by a single ovoid nucleus and bipolar tails of cytoplasm creating a fibrillar background. Nuclear staining varies from normal to slightly hyperchromatic. Note the absence of endothelial proliferation, marked pleomorphism and necrosis. (H & E).

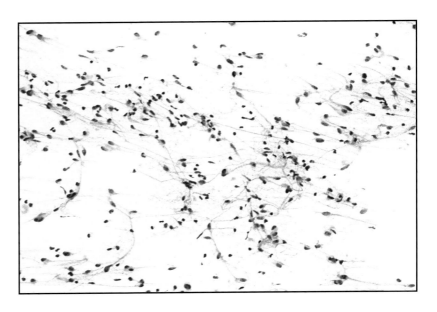

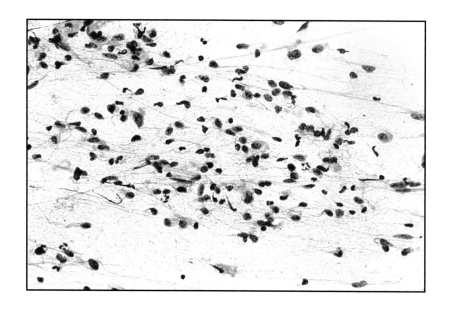

Image 3.79
Some of the neoplastic astrocytes from this low-grade astrocytoma have a plumper or rounder appearance, whereas others have a slender bipolar configuration. Most of the nuclei are small and uniform. (H & E).

A   B

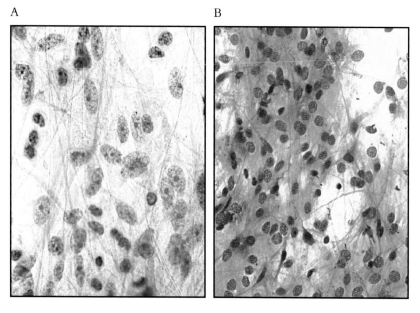

Image 3.80
A Aspirate of a low-grade cystic astrocytoma. The glial nuclei are uniform with thin smooth nuclear membranes, fine chromatin, and small nucleoli. Note the well-formed elongated cell processes. (Papanicolaou).
B Aspirate of a low-grade astrocytoma. The smear is hypercellular and composed of cells with uniform nuclei and indistinct cell borders. Cell processes are evident. (Romanowsky).

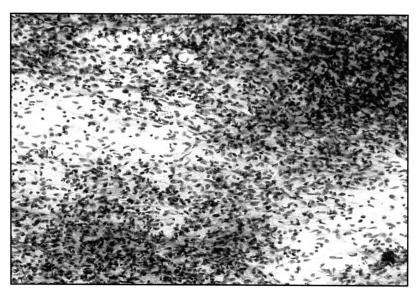

Image 3.81
Obviously marked cellularity in an anaplastic astrocytoma. Hyperchromasia is evident but little in the way of pleomorphism is seen in this field. (H & E).

Image 3.82
Anaplastic astrocytoma (see Image 3.80). It demonstrates marked endothelial cell proliferation; many of these elements have elongated and slender nuclei. In addition, dispersed neoplastic astrocytes are present. (H & E).

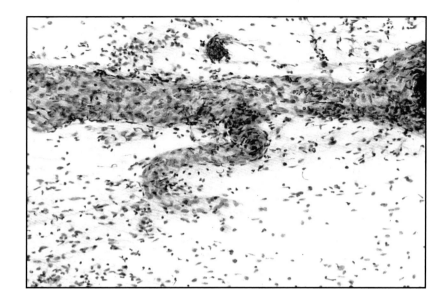

Image 3.83
Crush smear of a glioblastoma. As in Image 3.80, the cellularity of this neoplasm is markedly accentuated. Also note the endothelial cell proliferation within the center of the field. (H & E).

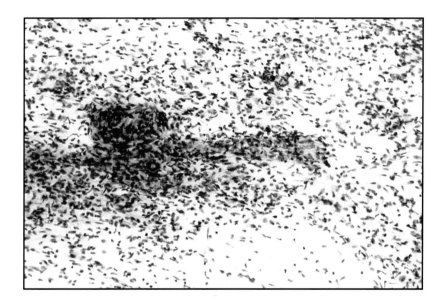

Image 3.84
Anaplastic astrocytoma (see Image 3.80). A moderate level of pleomorphism is noted among the neoplastic astrocytes. Note the persistence of reactively delicate fibrillar cytoplasm. (H & E).

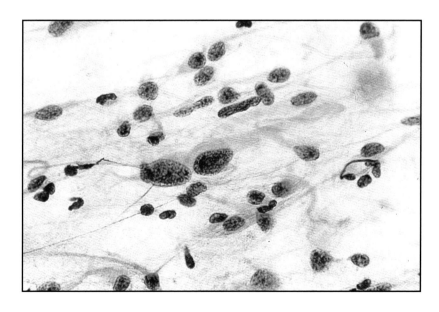

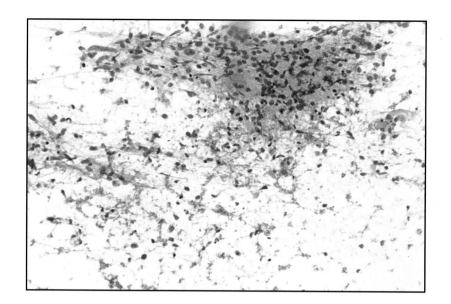

Image 3.85
Much of the field of this crush preparation of a glioblastoma is occupied by necrotic tumor tissue. (H & E).

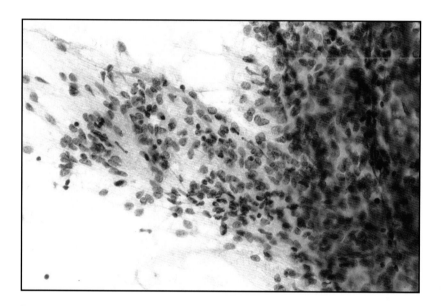

Image 3.86
Crush preparation of an ependymoma from the 4th ventricle of a 1-year-old boy. In the thinner portion of the smear, the neoplastic nuclei can be seen as relatively small, round and uniform. The formation of a large pseudorosette is suggested by the nuclear alignments and the abundant pink-staining cytoplasm. (H & E).

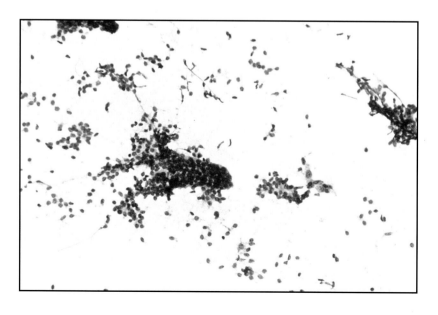

Image 3.87
Crush smear of choroid plexus papilloma from a 1-year-old child. Both 3-dimensional papillary structures and monolayers of tumor cells are apparent. (H & E).

Image 3.88
Gliobastoma (see Image 3.85). Note that the nuclei are small, uniform and bland. (H & E).

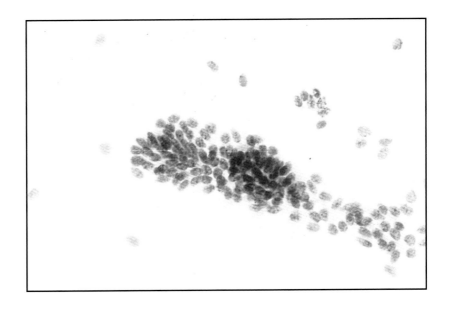

Image 3.89
Crush smear of a medulloblastoma. It is obviously hypercellular and composed of small, uniform neoplastic cells with hyperchromatic nuclei and little in the way of cytoplasm. Note the presence of foci of calcification and the absence of a fibrillar background. (H & E).

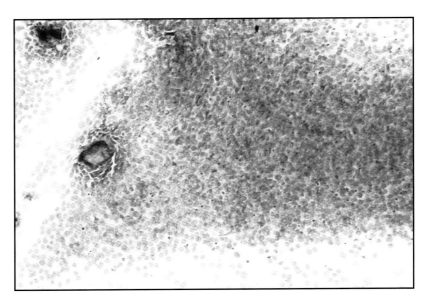

Image 3.90
Medulloblastoma (see Image 3.89). Each tumor cell has a solitary round nucleus with evenly distributed chromatin and a high N/C ratio. Rosette formation is suggested by a concentric arrangement of the neoplastic nuclei. (H & E).

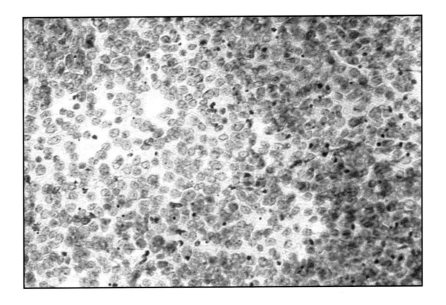

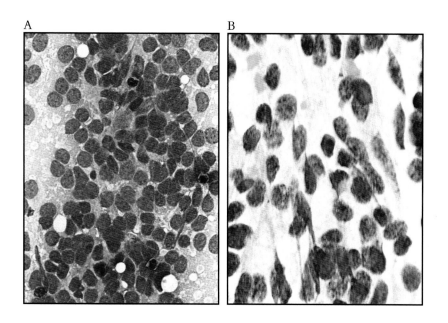

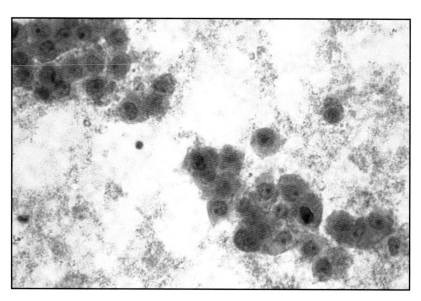

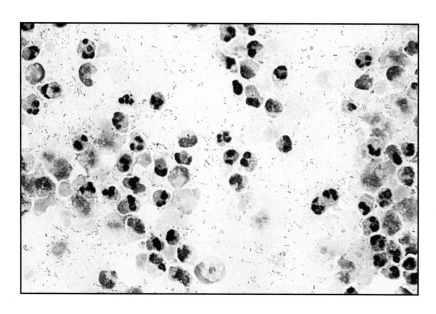

Image 3.91
A Numerous small and uniform malignant cells with high N/C ratio are present in this Diff-Quik–stained aspirate of a medulloblastoma. Nucleoli are poorly developed. Primitive pseudorosette formation is suggested.
B Papanicolaou-stained aspirate of medulloblastoma. Chromatin is finely granular and evenly distributed. Some nuclei are "carrot-shaped."

Image 3.92
Uniform-appearing neoplastic cells in aspirate of the suprasellar region in a child. Each tumor cell from this chromophobe adenoma has a moderate volume of somewhat granulated cytoplasm and a solitary central nucleus. The latter are round with vesicular chromatin and small nucleoli. (Papanicolaou). (Case courtesy of Dr B Naylor).

Image 3.93
This is an aspirate of a brain abscess in a child. Numerous neutrophils are evident. Gram-positive cocci are present in the background. (Romanowsky).

Image 3.94
CT scan of a child with a cerebral abscess infected with *Aspergillus.*

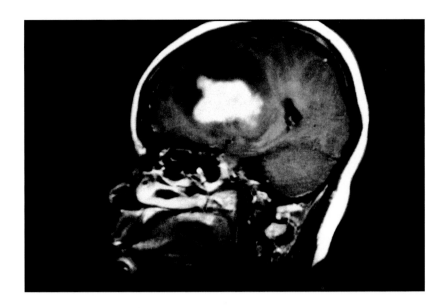

Image 3.95
The Diff-Quik–stained aspirate shows the "negative-image" staining of the hyphae of *Aspergillus.* Note the acute angle branching.

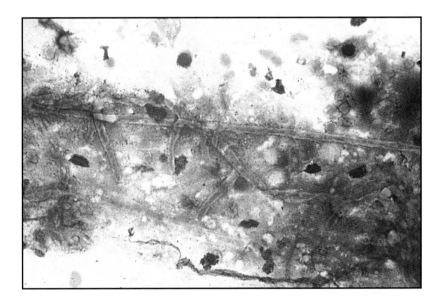

References

1. Bigner SH, Johnston WW. Cytopathology of the central nervous system. American Society of Clinical Pathologists Press, 1994, Chicago.
2. Rosenthal DL. Cytology of the central nervous system. Karger, Basel, 1984.
3. Geisinger KR, Hajdu SI, Helson L. Exfoliative cytology of non-lymphoreticular neoplasms in children. *Acta Cytol* 28:16-28, 1984.
4. Bigner SH. Cerebrospinal fluid (CSF) cytology: current status and diagnostic applications. *J Neuropathol Exp Neurol* 51:235-245, 1992.
5. Gondos B. Millipore filter vs. cytocentrifuge for evaluation of cerebrospinal fluid. *Arch Pathol Lab Med* 110:687-688, 1986.
6. Kjeldsberg CR, Knight JA. Body fluids: Laboratory Examination of Amniotic Cerebrospinal, Synovial, and Serous Fluids. American Society of Clinical Pathologists Press, Chicago, 1993.
7. Portnoy JM, Olson LC. Normal cerebrospinal fluid values in children: another look. *Pediatrics* 75:484-487, 1985.
8. Dalens B, Bezou M-J, Coulet M, Raynard E-J. Cerebrospinal fluid cytomorphology in neonates. *Acta Cytol* 26:395-400, 1982.
9. Pappu LD, Purohit DM, Levkoff AH, Kaplan B. CSF cytology in the neonate. *Am J Dis Child* 136:297-298, 1982.
10. Bonadio WA. Bacterial meningitis in children whose cerebrospinal fluid contains polymorphonuclear leukocytes without pleocytosis. *Clin Ped* 27:198-200, 1988.
11. Wilkins RH, Odom GL. Ependymal-choroidal cells in cerebrospinal fluid. Increased incidence in hydrocephalic infants. *J Neurosurg* 41:555-560, 1974.
12. Woodruff KH. Cerebrospinal fluid cytomorphology using cytocentrifugation. *Am J Clin Pathol* 60:621-627, 1973.
13. Craver RD, Carson TH. Hematopoietic elements in cerebrospinal fluid in children. *Am J Clin Pathol* 95:532-535, 1991.
14. Fischer JR, Davey DD, Gulley ML, Goeken JA. Blast-like cells in cerebrospinal fluid of neonates. Possible germinal matrix origin. *Am J Clin Pathol* 91:255-258, 1989.
15. Takeda M, King DE, Choi HY, Gromik, Lang WR. Diagnostic pitfalls in cerebrospinal fluid cytology. *Acta Cytol* 25:245-250, 1981.
16. Diagnosis and management of meningitis. *Pediatrics* 78(suppl):959-982, 1986.
17. Adams WG, Deaver KA, Cochi SL, Plikaytis BD, Zell ER, Broome CV, Wenger JD. Decline of childhood *Haemophilus influenza* type b (Hib) disease in the Hib era. *JAMA* 269: 221-226, 1993.
18. Broadhurst LE, Erickson RL, Kelley PW. Decreases in invasive *Haemophilus influenza* diseases in U.S. Army children, 1984 through 1991. *JAMA* 269: 227-231, 1993.
19. Bonadio WA, Smith D. Cerebrospinal fluid changes after 48 hours of effective therapy for *Haemophilus influenza* type B meningitis. *Am J Clin Pathol* 94:426-428, 1990.
20. Bonadio WA, Smith DS, Goddard S, Burroughs J, Khaja G. Distinguishing cerebrospinal fluid abnormalities in children with bacterial meningitis and traumatic lumbar puncture. *J Infect Dis* 162:251-254, 1990.

21. Amir J, Harel L, Frydman M, Handsher R, Varsano I. Shift of cerebrospinal polymorphonuclear cell percentage in the early stage of aseptic meningitis. *J Pediatrics* 119:938-941, 1991.

22. Baker RC, Lenane AM. The predictive value of cerebrospinal fluid differential cytology in meningitis. *Ped Infect Dis J* 8:329-330, 1989.

23. Chesney PJ, Katcher ML, Nelson DB, Horowitz SD. CSF eosinophilia and chronic lymphocytic choriomeningitis virus meningitis. *J Peds* 94: 750-752, 1979.

24. Saigo P, Rosen PP, Kaplen MK, Solan G, Melamed MR. Identification of *Cryptococcus neoformans* in cytologic preparations of cerebrospinal fluid. *Am J Clin Pathol* 67: 141-145, 1977.

25. Hamilton SR, Gupta PK, Marshall ME, Donovan PA, Wingard JR, Zaatari GS. Cerebrospinal fluid cytology in histiocytic proliferative disorders. *Acta Cytol* 26: 22-28, 1982.

26. Wolfson WL. Cytopathologic presentation of cerebral histiocytosis. *Acta Cytol* 23: 392-398, 1979.

27. Bigner SH, Elmore PD, Dee AL, Johnston WW. The cytopathology of reactions to ventricular shunts. *Acta Cytol* 29: 391-396, 1985.

28. Traynelis VC, Wilson CD, Follett KA, Chambers J, Schorhet SS, Jr, Kaufman HH. Millipore analysis of valvular fluid in sterile valve malfunctions. *Neurosurgery* 28: 848-852, 1991.

29. Kontopolous E, Minns RA, O'Hare AE, Eden OB. Sedimentation cytomorphology of the CSF in ventriculitis. *Dev Med Child Neurol* 28:213-219, 1986.

30. Tzvetanova EM, Tzekov CT. Eosinophilia in the cerebrospinal fluid of children with shunts implanted for the treatment of internal hydrocephalus. *Acta Cytol* 30:277-280, 1986.

31. Traynelis VC, Powell RG, Koss W, Schochet SS Jr., Kaufman HH. Cerebrospinal fluid eosinophilia and sterile shunt malfunction. *Neurosurgery* 23: 645-649, 1988.

32. Hollman JR, Geisinger KR. Cytology of fluids from pleural, peritoneal and pericardial cavities. A comprehensive survey. *Acta Cytol* 38:209-217, 1994.

33. Heideman RL, Packer RJ, Albright LA, Freeman CR, Rorke LB. Tumors of the central nervous system. In: Principles and Practice of Pediatric Oncology. PA Pizzo, DG Poplack, eds. JB Lippincott, Philadelphia, 1989, p. 505-553.

34. Packer RJ, Siegel KR, Sutton LN, Litmann P, Bruce DA, Schut L. Leptomeningeal dissemination of primary central nervous system tumors of childhood. *Ann Neurol* 18:217-221, 1985.

35. Eade OE, Urich H. Metastasizing gliomas in young subjects. *J Pathol* 103:245-256, 1971.

36. Kocks W, Kalff R, Reinhardt V, Grote W, Hilke J. Spinal metastasis of pilocystic astrocytoma of the chiasma opticum. *Child's Nerv Syst* 5:118-120, 1989.

37. Nishio S, Korosue K, Tateishi J, Fukui M, Kitamuro K. Ventricular and subarachnoid seeding of intracranial tumors of neuroectodermal origin - a study of 26 consecutive autopsy cases with reference to focal ependymal defect. *Clin Neuropathol* 1:83-91, 1982.

38. Shapiro K, Shulman K. Spinal cord seeding from cerebellar astrocytomas. *Child's Brain* 2:177-186, 1976.

39. Ilgren EB, Stiller CA. Cerebellar astrocytomas. Clinical characteristics and prognostic indices. *J Neuro-Oncol* 4:293-308, 1987.

40. Russell DS, Rubinstein LJ. Pathology of Tumors of the Nervous System. 5th ed. Williams and Wilkins, Baltimore, 1989, p 421-448.

41. Deutsch M. Medulloblastoma: staging and treatment outcome. *Int J Rad Oncol Biol Phys* 14:1103-1107, 1988.

42. Finlay JL, Goin SC. Brain tumors in children. I. Advances in diagnosis. *Am J Ped Hematol Oncol* 9:246-255, 1987.

43. Flannery AM, Tomita T, Radkowski M, McLone DG, Medulloblastoma in childhood: postsurgical evaluation with myelography and cerebrospinal fluid cytology. *J Neuro-Oncol* 8:149-151, 1990.

44. Garton GR, Schomberg PJ, Scheithauer BW, Shaw EG, Ilstrup DM, Blackwell CR, Laws GR Jr., Earle JD, Medulloblastoma - prognostic factors and outcome of treatment: review of the Mayo Clinic experience. *Mayo Clin Proc* 65:1077-1086, 1990.

45. Schiffer D, Giordana MT, Vigliani MC, Brain tumors of childhood: nosological and diagnostic problems. *Child's Nerv Syst* 5:220-229, 1989.

46. Cappellari JO, Geisinger KR, Challa VR. Pineal parenchymal tumors: cytomorphologic, immunohistochemical, and cytometric observations. *Acta Cytol* 34:727, 1990.

47. Choucair AK, Levin VA, Gutin PH, Davis RL, Silver P, Edwards MSB, Wilson CB. Development of multiple lesions during radiation therapy and chemotherapy in patients with gliomas. *J Neurosurg* 65:654-658, 1986.

48. Naylor B. The cytologic diagnosis of cerebrospinal fluid. *Acta Cytol* 8: 141-148, 1964.

49. Watson CW, Hajdu SI. Cytology of primary neoplasms of the central nervous system. *Acta Cytol* 21: 40-47, 1977.

50. Auer RN, Rice GPA, Hinton GG, Amacher AL, Gilbert JJ. Cerebellar astrocytoma with benign histology and malignant clinical course. *J Neurosurg* 54:128-132, 1981.

51. Obana WG, Cogen PH, Davis RL, Edwards MSB. Metastatic juvenile pilocytic astrocytoma. Case report. *J Neurosurg* 75:972-975, 1991.

52. McLaughlin JE. Juvenile astrocytomas with subarachnoid spread. *J Pathol* 118:101-107, 1976.

53. Kandt RS, Shinnar S, D'Souza BJ, Singer HS, Wharam MD, Gupta PK. Cerebrospinal metastases in malignant childhood astrocytomas. *J Neuro-Oncol* 2:123-128, 1984.

54. Grant R, Naylor B, Junck L, Greenberg HS. Clinical outcome in aggressively treated meningeal gliomatosis. *Neurology* 42:252-254, 1992.

55. Buchino JJ, Mason KG. Choroid plexus papilloma. Report of a case with cytologic differential diagnosis. *Acta Cytol* 36:95-97, 1992.

56. Kim K, Greenblatt SH, Robinson MG. Choroid plexus carcinoma. Report of a case with cytopathologic differential diagnosis. *Acta Cytol* 29:846-849, 1985.

57. Packer RJ, Perilongo G, Johnson D, Sutton LN, Vezina G, Zimmerman RA, Ryan J, Reaman G, Schut L. Choroid plexus carcinoma of childhood. *Cancer* 69:580-585, 1992.

58. Edwards MSB, Hanigan WC, Kalyan-Raman UP. Radiological and pathological findings in three cases of childhood pineocytomas. *Child's Nerv System* 2: 297-300, 1986.

59. Black P McL. Brain tumors. *New Engl J Med* 324:1555-1564, 1991.

60. Packer RJ, Sutton LN, Rosenstock JG, Rorke LB, Bilaniuk LT, Zimmerman RA, Littman PA, Bruce DA, Schut L. Pineal region tumors in childhood. *Pediatrics* 74: 97-102, 1984.

61. Edwards MSB, Davis RL, Laurent JP. Tumor markers and cytologic features of cerebrospinal fluid. *Cancer* 56:1773-1777, 1985.

62. Kun LE, D'Souza B, Tefft M. The value of surveillance testing in childhood brain tumors. *Cancer* 56:1818-1823, 1985.

63. Ho DM, Liu H-C. Primary intracranial germ cell tumor. Pathologic study of 51 patients. *Cancer* 70: 1577-1584, 1992.

64. Chapman PH, Linggood RM. The management of pineal area tumors: a recent reappraisal. *Cancer* 46: 1253-1257, 1980.

65. Hajdu SI, Nolan MA. Exfoliative cytology of malignant germ cell tumors. *Acta Cytol* 19: 255-260, 1975.

66. Gindhart TD, Tsukahara YC. Cytologic diagnosis of pineal germinoma in cerebrospinal fluid and sputum. *Acta Cytol* 23: 341-346, 1979.

67. Zaharopolos P, Wong JY. Cytology of common primary midline brain tumors. *Acta Cytol* 24: 384-390, 1980.

68. Kamiyama M, Tateyama H, Fujiyoshi Y, Tata T, Eimote T, Shibata H, Hashizume Y. Cerebrospinal fluid cytology in immature teratoma of the central nervous system. A case report. *Acta Cytol* 35: 757-760, 1991.

69. Donaldson SS, Egbert PR. Retinoblastoma. In: Principle and Practice of Pediatric Oncology. PA Pizzo, GD Poplack, eds. JB Lippincott, Philadelphia, 1989, p 555-568.

70. Greenberg ML, Goldberg L. The value of cerebrospinal fluid cytology in the early diagnosis of metastatic retinoblastoma. *Acta Cytol* 21: 735-738, 1978.

71. Pratt CB, Meyer D, Chenaille P, Crom DB. The use of bone marrow aspirations and lumbar puncture at the time of diagnosis of retinoblastoma. *J Clin Oncol* 7: 140-143, 1989.

72. Helson L, Krochmal P, Hajdu SI. Diagnostic value of cytologic specimens obtained from children with cancer. *Ann Clin Lab Sci* 5: 294-297, 1975.

73. Farr GH, Hajdu SI. Exfoliative cytology of metastatic neuroblastoma. *Acta Cytol* 16: 203-206, 1972.

74. Tomei G, Grimoldi N, Cappricci E, Sganzerla EP, Gain SM, Villani R, Masini B. Primary intracranial rhabdomyosarcoma: report of two cases. *Child's Nerv Syst* 5: 246-249, 1989.

75. Jolles CJ, Karayianis S, Smotkin D, DeLia JE. Advanced ovarian dysgerminoma with cure of tumor persistent in meninges. *Gynecol Oncol* 33: 389-391, 1989.

76. Packer RJ, Allen J, Nielsen S, Petito C, Deck M, Jereb B, Brainstem glioma: clinical manifestations of meningeal gliomatosis. *Ann Neurol* 14: 177-182, 1983.

77. Schmitt HP, Wowra B, Sturm V. Diagnostic value of the stereotactic approach to focal lesions in the deep brain of children and adolescents. *Brain Dev* 10: 305-311, 1988.

78. Liwnicz BH, Henderson KS, Masukawa T, Smith RD. Needle aspiration cytology of intracranial lesions. A review of 84 cases. *Acta Cytol* 26: 779-786, 1982.

79. Willems JGMS, Alva-Willems JM. Accuracy of cytologic diagnosis of central nervous system neoplasms in stereotactic biopsies. *Acta Cytol* 28: 243-249, 1984.

80. Cahill EM, Hidvegi DF. Crush preparations of lesions of the central nervous system. A useful adjunct to the frozen section. *Acta Cytol* 29: 279-285, 1985.

81. Silverman JF. Cytopathology of fine-needle aspiration biopsy of the brain and spinal cord. *Diagn Cytopathol* 2: 312-319, 1986.

82. Mouriquand C, Benabid AL, Breyton M. Stereotactic cytology of brain tumors. Review of an eight-year experience. *Acta Cytol* 31: 756-764, 1987.

83. Nguyen G-K, Johnson ES, Mielke BW. Cytology of neuroectodermal tumors of the brain in crush preparations. A review of 56 cases of deep-seated tumors sampled by CT-guided stereotactic needle biopsy. *Acta Cytol* 33: 67-73, 1989.

84. Chandrasoma PT, Apuzzo MLJ. Stereotactic Brain Biopsy. Igaku-Shoin Medical Publishers Inc, New York, 1989.

85. Cappabianca P, Spaziante R, Caputi F, Pettinato G, Del Basso De Caro M, Carrabs G, de Diuitiis E. Accuracy of the analysis of multiple small fragments of glial tumors obtained by stereotactic biopsy. *Acta Cytol* 35: 505-511, 1991.

86. Pennelli N, Montaguti A, Carteri A, Midena E, Boccato P. Juvenile pilocytic astrocytoma of the optic nerve diagnosed by fine needle aspiration biopsy. *Acta Cytol* 32: 395-398, 1988.

87. Altermatt HJ, Scheithauer BW. Cytomorphology of subependymal giant cell astrocytoma. *Acta Cytol* 36: 171-175, 1992.

88. Silverman JF, Timmons RL, Leonard JR, Hardy IM, Harris LS, O'Brien K, Norris HT. Cytologic results of fine-needle aspiration biopsies of the central nervous system. *Cancer* 58: 1117-1121, 1986.

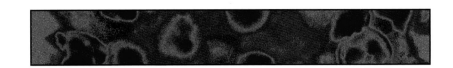

CHAPTER FOUR

Serous Effusions

The clinical value of exfoliative cytopathology of serous effusions is well recognized.[1-4] Yet, almost all of these descriptions and data have been derived from serous effusions in adult patients. Very little information exists that specifically concentrates on serous effusions in children. As in adults, serous effusions in children may be either transudates or exudates. Also, as with adults, it is the exudate that is more apt to be examined cytologically. In all age groups, exudates are usually the consequence of either inflammation, both infectious and noninfectious, or malignant neoplasms.

Acute Inflammation

Effusions secondary to inflammatory causes far outnumber those due to neoplasms.[5-7] A large proportion of these, especially pleural effusions, are related to an acute inflammatory process.[6,7] As would be expected, neutrophils predominate and may reveal a spectrum of degenerative changes (Image 4.1). They may be so numerous as to obscure evaluation of other cell types (Image 4.2). Both histiocytes and mesothelial cells may occur sparsely. If the sediment is stained with a Gram or Romanowsky stain, bacteria and other organisms may be recognized in both intracellular and extracellular sites (Image 4.3). In the series of Wolfe et al, pneumonia was the most frequent stimulus to a pleural effusion.[6]   In their report from a large children's hospital, Kmetz and Newton found 77% of their satisfactory specimens were nonneoplastic, but these were not further broken down as to microscopic pattern or etiology.[5]   In the review of Hallman and Geisinger, a large proportion of pleural fluid specimens were dominated by neutrophils and were related to pneumonia.[7] A smaller proportion of ascitic fluids were so involved and were associated with a number of conditions, eg, pancreatitis and perforated viscus.   That series also included an example of neutrophils admixed with extracellular stellate masses that are marked by a yellow, almost refractile color consistent with bile (Image 4.4). This occurred in a young child with a traumatically injured bile duct.[7] None of their pericardial specimens were acutely inflamed.

Chronic Inflammation

The list of etiologies associated with chronically inflamed effusions is quite long.   Microscopically, the picture is quite variable, but most frequently small, mature-appearing lymphocytes predominate and may be numerous (Image 4.5).[1-4]   They may be admixed with mesothelial cells and histiocytes.   The latter cell type may be well represented and may include multinucleated inflammatory giant cells.   In the series reported by Wolfe and colleagues, tuberculosis was a frequent cause of pleural effusion.[5,6]   However, their series reported on the years 1952 through 1967.   In tuberculosis effusions one typically sees an almost pure population of small lymphoid cells with only rare mesothelial elements,   although in many patients, a more variable picture with neutrophils and/or prominent mesothelial cells may be found.[2,3,8]   In more recent experience, tuberculosis did not play a prominent role in the production of effusions.[7]   We have seen several examples of pleural effusions associated with systemic lupus erythematosus in children.[7] Although a mixed inflammatory pattern was present, the small lymphocyte was the major cell type.   In pediatric patients, we have not identified lupus erythematosus cells in the fluid specimens.   Infrequently, we have seen chronic inflammatory cell infiltrates in pericardial fluid specimens from children, some of which could be ascribed to the postpericardiotomy syndrome and viral pericarditis.

Serous effusion specimens with a predominance of chronic inflammatory cells may be seen in a number of infectious states.   Most often, these are related to systemic viral infections in which the cytomorphologic features of fluid specimens are totally nonspecific.   Very infrequently, during the course of a systemic infection, herpes virus may infect mesothelial cells (Image 4.6).[2,4,9,10]   The resultant effusion may contain exfoliated mesothelial cells with the classic nuclear cytopathologic alterations.   Even more rarely, cytomegalovirus may infect mesothelial cells producing recognizable cellular changes in exfoliated cells in effusions.   Apparently, such viral-induced cellular changes are exceedingly rare in children.   Also rare are various types of fungi in serous effusion specimens.   *Candida* and *Aspergillus* are the two most frequent types.   We have seen an example of congenital toxoplasmosis

In tuberculosis effusions one typically sees an almost pure population of small lymphoid cells with only rare mesothelial elements

in a newborn boy with failure to thrive and progressive ascites.[7] The first indication that the patient had toxoplasmosis was the examination of the peritoneal fluid, which contained an intense mixed inflammatory cell reaction. In addition, numerous trophozoites, both extracellularly and intracellularly, were present (Image 4.7). These measured approximately 2 μm and had the contours of a banana. An aliquot of the ascitic fluid was examined by transmission electron microscopy. The structures had features fully consistent with those of the trophozoites of *Toxoplasma gondii*. Although it is recognized that congenital toxoplasmosis may rarely present as ascites, diagnosis has usually been based on serologic studies and not on cytomorphologic findings.[11]

Grossly, chylous effusions have a cloudy, milky-white appearance due to the presence of numerous chylomicrons (Image 4.8). Most such effusions occur in neonates, but we have seen them in older children as well.[7,11-14] Microscopically, the fluids contain an almost pure population of small, mature-appearing lymphocytes (Image 4.9). Only rare mesothelial cells and histiocytes are also present. With the Papanicolaou technique, the chylomicrons, of course, are not visualized. Some of these cases have been associated with injuries or abnormalities of the thoracic duct, although many have been idiopathic.

Meconium peritonitis is a form of chemical inflammation secondary to perinatal perforation of the gastrointestinal tract. This inflammatory state may be associated with the production of serous effusions. Rarely, a cytologic diagnosis of meconium peritonitis or pleuritis has been reported.[15] Cytomorphologic features include anucleated squamous cells, fecal debris, hemosiderin granules, and a mixed inflammatory cell reaction (Image 4.10).

We have reported a small handful of cases of serous effusions in children that contained infiltrates of numerous cytologically atypical lymphocytes and other mononuclear inflammatory cells.[16] Acute leukemias and malignant lymphomas comprise a very large proportion of all childhood cancers, and thus, benign but atypical lymphocytosis raises a critical differential diagnosis in serous effusion cytology. We have seen three such specimens in peritoneal fluids. The oldest child was 2 years old, but the others were less than 2 months old. The lymphocytes were somewhat heterogenous in size and appearances (Images 4.11 through 4.13). A number had relatively vesicular nuclei and an occasional prominent nucleolus. Chromatin was variably clumped and the contours of the nuclei ranged from round and smooth to complex and irregular. In 2 children, these markedly atypical cytologic features led to an initial misdiagnosis of malignant neoplasm. Underlying etiologies included hereditary tyrosinemia with cirrhosis, omental cystic lymphangioma and "unknown."[16] We have also seen an example of a very atypical lymphocytosis in the pleural fluid in a 4-year-old girl with autoimmune hepatitis. Cytologic features included numerous blasts and plasmacytoid cells (Images 4.14 and 4.15). The cytologic features were so bizarre and unusual that it led to a consideration of malignant lymphoma. Clinical follow-up with a resolution of the effusions in these patients has confirmed the benign nature of these cytologically atypical effusions. It has been our experience that the use of flow cytometry with cell surface markers for lymphoid lineage has been helpful, as has immunocytochemistry. The results of these studies show

The use of flow cytometry with cell surface markers for lymphoid lineage has been helpful, as has immunocytochemistry

a heterogenous mixture of T and B lymphocytes with a preponderance of T cells. We have seen a case of familial hemophagocytic syndrome presenting initially as a peritoneal effusion with very atypical cells (Image 4.16).[17]

Eosinophilic pleural effusions contain large numbers of eosinophilic leukocytes within the fluid (Image 4.17).[2,3] The actual percentage of cells represented by eosinophils is variable from report to report. Many conditions have been associated with the production of an eosinophilic pleural effusion; a common occurrence is pneumothorax. Most reported examples of eosinophilic pleural effusions have been in adults. This is apparently a rare condition in children.[18]

Noninflammatory Fluids

A number of conditions in children are associated with serous effusions that are dominated by mesothelial cells, with little or no inflammatory infiltrate. Many of these are transudates. Major causes include congenital heart disease with cardiac failure (pleural) and liver failure (peritoneal). Usually, a benign cytologic diagnosis is straightforward (Image 4.18).

Malignant Effusions

A significant and very important minority of serous effusions in children contain neoplastic cells. Except for cerebrospinal fluid, serous effusions are the specimen type that most often contain tumor cells.[18,19] The distribution of tumor types varies according to patient age and specific serous cavity involved.

Clinical Features

Published studies from cancer hospitals have reported that the majority of serous effusions in children are positive for tumor cells.[19,20] Helson has provided one of the most comprehensive reports.[19] During a 2-year period at Memorial Sloan-Kettering Cancer Center, 65% of all serous effusions examined microscopically were positive. The vast majority of the pleural fluids contained tumor cells, most often derived from osteosarcomas and rhabdomyosarcomas; neuroblastoma, nephroblastoma and malignant lymphoreticular neoplasms also yielded high proportions of positive results. Neuroblastoma and the malignant germ cell tumors were the most likely to produce positive ascitic specimens. A pericardial fluid from one child contained osteosarcoma cells.

When combining all of our personal experiences with effusion cytology, we have found the following relative distribution of tumor types according to specimen types.[20] The most common causes of positive pleural effusions in children included the malignant lymphomas, nephroblastoma (Wilms' tumor) and the bone sarcomas. Both osteosarcoma and Ewing's sarcoma may metastasize to the pleura, producing positive effusions. The most common causes of positive peritoneal fluids include the malignant lymphomas, neuroblastoma and the germ cell tumors. Of the latter, the majority are ovarian in origin. It is of interest to note that very rarely primary brain tumors may metastasize to the serous cavities, producing cytologically positive effusions.[19] Although quite uncommon in our experience, the most frequent causes of a positive pericardial effusion are leukemias and lymphomas.

In our review of 144 children with nonlymphoreticular neoplasms from Memorial Hospital we found distinctive patterns of distribution according to patient age.[20] We evaluated this by using the age of the patients at the time of the first positive exfoliative specimen. 77% of the children with neuroblastoma were 4 years old or younger and two-thirds with Wilms' tumor were less than 9 years. Conversely, 77% with the germ cell tumors were 9 years or older. 90% of the children with osteosarcoma were 9 years or older with the youngest patient being 6. The femur was the most common primary site. This age pattern was mirrored by the 10 children with Ewing's sarcoma. Rhabdomyosarcoma was relatively evenly distributed among the different age groups. This pattern of distribution, of course, basically reflects the peak ages at which children develop these different types of neoplasm. In our series, the germ cell tumors and Wilms' tumor were the only two neoplasms which predominated in girls.

In the 15-year series reported by Wolfe et al, cancer was the second most common cause of a pleural effusion.[6] However, only a minority (20%) of this subset of patients had specimens that contained neoplastic cells. These were mostly derived from malignant lymphomas and acute leukemias. This has also been our more recent experience from a large general hospital.[7] The study of Kmetz and Newton, which is one of the earliest pediatric reports, came from a large children's hospital.[5] The most common cause of a malignant serous effusion in their institution was Wilms' tumor.

In the vast majority of instances in which a serous fluid from a child contains malignant cells, the diagnosis of a specific primary tumor has already been established on biopsied or surgically resected neoplasm. For instance, in the large reported series, most children with positive serous effusions carry a known neoplastic diagnosis.[19,20] From a practical point of view, therefore, the cytologist is not compelled to identify specifically the exact tumor type in the cytologic material. The pathologist merely needs to report the presence of tumor cells. For example, in a patient with treated neuroblastoma, the appearance of cohesive small malignant cells in a subsequent peritoneal fluid specimen can be diagnosed simply as: "small malignant cells consistent with neuroblastoma are present."

There are several circumstances in which one might pursue the exact cell type in a cytologic preparation, such as the rare instances in which neoplasm in a pediatric patient first presents as an effusion. Here, aggressive attempts to classify the neoplastic elements is warranted. A minority of children with cancer will develop a second primary

There are several circumstances in which one might pursue the exact cell type in a cytologic preparation, such as the rare instances in which neoplasm in a pediatric patient first presents as an effusion

neoplasm, either spontaneously or in relation to therapy for the first malignancy. If a new tumor is suspected on either clinical or morphologic grounds, then tumor typing is recommended. Finally, tumor typing for academic purposes is done. In these instances we prefer to use immunocytochemistry, especially if a good cell block is available. The exact antibodies used may be specifically tailored for each clinical situation, but in the absence of a prior primary diagnosis, a panel of antibodies is the preferred initial approach. Transmission electron microscopy may also be utilized but is generally less effective, as sampling error is more likely in ultrastructural studies. Also, it is generally more expensive and less readily available than immunocytochemistry. Cytogenetic and DNA ploidy analyses can also be performed on effusion and other cytologic specimens.

A morphologic hallmark of the non-lymphoreticular neoplasms is the presence of intercellular cohesion with the formation of true cellular aggregates

Cytomorphology

There are morphologic clues, sometimes rather subtle, which may suggest a specific tumor or group of tumors. As stated in the introductory chapter, pediatric neoplasms can be crudely separated into two groups, the more common being the small cell tumor group.[20] For cytologic purposes, this can be further divided into the lymphoreticular and nonlymphoreticular categories. The former, which includes both acute leukemias and lymphomas, present in fluids as individually dispersed malignant cells (Images 4.19 through 4.26). That is, there is no recognizable intercellular cohesion; even in highly cellular smears the blasts barely contact one another. A morphologic hallmark of the nonlymphoreticular neoplasms is the presence of intercellular cohesion with the formation of true cellular aggregates (Images 4.27 through 4.33). As a result, some cells will usually form chains, small sheets, and spheres, in which molding may be apparent. By focusing up and down, one may be able to recognize pseudorosettes within cellular clusters.[5,20,21] These structures are not specific; in addition to their possible presence in neuroblastoma, they may also be seen in Ewing's sarcoma and in the very rarely metastasizing hepatoblastoma and primary brain tumors. In our experience and that of others, specific organoid structures, ie, tubule formation, are exceedingly rare in exfoliated Wilms' tumor cells.[20,22] Much more often, small nondescript cellular spheres are present, admixed with individually dispersed tumor cells (Image 4.33). A characteristic biphasic population of round and plump elongated cells have been described for this tumor, but this is actually uncommon and focal in smears (Image 4.32).[19] As stated above, reactive lymphoid cells need to be distinguished from both lymphoreticular and nonlymphoreticular small cell tumors.[23]

Embryonal rhabdomyosarcoma is generally classified as a small cell tumor. However, many neoplastic cells may have a moderate volume cytoplasm and multinucleation is not infrequent. This is one malignancy for which exfoliated cells may be quite distinctive in fluid specimens.[18,21,22] Intercellular cohesion is not as well developed as in neuroblastoma and organoid arrangements do not occur. Isolated tumor cells predominate in many examples. Pleomorphism is greater than in other small cell tumors and may be recognized by a wider range of cell size and more variable nuclear-cytoplasmic (N/C) ratios (Image 4.34). The contours of the nuclear membranes may be more irregular than in most other small cell tumors. Small notches and even deep indentations may occur within these membranes. Nucleoli are also better developed. Finally, tumor cells may display 2 or more nuclei (Image 4.35). In binucleated cells, the 2 nuclei are often polarized to 1 end of the cell and may be arranged so as to form a characteristic acute angle. Immunostaining for muscle markers and electron microscopy might be helpful.[24]

Another neoplasm that may provide overlapping morphologic features is the recently described entity, intraabdominal desmoplastic small round cell tumor.[25] This cancer typically occurs in adolescent boys who present with enlarged, thickened omentums, ascites and no obvious visceral mass lesions. These tumors usually grow as distinct nests of small malignant cells with high N/C ratios and little in the way of differentiation at the conventional light microscopic level. A prominent desmoplastic response is incited. By immunohistochemical and ultrastructural studies, these neoplasms demonstrate multilineage differentiation.[25,26]

We have seen peritoneal fluid specimens from a 16-year-old boy with this peculiar entity.[27] Both aggregated and dispersed single malignant cells were visible against the background of numerous benign mesothelial elements (Image 4.36). The tumor cells were relatively monomorphic, small round cells with scanty to moderate dense volumes of cyanophilic cytoplasm, a round to oval nucleus, and a high N/C ratio. Nuclei were densely hyperchromatic with finely granular chromatin, inconspicuous nucleoli and generally irregular nuclear membranes. Nuclear molding was present within the cellular aggregates, some of which also had a suggestion of acinar arrangements. The major differential diagnostic points considered, in context with the clinical impression of no visceral mass lesion, was malignant mesothelioma versus poorly differentiated adenocarcinoma.[28] Ultrastructurally, features consistent with adenocarcinoma were present, including intercellular junctions, villi and extracellular lumina (Images 4.37 and 4.38). As is typical of this new entity, the immunostains were positive for cytokeratin, epithelial membrane antigen, neuron specific enolase, desmin, vimentin and Leu-M1. Overall, on a cell-for-cell basis, this neoplasm could be considered a small cell neoplasm. However, cytomorphologic features suggestive of glandular development, ultrastructural findings, and immunochemical features were more suggestive of a large cell neoplasm. An alternative diagnostic term for this entity is mesothelioblastoma.[25]

Osteosarcoma is the prototype of the less frequent large cell tumor group. Positive serous effusions, usually pleural, are generally moderately cellular at best, but the malignant cells are usually easily recognizable.[20] Smears contain individual malignant osteoblasts as well as small poorly cohesive clusters. Cellular pleomorphism is a striking feature (Image 4.39). Most cells are round with a highly variable amount of dense eosinophilic cytoplasm. Nuclei are round to irregular and darkly hyperchromatic with prominent nucleoli, numbering from 1 to several per cell (Images 4.40 through 4.42). Degenerative changes may be well developed, perhaps reflecting on-going chemotherapy. Contrary to findings in fine needle aspiration biopsy specimens, osteoid will not be present in effusions.

Only uncommonly do atypical reactive mesothelial cells pose a diagnostic challenge in pediatric cytopathology. Yet, it is well known that chemotherapy may produce bizarre, pseudo-malignant appearances in benign mesothelial cells and that such therapy may also initiate or promote serous effusions.[29] We have seen rare examples of highly atypical reactive changes which caused confusion diagnostically with metastatic osteosarcoma in pericardial fluids and with ovarian neoplasms in peritoneal specimens. In osteosarcoma, the use of immunocytochemistry with antibodies against cytokeratin and other epithelial markers would resolve the problem.

It is somewhat surprising that cells from primary hepatic cancers only rarely involve serous effusions in children and adults.[20] In ascitic fluid, neoplastic hepatocytes from hepatocellular carcinomas are large with obviously malignant nuclei and variable N/C ratios. Granular eosinophilic cytoplasm is apparent in most cells, as are macronucleoli. Distinct cellular arrangements, eg, trabeculae, have not been recognized. We are unaware of a report of hepatoblastoma cells in a serous effusion specimen.

The germ cell tumors comprise a fascinating collection of benign and malignant neoplasms.[30-34] As in adults, they arise most often in the gonads, but may also originate in extragenital sites as well. According to Kapila et al, ovarian germ cell tumors most often occur in ascitic fluids, whereas pleural fluids are the most common sites for metastatic testicular and mediastinal neoplasms.[31] Most common in both sexes is the germinoma. These malignancies produce a characteristic exfoliative picture.[20,30-32] As expected from the histology, tumor cells are uniform and large with a single huge round nucleus that contains one or more well developed nucleoli (Images 4.43 and 4.44). The latter stand out especially well as the chromatin is very finely granular and evenly dispersed throughout the nucleus creating a clear to vesicular pattern (Table 3.6). Cytoplasm is moderate in volume and is either clear, granular or finely vesicular in appearance. Characteristically, within fluid specimens, germinoma cells are dispersed as single elements with little inclination to form clusters. When they do aggregate, they occur in small flat arrays or sheets. Kashimura et al found numerous lymphocytes in the smear background of peritoneal fluid specimens.[32]

From a purely cytomorphologic view, the major differential diagnostic distinction is large cell malignant lymphoma. In both lymphoma and germinoma, large isolated tumor cells with prominent nucleoli occur in serous effusions. In lymphomas, nuclear contours tend to be much more irregular and tumor cell aggregation is never seen. Germinomas would be negative for leukocyte common antigen by immunocytochemistry and for lymphoid surface markers by flow cytometry. Another differential diagnostic point could be germinoma versus ovarian adenocarcinomas, including embryonal carcinomas. In girls, especially adolescents, who present with a pelvic mass and ascites, this distinction may be important. According to Kashimura and colleagues, dysgerminoma cells, when compared to adenocarcinoma, more fre-

We have seen rare examples of highly atypical reactive changes which caused confusion diagnostically with metastatic osteosarcoma in pericardial fluids and with ovarian neoplasms in peritoneal specimens

quently occur singularly and in small flat sheets, have less well-developed cytoplasmic vacuoles, have less thickening of the nuclear membranes and more often have multiple nucleoli.[32] To this we would add that nuclei are more often centrally placed within their cytoplasm in germinoma cells. Embryonal carcinoma presents a cytomorphologic picture of a rather poorly differentiated adenocarcinoma with 3-dimensional papillary and glandular structures in exfoliated specimens.[30,31] The malignant cells have eccentric hyperchromatic nuclei and high N/C ratios. In serous effusions, they would be difficult to distinguish from a yolk sac tumor or other adenocarcinomas. Morimoto et al reported the cytologic findings from 2 patients with ovarian yolk sac tumors in ascitic fluids.[33] In addition to small homogeneous malignant cells in glandular groupings, dense globules, both intracytoplasmic and extracellular, were recognized with the periodic acid-Schiff and Romanowsky stains, but not with the Papanicolaou stain.

We have seen an interesting specimen from an 11-year-old girl who presented with a pelvic mass, massive ascites, and pleural effusions.[20] Her tumor was a high-grade immature teratoma of the ovary with extensive neuroblastic elements. A pleural fluid specimen contained numerous small malignant cells consistent with an origin from the primitive neural component of the neoplasm. They were small uniform cells each with a single hyperchromatic nucleus and a high N/C ratio. Many were present in cohesive aggregates, including pseudorosette formation.

Cobb et al reported the case of a 15-year-old boy who presented acutely with chest pain, respiratory distress and pleural effusions, secondary to the rupture of a benign cystic teratoma of the anterior mediastinum.[34] The serous cytology specimen included mature nucleated and anucleated squamous cells, mature glandular elements (none with cilia), hairs, psamomma bodies and cholesterol crystals, all present against a background of an intense mixed inflammatory reaction (Image 4.45). As this situation constitutes a medical emergency, caution was taken against misinterpreting these features as contaminants. As always, a close and careful correlation with the clinical picture aids in arriving at the correct and accurate cytologic diagnosis.

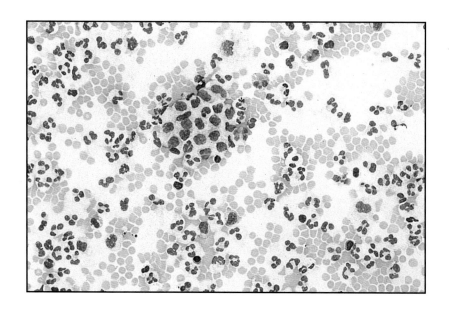

Image 4.1
This is a peritoneal fluid specimen from a young girl who had acute appendicitis. Grossly, the fluid appeared purulent and this was confirmed microscopically. In the center of the field is a cohesive cluster of uniform mesothelial cells, each with a single round nucleus and abundant cytoplasm. However, the predominant cellular element is the neutrophilic leukocyte. The smear background is remarkably clean. (Romanowsky).

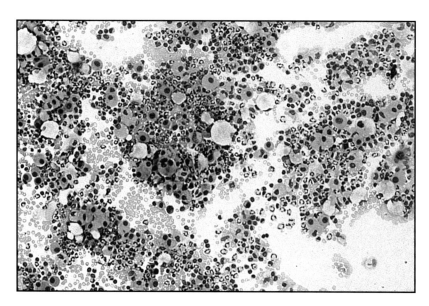

Image 4.2
This is a pleural fluid from a boy with bacterial pneumonia. Neutrophils are so numerous that they form sheets interrupted by solitary mesothelial cells. (Romanowsky).

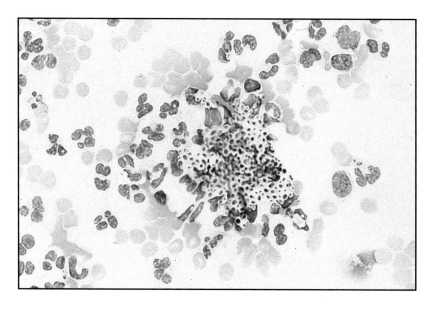

Image 4.3
Neutrophils predominate in this ascitic fluid specimen from a child with a perforated viscus, which produced *Candida* peritonitis. Note that many yeast forms have been phagocytized. (Romanowsky).

Image 4.4
Bile peritonitis. Mesothelial cells, neutrophils and mononucleated inflammatory elements are embedded in a background of brilliant yellow pigment. This picture is basically pathognomonic of biliary tract or liver injury. (Papanicolaou).

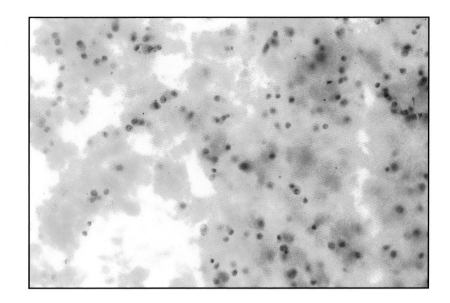

Image 4.5
This fluid specimen is from a pericardial effusion in a young boy with the clinical impression of myocarditis, probably of viral etiology. Mature-appearing small lymphocytes are the major cell type present. (Papanicolaou).

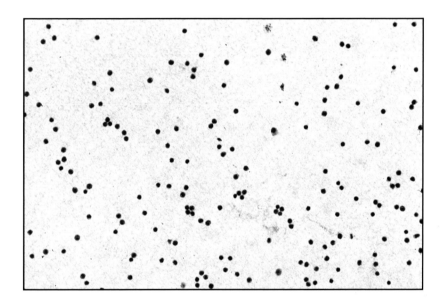

Image 4.6
Ascitic fluid specimen from a 19-year-old man with a systemic viral infection following herpes proctitis. Multiple molded enlarged nuclei occupy most of the cytoplasm of this mesothelial cell. Their chromatin has the characteristic "ground glass" appearance. (Papanicolaou).

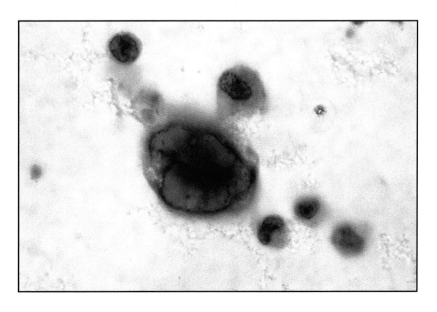

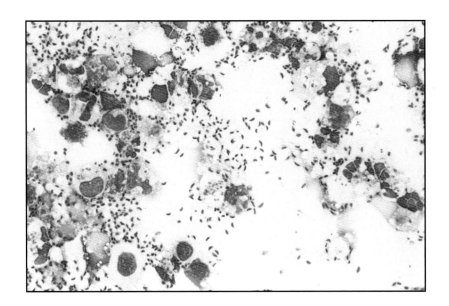

Image 4.7
Spontaneous ascitic fluid in a new-born boy with congenital toxoplasmosis. Degenerative changes are well developed among the cells of the mixed inflammatory infiltrate. Numerous trophozoites are obvious. Although some have been phagocytized, many others are extracellular. (Romanowsky).

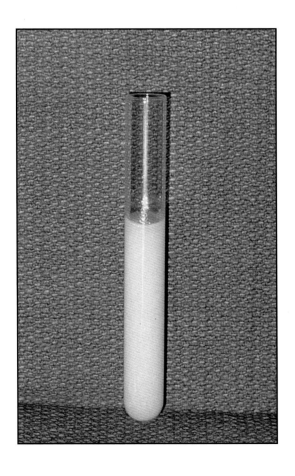

Image 4.8
Pleural fluid from a 1-day-old neonate with idiopathic chylothorax. Its creamy appearance is due to the myriad of chylomicrons.

Image 4.9

In chylothorax, one sees a predominance of small mature-appearing lymphocytes. Each has a smooth round nucleus with dense chromatin and a very high N/C ratio. Nucleoli are not apparent. (Papanicolaou).

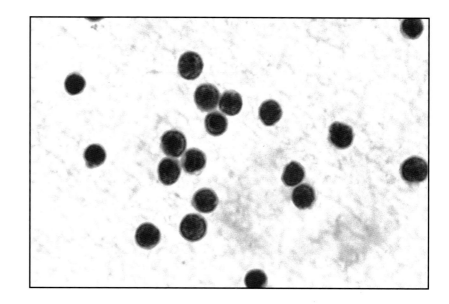

Image 4.10

A Meconium pleuritis. Histiocytes and neutrophils are mixed with amorphous fecal type debris. Degenerative changes are well developed. (Papanicolaou).

B Fragments of meconium are present in this cell block preparation. (H&E).

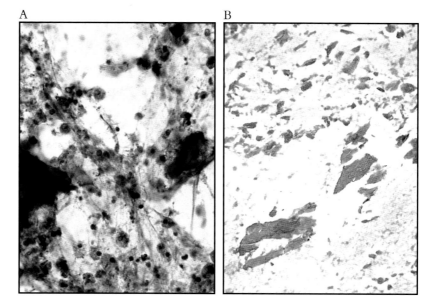

Image 4.11

Atypical lymphocytosis in ascitic fluid from an infant with tyrosinemia. In addition to mesothelial cells there are numerous somewhat heterogenous lymphoid elements. Some of the latter have prominent nucleoli and complex nuclear envelopes. (Papanicolaou).

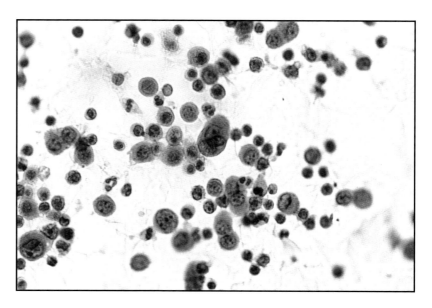

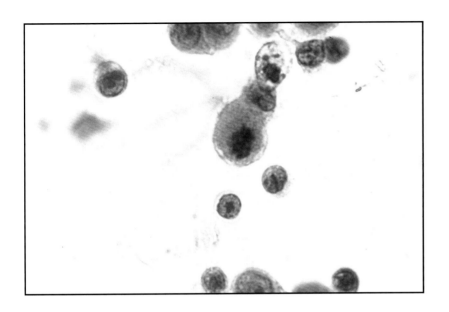

Images 4.12
Atypical lymphocytosis in ascitic fluid (see Image 4.11). Several of the lymphocytes have vesicular chromatin and one large central nucleolus. Others have very irregularly contoured nuclei. These features led to an impression of a malignant lymphoreticular neoplasm. (Papanicolaou).

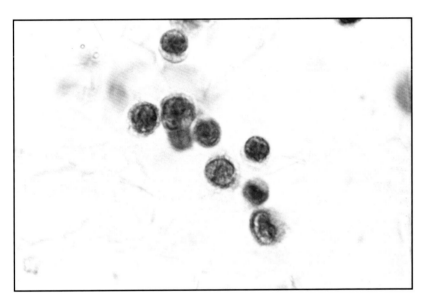

Image 4.13
Atypical lymphocytosis in ascitic fluid, as in Image 4.12 (Papanicolaou).

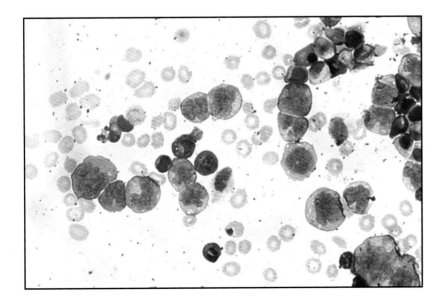

Image 4.14
Pleural fluid from a 4-year-old girl with severe autoimmune hepatitis. It is highly cellular with numerous lymphoid cells demonstrating a very wide spectrum of morphologic appearances. Small mature-appearing lymphocytes with small round nuclei and dense chromatin are present, as are large cells with bizarre-appearing nuclei and huge nucleoli and plasmacytoid lymphocytes. (Romanowsky).

Image 4.15
Pleural fluid in a case of severe autoimmune hepatitis (see Image 4.14). A minority of the lymphocytes have highly complex (cloverleaf-like) nuclei with finely reticulated chromatin. Note the range in appearances. (Romanowsky).

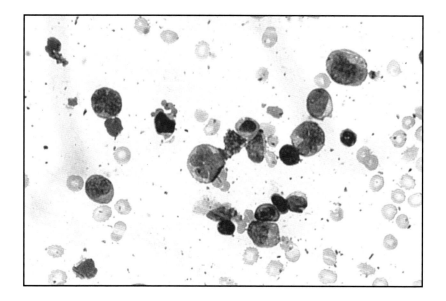

Image 4.16
Peritoneal fluid from a newborn boy who died within weeks of the development of ascites. Highly atypical cytologic features in the mononuclear inflammatory cells led to an incorrect suspicion of a malignant lymphoreticular neoplasm. He (and later his brother) died secondary to familial hemophagocytic syndrome. (Papanicolaou).

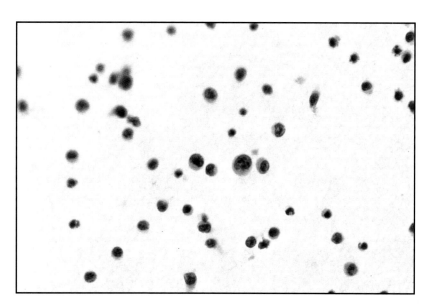

Image 4.17
A Spontaneous idiopathic eosinophilic pleuritis. Eosinophilic leukocytes overwhelmingly outnumber the other nucleated cells. (Romanowsky).
B Eosinophilic ascites in a 16-year-old boy with hydatid disease (echinococcosis) in which numerous eosinophils stand out. (H & E). (Courtesy of Dr B Naylor).

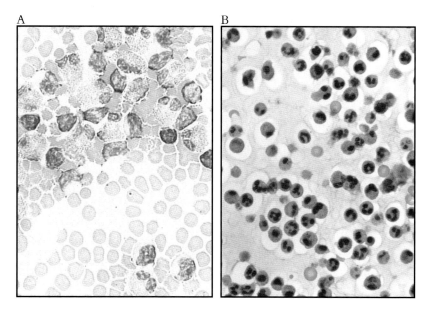

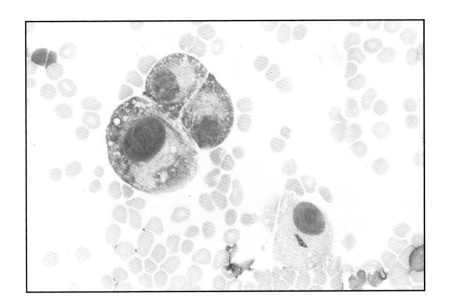

Image 4.18
Mesothelial cells are characterized by a single often perfectly round nucleus and abundant cytoplasm, leading to relatively low N/C ratios. When they articulate with one another, a narrow slit-like space (or "window") due to numerous long microvilli, is typically found. (Romanowsky).

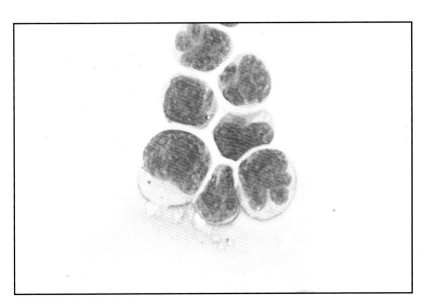

Image 4.19
Pleural fluid from a child with relapsed ALL-L$_2$. Features of the blasts include complex irregularities of the nuclear membranes, prominent nucleoli and high N/C ratios. Morphologically, this could not be distinguished from lymphoblastic lymphoma, although nucleoli are better developed in the L$_2$ form of ALL. (Romanowsky).

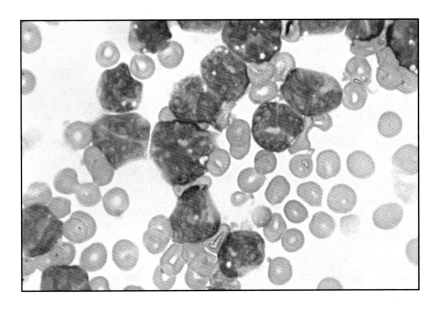

Image 4.20
ALL-L$_2$ in a serous effusion. Note the extremely complex nuclear contours and the very high N/C ratio. (Romanowsky).

Image 4.21
Numerous blasts are disseminated as a single cell suspension in this pleural fluid. This is a serous effusion specimen from a child undergoing therapy for AML. Although the cells are quite crowded, intercellular cohesion is absent. Degenerative changes, probably secondary to chemotherapy, are readily apparent. (Romanowsky).

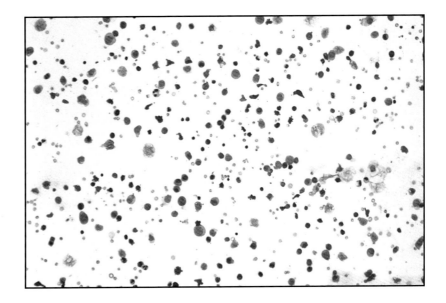

Image 4.22
Although Burkitt's lymphoma cells are more often seen in ascitic fluid, these are in a pleural specimen overrun by numerous blasts in a child receiving chemotherapy. Although the blasts are closely packed, intercellular cohesion is absent. Even at this low magnification, cytoplasmic vacuoles are evident. (Romanowsky).

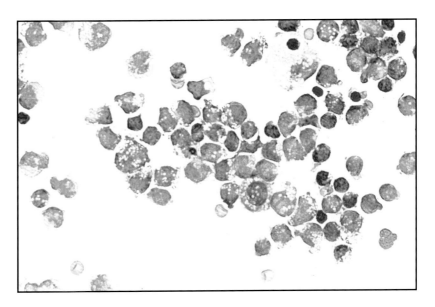

Image 4.23
Ascitic fluid positive for Burkitt's lymphoma. Each tumor cell has a single rather round nucleus with finely reticulated chromatin and one or more obvious nucleoli. Basophilic cytoplasm is evident, as are degenerative changes. (Romanowsky).

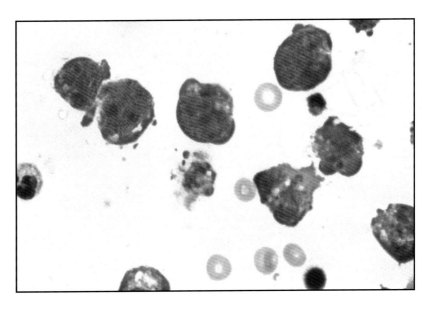

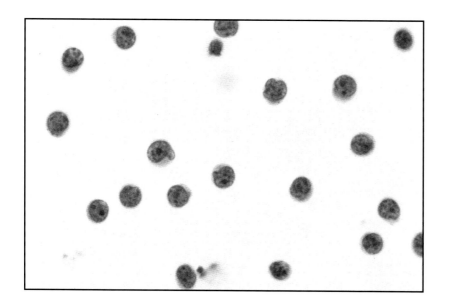

Image 4.24
This pleural fluid shows the classic appearance of lymphoblastic lymphoma. The individually dispersed malignant cells have distinct and often quite irregular nuclear membranes, finely granular chromatin, and very high N/C ratios. Nucleoli are inconspicuous. (Papanicolaou).

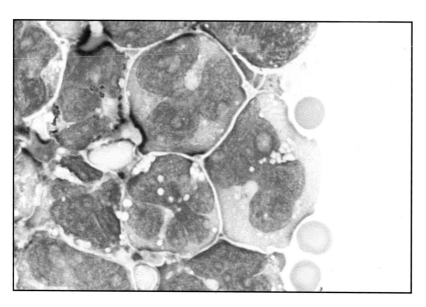

Image 4.25
Large cell lymphoma in a pleural fluid. Highly complex nuclear contours are evident, as are huge nucleoli. Although densely packed in the cytospin preparation, there is no cohesion. Cytoplasmic vacuoles are not limited to the cells of Burkitt's lymphoma. (Romanowsky).

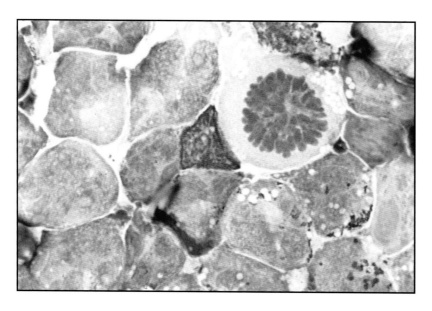

Image 4.26
Large cell lymphoma in a pleural fluid specimen (see Image 4.25). In addition to vacuoles, some cells have magenta cytoplasmic structures that are thought to be lysosomes. A tumor cell is in mitosis. (Romanowsky).

Image 4.27
In serous effusions, intercellular cohesion is a hallmark of nonlymphoreticular tumor cells, as seen in this ascitic fluid positive for neuroblastoma. Rosette formation is suggested. Each tumor cell has a single round hyperchromatic nucleus that resembles that of its neighbors. Chromatin is very finely granular and evenly dispersed, and nucleoli are small but distinct. N/C ratios are high. (Papanicolaou).

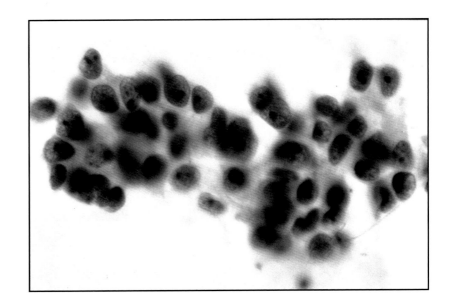

Image 4.28
Although definitive diagnostic features of neuroblastoma are not evident in this Diff-Quik–stained fluid specimen, molding of their nuclei is apparent.

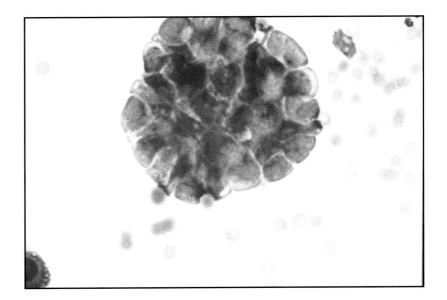

Image 4.29
Neuroblastoma cells may present in fluids as single cells. On a cell-for-cell basis, they may be very difficult to distinguish from leukemic blasts, although the nuclear membranes are very smooth. (Papanicolaou).

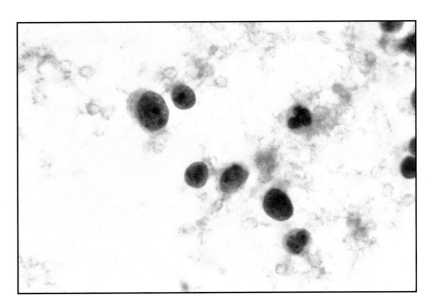

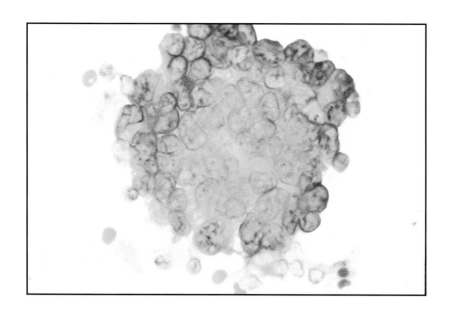

Image 4.30
Immunocytochemical reactions may be performed directly on serous effusion smears. Here we seen an intense cytoplasmic decoration of neuroblastic cells by neuron-specific enolase.

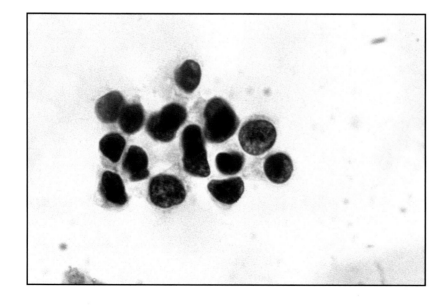

Image 4.31
Pleural fluid specimen from a 15-year-old girl with metastatic Ewing's sarcoma. These tumor cells show no specific differentiation. Within this loosely cohesive aggregate, each cell resembles its neighbors closely with a single hyperchromatic nucleus and a very high N/C ratio. Chromatin is densely clumped and nucleoli are not evident. Very small notches or angulations of the nuclear membranes are present. (Papanicolaou).

Image 4.32

A Pleural fluid positive for metastatic Wilms' tumor. Tumor cells are small with high N/C ratios, some having rounded contours and others being elongated or spindled, creating a biphasic appearance. (Papanicolaou).

B Ascitic fluid from a 5-year-old boy with nephroblastoma. Tubule formation is strongly suggested within these aggregates of small uniform cells with round nuclei and little in the way of cytoplasm. (Papanicolaou).

C A cell block of the same ascitic fluid as in B. Although some clusters appear undifferentiated (blastema), others contain neoplastic tubules. (H & E). (B & C courtesy of Dr B Naylor).

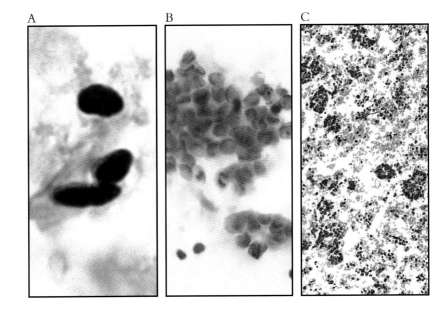

Image 4.33

Nondescript aggregates of small relatively uniform malignant cells occur much more frequently in serous effusions positive for Wilms' tumor than the biphasic appearance seen in Image 4.32. Although this cellular mass is obviously neoplastic and consistent with a small cell tumor, no specific lineage is suggested. (Papanicolaou).

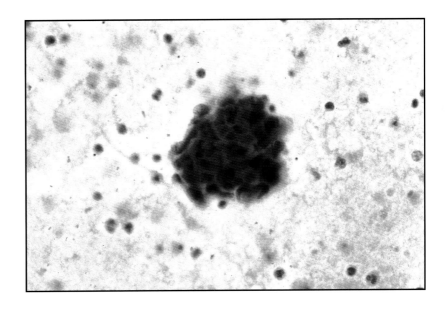

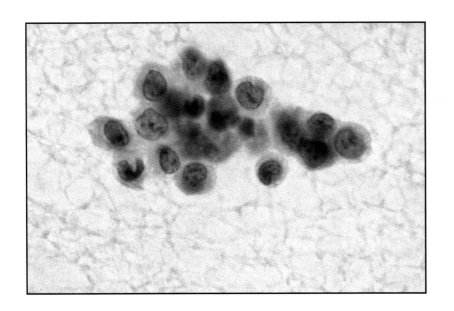

Image 4.34
This ascitic fluid specimen contains tumor cells from a pelvic embryonal rhabdomyosarcoma. Most of the cells have a single somewhat eccentrically placed nucleus and a reactively scanty volume of cytoplasm. Deep notches and other irregularities of the nuclear envelope are characteristic. (Papanicolaou).

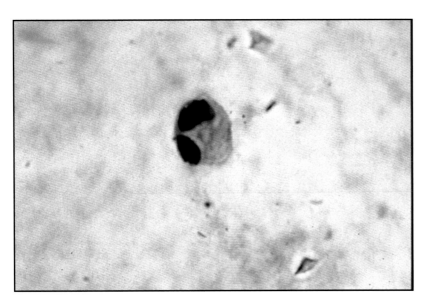

Image 4.35
Occasionally, rhabdomyosarcoma cells have greater volumes of cytoplasm and two or more nuclei. As seen here, the formation of an acute angle between the two nuclei is typical of sarcomas. (Papanicolaou).

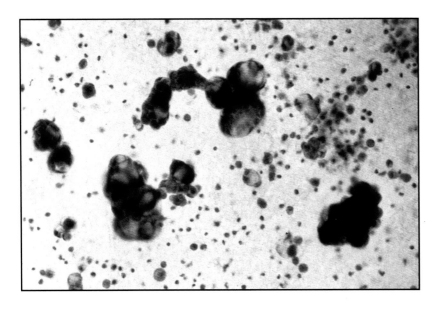

Image 4.36
This ascitic fluid specimen is positive for tumor cells derived from an intra-abdominal desmoplastic small round cell tumor. Large 3-dimensional cellular aggregates, some of which are suggestive of papillary formation, are present. The individual neoplastic cells within the aggregates are characterized by a solitary hyperchromatic nucleus and a moderate volume of cytoplasm, sometimes appearing to be vacuolated. Isolated small tumor cells are also present dispersed within the fluid. (Papanicolaou).

Image 4.37
Electron micrograph of an aliquot of ascitic fluid (see Image 4.36). The two tumor cells form part of the circumference of a gland-like structure containing a central lumen. Intercellular junctions, however, are quite primitive and microvilli are poorly developed.

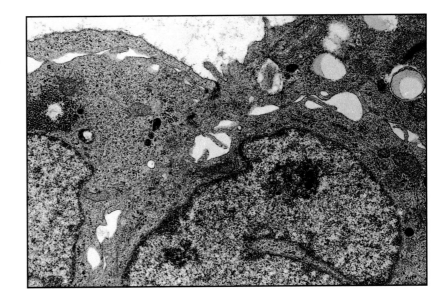

Image 4.38
Electron micrograph of an aliquot of ascitic fluid (see Image 4.36). No evidence of specific cellular lineage is evident. One malignant cell has a wavy bundle of intermediate filaments within its cytoplasm. This may correspond to the desmin positivity seen immunohistochemically.

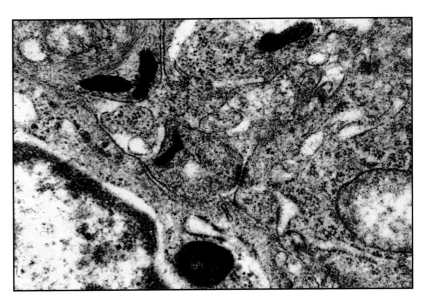

Image 4.39
Marked pleomorphism is characteristic of osteosarcoma, as seen in this pleural fluid specimen. Nuclei are very often hyperchromatic or almost pyknotic, and range from round to quite irregular in contour. N/C ratios are also quite variable. Nucleoli may be prominent. (Papanicolaou).

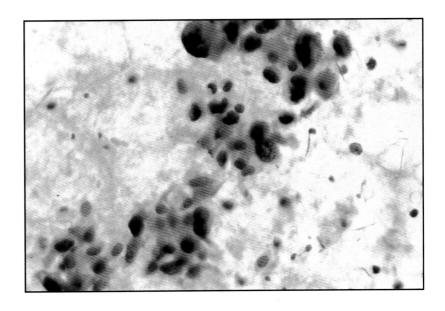

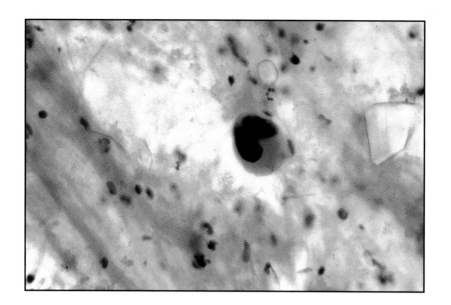

Image 4.40
Multinucleation is common in osteosarcoma. In binucleated tumor cells, an acute angle is often formed between the two nuclei. Note the marked hyperchromasia. (Papanicolaou).

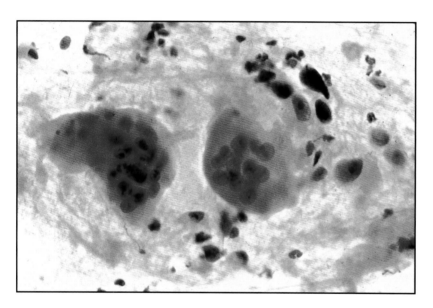

Image 4.41
In addition to the obviously malignant mononucleated tumor cells, two osteoclast-like giant cells are present in this pleural specimen. Their nuclei are round, uniform and relatively bland. (Papanicolaou).

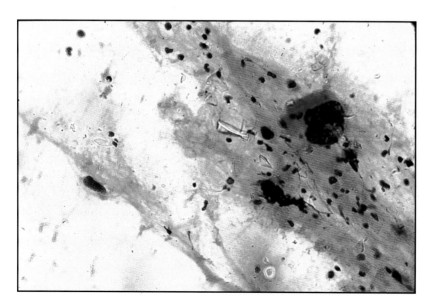

Image 4.42
A massive tumor giant cell is present among inflammatory elements and proteinaceous fluid. (Papanicolaou).

Image 4.43
Ascitic fluid specimen. Dysgerminoma cells are usually dispersed as single cellular elements. Each has a large vesicular nucleus with one or more prominent nucleoli and thick (and usually smooth) nuclear membranes. A thin rim of pale cytoplasm is evident. (Papanicolaou).

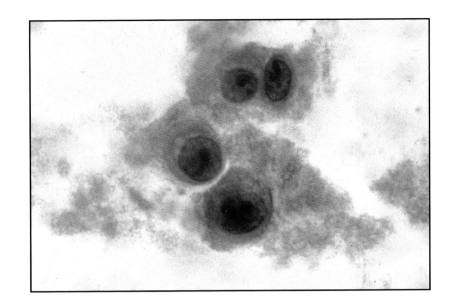

Image 4.44
Ascitic fluid specimen. (Papanicolaou).

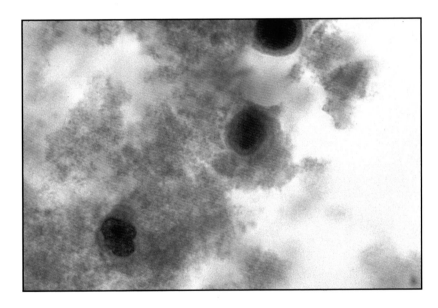

Image 4.45
Pelvic wash specimen from a teenage girl with a ruptured ovarian cystic teratoma. Clusters of mesothelial cells are present against a background of mature-appearing squamous cells. (Papanicolaou).

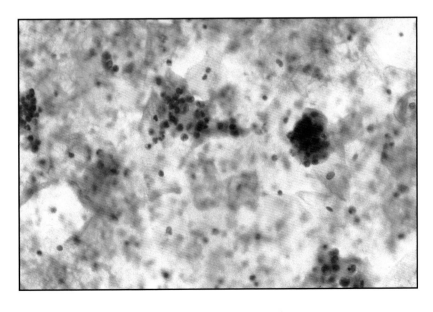

References

1. Kjeldsberg CR, Knight JA. Body Fluids. Laboratory Examination of Amniotic Cerebrospinal, Synovial, and Serous Fluids. American Society of Clinical Pathologists Press, Chicago, 1993.
2. Naylor B. Pleural, Peritoneal and Pericardial Fluids in Comprehensive Cytopathology. M. Bibbo, ed. WB Saunders, Philadelphia, 1991.
3. Koss LG. Diagnostic Cytology and Its Histopathologic Bases. 4th ed. JB Lippincott, Philadelphia, 1992.
4. Nance KV, Silverman JF. The cytology of serous effusions. *Cytopath Ann* 2:147-180, 1993.
5. Kmetz Dr, Newton WA. The role of clinical cytology in a pediatric institution. *Acta Cytol* 7:207-210,1963.
6. Wolfe WG, Spock A, Bradford WD. Pleural fluid in infants and children. *Am Rev Respir Dis* 98:1027-1032,1968.
7. Hallman JR, Geisinger KR. Cytology of fluids from pleural, peritoneal and pericardial cavities in children. A comprehensive survey. *Acta Cytol* 38:209-217, 1994.
8. Nance KV, Shermer RW, Askin FB. Diagnostic efficacy of pleural biopsy as compared with that of pleural fluid examination. *Mod Pathol* 4:320-324,1991.
9. Goodman ZD, Gupta PK, Frost JK, Erozan YS. Cytodiagnosis of viral infections in body cavity fluids. *Acta Cytol* 23:204-208,1979.
10. McCalmont TH, McLeod DL, Kerr RM, Hopkins MB, Geisinger KR. Fatal disseminated herpesvirus infection with hepatitis. A peritoneal fluid cytologic warning. *Arch Pathol Lab Med* 118:566-567, 1994.
11. Griscom NT, Colodny AH, Rosenberg HK, Fliegel CP, Hardy BE. Diagnostic aspects of neonatal ascites: report of 27 cases. *Am J Roentgenol* 128:961-970,1977.
12. Van Aerde J, Campbell AN, Smyth JA, Lloyd D, Bryan MH. Spontaneous chylothorax in newborns. *Am J Dis Child* 138:961-964,1984.
13. Edelman KA, Levine AB, Chitkara U, Berkowitz RL. Reliability of pleural fluid lymphocyte counts in the antenatal diagnosis of congenital chylothorax. *Obstet Gynecol* 78:530-532,1991.
14. Weber AM, Philipson EH. Fetal pleural effusion: a review and meta-analysis for prognostic indicators. *Obstet Gynecol* 79:281-286,1992.
15. Silverman JF, Kopelman AE. Meconium pleuritis: cytologic diagnosis in a neonate with perforated sigmoid colon and diaphragmatic hernia. *Ped Pathol* 6:325-333,1986.
16. Collins Orris KA, Geisinger KR, Cappellari JO, Hopkins MB III. Atypical lymphocytosis in ascitic fluid in young children: a potential diagnostic challenge. *Acta Cytol* 36:597,1992.
17. Silverman JF, Singh HK, Joshi VV, Holbrook CT, Chauvenet AR, Harris LS, Geisinger KR. Cytomorphology of familial hemophagocytic syndrome. *Diagn Cytopathol* 9:404-410, 1993.
18. Krishnan S, Statsinger AL, Kleinman M, Bertoni MA, Sharma P. Eosinophilic pleural effusion with Charcot-Leyden crystals. *Acta Cytol* 27:529-532,1983.
19. Helson L, Krochmal P, Hajdu SI. Diagnostic value of cytologic specimens obtained from children with cancer. *Ann Clin Lab Sci* 5:294-297,1975.

20. Geisinger KR, Hajdu SI, Helson L. Exfoliative cytology of non-lymphoreticular neoplasms in children. *Acta Cytol* 28:16-28,1984.
21. Farr GH, Hajdu SI. Exfoliative cytology of metastatic neuroblastoma. *Acta Cytol* 16:203-206,1972.
22. Hajdu SI. Exfoliative cytology of primary and metastatic Wilms' tumor. *Acta Cytol* 15:339-342,1971.
23. Hajdu SI, Koss LG. Cytologic diagnosis of metastatic myosarcomas. *Acta Cytol* 13:545-551,1969.
24. Allsbrook WC Jr, Stead NW, Pantazis CG, Houston JH, Crosby JH. Embryonal rhabdomyosarcoma in ascitic fluid. Immunocytochemical and DNA flow cytometric study. *Arch Pathol Lab Med* 110:847-849,1986.
25. Gerald WL, Miller HK, Battifora H, Miettinen M, Silva EG, Rosai J. Intra-abdominal desmoplastic small round-cell tumor. Report of 19 cases of a distinctive type of high-grade polyphenotypic malignancy affecting young individuals. *Am J Surg Pathol* 15:499-513,1991.
26. Bian Y, Jordan AG, Rupp M, Cohn H, McLaughlin CJ, Miettinen M. Effusion cytology of desmoplastic small round cell tumor of the pleura. A case report. *Acta Cytol* 37:77-82, 1993.
27. Thompson EN III, Teot LA, Geisinger KR. Exfoliative and aspiration cytomorphology of intraabdominal desmoplastic small-round cell tumor. The first reported case. *Acta Cytol* 36:599, 1992.
28. Armstrong GR, Raafat F, Ingram L, Mann JR. Malignant peritoneal mesothelioma in childhood. *Arch Pathol Lab Med* 112:1159-1162, 1988.
29. Geisinger KR, Ng LW, Hopkins MB III, Barrett RJ, Welander CE, Homesley HD. Tenckhoff catheter cytology in patients with ovarian cancer. *Cancer* 62:1582-1585, 1988.
30. Hajdu, SI, Nolan MA. Exfoliative cytology of malignant germ cell tumors. *Acta Cytol* 19:255-260, 1975.
31. Kapila K, Hajdu SI, Whitmore WF, Golbey RB, Beattie EJ. Cytologic diagnosis of metastatic germ cell tumors. *Acta Cytol* 27:245-251, 1983.
32. Kashimura M, Tsukamoto N, Matsuyama T, Kashimura Y, Sugimori H, Taki I. Cytologic findings of ascites from patients with ovarian dygerminoma. *Acta Cytol* 27:59-62, 1983.
33. Morimoto N, Ozawa M, Amano S. Diagnostic value of hyaline globules in endodermal sinus tumor. Report of two cases. *Acta Cytol* 25:416-420, 1981.
34. Cobb CJ, Wynn J, Cobb SR, Duane GB. Cytologic finding in an effusion caused by rupture of a benign cystic teratoma of the mediastinum into a serous cavity. *Acta Cytol* 29:1015-1020, 1985.

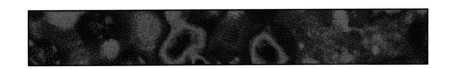

CHAPTER FIVE

Cervicovaginal Cytology

Worldwide, cytopathology gained its diagnostic foundation with the development and widespread usage of the cervicovaginal (Pap) smear. Of course, this test is very well known to the medical profession, and discussion will be limited to considerations for the pediatric patient. The major purpose of the Pap smear is to screen for premalignant alterations in the epithelium of the cervix and vagina with a relatively simple, nontraumatic procedure. Such smears may also reliably detect genital infections. Furthermore, properly obtained and prepared vaginal specimens may be used to address hormonal maturation in girls. Recently, Koss eloquently reviewed the advantages and limitations of the Papanicolaou test.[1]

The most important function of the cervicovaginal smear is the detection of proliferative lesions in the squamous epithelium of the cervix and vagina. The nomenclature for entities is varied and somewhat controversial. Most recently, the Bethesda system's classification scheme has been widely embraced in the United States.[2-4] It divides premalignant changes into two groups, low- and high-grade squamous intraepithelial lesions. During the past decade, there has been an explosion of data demonstrating a strong association of these preinvasive proliferations, as well as invasive carcinoma, to prior infection by several different types of human papilloma viruses (HPV).[5-14]

The last 10 years or so have also witnessed a marked downward shift in the mean age at which these diseases develop, resulting in a significant increase in the detection of HPV-related lesions in the pediatric population.[5-12] This is especially true in adolescent girls in whom rare invasive squamous cell carcinomas have been diagnosed.[5-9] Mild dysplasias and condylomas (low-grade squamous intraepithelial lesions) are much more frequently detected and can be treated adequately. Of course, long-term follow-up is mandatory due to the relatively high recurrence rates for these infections. In very young girls, vulvar condylomas are being seen more often as well. In the 1st year or 2 of life, these may be related to perinatal, transvaginal exposure to virus from the mother.[10,11] In older patients, sexual transmission is the most likely mode. Vulvar condylomas are not infrequently associated with abnormal proliferations more proximally (vagina and/or cervix), necessitating evaluation of these sites, at least with a Pap smear, whenever possible.

In the series of sexual active adolescent patients reported by Rosenfeld and colleagues, HPV DNA was found by Southern blot hybridization in 38% of the patients.[7] 8% of the patients in this series also were found to have cytologic abnormalities in their cervicovaginal cytologic smears. Such cellular abnormalities were much more likely (17% vs 3%) in adolescents positive for HPV. Adolescent women with multiple sexual partners were much more likely to be positive for presence of this virus. Similarly, Moscicki et al found multiple sexual partners to be the only significant risk factor for HPV positivity in their very large series of sexually active adolescent women.[9] Overall 15% of their patients were positive for HPV DNA by dot blot hybridization. Importantly, greater than 60% of these positive patients were found to have one of the more oncogenic viral types. Martinez et al evaluated cervicovaginal cytologic findings and HPV DNA, as determined by Southern blot hybridization, in a series of adolescent patients.[6] Nearly half (48%) of the patients with abnormal Pap smears harbored HPV DNA sequences. Only 3% of the patients with normal cytologic smears were positive for HPV.

Only a very terse overview of the cytomorphology of squamous intraepithelial lesions will be presented here, as they have been very well detailed elsewhere.[13,14] Nuclei of the dysplastic cells comprising these lesions are abnormal (Images 5.1 through 5.7). They are larger than normal, hyperchromatic, and have variably sized chromatin granules. Although the chromatin may range from finely to coarsely granular, it is usually uniformly distributed throughout the confines of the nucleus. Nuclear membranes are distinct, except in condyloma cells, and may be smooth and regular to angulated or manifest other abnormalities of contour. Generally, nucleoli are not visible. N/C ratios are always elevated, and in general, increase as the degree of dysplasia increases from mild to moderate to severe (Images 5.1 through 5.3). Within the smears, these abnormal cells are present both singly and in cohesive aggregates. As the lesions approach a full thickness change (carcinoma-in-situ), intercellular borders become indistinct so that the cellular clusters resemble syncytia (Image 5.4). At the other end of the spectrum, the nuclei in condyloma cells (koilocytes) have homogeneous or smudged, evenly spread, dark chromatin with little texture or structure (Images 5.5 through 5.7). These nuclei may also have contorted configurations (so-called "raisin-like" outline). Binucleation is common.

The cytoplasm in these cells varies in quantity and quality. In general, it parallels that found in normal stratified squamous epithelium with the mildly dysplastic elements having relatively abundant transparent cytoplasm (Image 5.1). With increasing levels of severity, cytoplasmic volume decreases and it becomes denser and more cyanophilic (Image 5.2 and 5.3). Some cells may have brilliantly orangeophilic, dense cytoplasm, reflecting the abnormal presence of keratin proteins. The classic cytologic component of the condyloma is the koilocyte (Image 5.5 and 5.6). This cell has a large amount of cytoplasm and a large abnormal (dyskaryotic) nucleus. Its distinguishing feature is the presence of a large perinuclear clear zone or halo. The interface of the halo and the more peripheral cytoplasm is crisp and distinct. A thickened cell membrane is another feature of an unequivocal koilocyte.

Another important feature of the Pap smear is the identification of pathogenic microbial organisms.[13-16] Most commonly, the fungus *Candida* is present, often but not always associated with a well developed acute inflammatory infiltrate. With the Pap stain, pseudohyphae appear as delicate, eosinophilic interconnected cylinders ("sausage-links"). Small round budding yeast cells may also be seen. Frequently, these organisms are intimately admixed with the squamous epithelial cells of the smear and may produce changes of inflammatory "atypia" which need to be distinguished from a low-grade squamous intraepithelial lesion. Herpes simplex virus is another pathogen identified with some frequency in the pediatric population. Classic cytopathic alterations include the formation of large squamous cells with multiple, molded nuclei. In some, the classic Cowdry-type A inclusions may be seen. In others, the chromatin has a refractile homogenous or "ground-glass" appearance. It is usually quite easy to distinguish these infected cells from dysplastic elements. In the large series of Pap smears from children reported by Diller et al, trichomonads were seen quite frequently.[15] *Trichomonas vaginalis* appears as oval, round, or pyramidal-shaped structures with a cyanophilic staining reaction (Image 5.8).[16] Each organism has a single round and generally eccentric, hypochromatic nucleus (Image 5.9). Faintly stained eosinophilic granules are found within the cytoplasm. They may be dispersed freely and attached to squamous cells. On occasion, a *Chlamydia* infection may be suggested in the smear (Image 5.10). Metaplastic squamous cells are infected and may contain cytoplasmic inclusion bodies. In early stages, one or more small granules are encased by vacuoles; often several of these appear closely clustered within the cell's cytoplasm. Later, these appear to fuse with the formation of a larger body also surrounded by a vacuole. Other pathogenic organisms are infrequently observed (Images 5.11 and 5.12).

Only infrequently have we been asked to assess the status of ovarian function in children via the use of vaginal cytology. The specimen must be derived from the lateral vaginal wall. We prefer to use a maturation index in which the ratio of parabasal to intermediate to superficial squamous cells is calculated.[17] In very young children, a parabasal cell predominance is normal, reflecting the absence of circulating ovarian steroid hormones. Several years prior to the menarche, an intermediate cell predominance is seen. With the onset of normal menses, a superficial cell picture will be present at mid cycle.

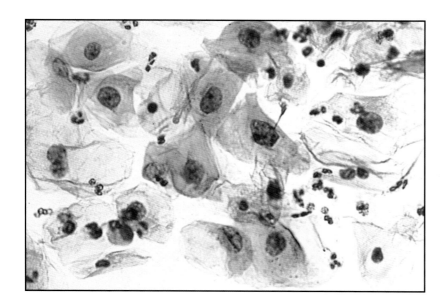

Image 5.1
In mild squamous dysplasia, nuclei are much larger than normal and are hyperchromatic. N/C ratio is definitely increased relative to normal epithelial cells. Cytoplasm is translucent with polygonal contours. (Papanicolaou).

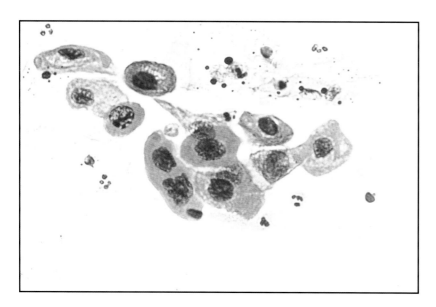

Image 5.2
In moderate squamous dysplasia, N/C ratio is increased compared to those in mild dysplasia, and cytoplasm is denser. Nuclei, however, are not particularly different. (Papanicolaou).

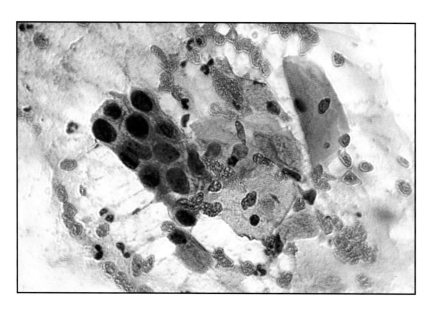

Image 5.3
N/C ratio is greatly increased in severe squamous dysplasia, as seen in this sheet of abnormal cells. Within this sheet, intercellular borders remain distinct. Also present are normal superficial and intermediate squamous cells: compare the sizes of the normal and dysplastic nuclei, and the differences in their N/C ratios. (Papanicolaou)

Image 5.4

In squamous carcinoma in situ, the cells often resemble those seen in severe dysplasia. A major difference, as seen here, is the arrangement of the abnormal cells into syncytia. Syncytia are cellular aggregates, at times 3-dimensional, with an apparent loss or reduction of both distinct cellular borders and nuclear polarity. (Papanicolaou).

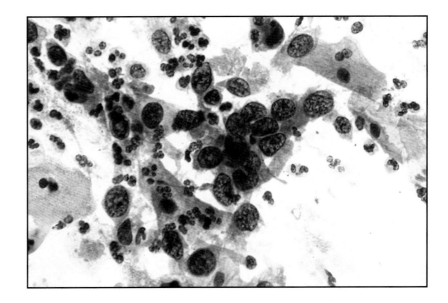

Image 5.5

The koilocyte is characterized by an enlarged nucleus that appears separated from the stained peripheral cytoplasm by a sizeable perinuclear halo or cavity. A sharp interface between the dense peripheral cytoplasm and the halo typifies this cell. Chromatin may be variable, but in this cell it is finely granular and pale. Compare the nuclei of the koilocyte and the normal superficial squamous cell. (Papanicolaou).

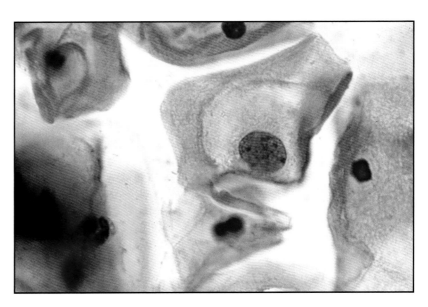

Image 5.6

Koilocytes readily stand out from the normal squamous cells due to their larger nuclei and crisp perinuclear halo. Note the clean smear background. (Papanicolaou).

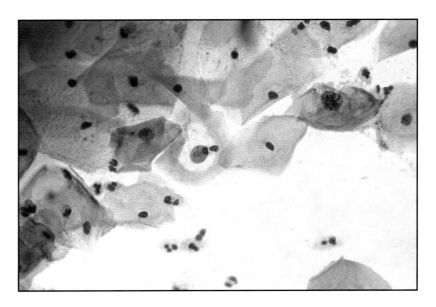

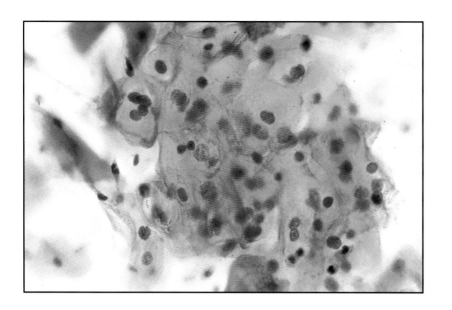

Image 5.7

In smears from patients with condyloma, dyskeratocytes are often more common than koilocytes. These cells have dense, frequently brilliant orangeophilic cytoplasm and relatively small but atypical nuclei. The latter may be vesicular or quite hyperchromatic and irregular in contour with smudged chromatin. Usually they are present in cohesive aggregates. (Papanicolaou).

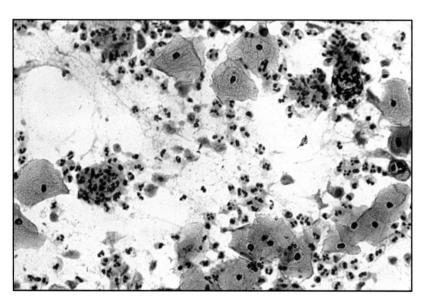

Image 5.8

As seen here, neutrophils are often numerous in smears of patients infected with *Trichomonas*. The organisms appear in the center of this field as small pyramidal pale blue staining structures. Most are freely dispersed, but a few appear to be attached to the surfaces of the squamous epithelial cells. The latter often take a rosy pink hue. (Papanicolaou).

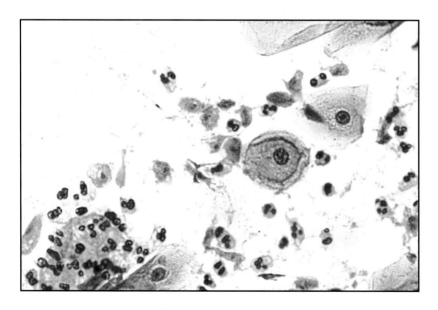

Image 5.9

Trichomonas infection (see Image 5.8). The trichomonads appear slightly larger than the adjacent neutrophils and have pale-staining small round nuclei. Several of them also demonstrate cytoplasmic granularity. Small perinuclear halos are present in several of the squamous cells secondary to the inflammatory reaction. These nonspecific changes should not be mistaken for koilocytic atypia. (Papanicolaou).

Image 5.10
Two metaplastic squamous cells contain multiple granule-containing cytoplasmic vacuoles. These features are suggestive, but in our opinion, not diagnostic of *Chlamydia* infection, as intracytoplasmic mucin and degenerative changes may appear similar. In the lower portion of the field are a small aggregate of endocervical glandular cells.

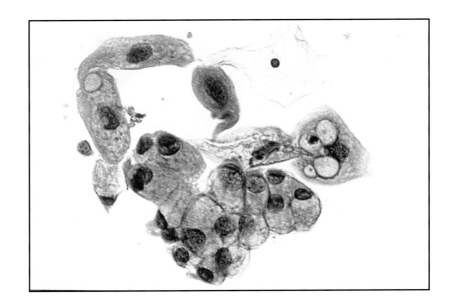

Image 5.11
Pap smear was from a 15-year-old alleged rape victim. Present is the egg of the pinworm (*Enterobius vermicularis*). Ova contain a larvae and demonstrate asymmetry of their long axes' contours. (Papanicolaou). (Courtesy of Dr B Naylor).

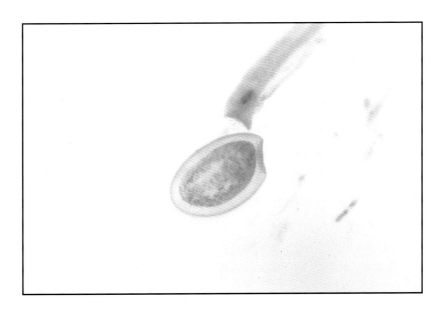

Image 5.12
A louse is present in this cervicovaginal smear. (Papanicolaou). (Courtesy of Dr B Naylor).

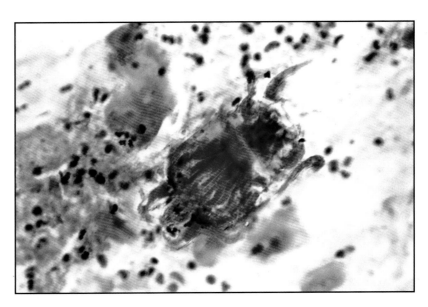

References

1. Koss LG. The Papanicolaou test for cervical cancer detection. A triumph and a tragedy. *JAMA* 261:737-743, 1989.
2. National Cancer Institute Workshop. The 1988 Bethesda system for reporting cervical/vaginal cytological diagnoses. *JAMA* 262:931-934, 1989.
3. Luff RD. The Bethesda system for reporting cervical/vaginal cytologic diagnoses. Report of the 1991 Bethesda workshop. *Am J Clin Pathol* 98:152-154, 1992.
4. Davey DD, Nielsen ML, Rosenstock W, Kline TS. Terminology and specimen adequacy in cervicovaginal cytology. The College of American Pathologists interlaboratory comparison program experience. *Arch Pathol Lab Med* 116:903-907, 1992.
5. Raymond CA. Cervical dysplasia upturn worries gynecologists, health officials. *JAMA* 257:2397-2398, 1987.
6. Martinez J, Smith R, Farmer M, Resqu J, Alger L, Daniel R, Gupta J, Shah K, Naghashfar Z. High prevalence of genital tract papillomavirus infection in female adolescents. *Pediatrics* 82:604-608, 1988.
7. Rosenfeld WD, Vermund SH, Wentz SJ, Burk RD. High prevalence rate of human papillomavirus infection and association with abnormal Papanicolaou in sexually active adolescents. *Am J Dis Child* 143:1443-1447, 1989.
8. Davis AJ, Emans SJ. Human papilloma virus infection in the pediatric and adolescent patient. *J Pediatr* 115:1-9, 1989.
9. Moscicki A-B, Palefsky J, Gonzales J, Schoolnik GK. Human papillomavirus infection in sexually active adolescent females. Prevalence and risk factors. *Pediatr Res* 28:507-513, 1990.
10. Cohen BA, Honig P, Androphy E. Anogenital warts in children. Clinical and virologic evaluation for sexual abuse. *Arch Dermatol* 126:1575-1580, 1990.
11. Franger AL. Condylomata acuminata in prepubescent females. *Adolesc Pediatr Gynecol* 3:38-41, 1990.
12. Krowchuk DP, Anglin TM. Genital human papillomavirus infections in adolescents: implications for evaluation and management. *Sem Dermatol* 11:24-30, 1992.
13. Meisels A, Morin C. Cytopathology of the Uterine Cervix. American Society of Clinical Pathology Press, Chicago, 1991.
14. Koss LG. Diagnostic cytology and its histopathologic bases. 4th ed. JB Lippincott, 1992, Philadelphia.
15. Diller C, Murphy G, Lauchlan SC. Cervicovaginal cytology in patients 16 years of age and younger. *Acta Cytol* 27:426-428, 1983.
16. Gupta PK. Microbiology, inflammation, and viral infections. In: Comprehensive Cytopathology. M Bibbo, ed. WB Saunders, Philadelphia 1991, 115-152.
17. Weid GL, Bibbo M, Keebler CM. Evaluation of endocrinologic condition by exfoliative cytology. In: Compendium on Diagnostic Cytology: The Tutorials of Cytology, 5th ed. GL Weid, LG Koss, Reagan JW, eds. Chicago, 1983.

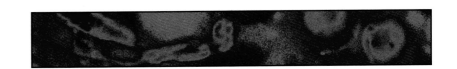

CHAPTER SIX

Respiratory Cytology

In adults, pulmonary cytologic specimens of both the exfoliative and aspiration types comprise a large percentage of all nongynecologic samples examined in many laboratories. Although the major goal of most specimens is to detect primary and metastatic neoplasms, increasing proportions of these samples are being utilized to diagnose potential infectious diseases.[1] As primary neoplasms of the lungs are very infrequent in children, cytologic examinations of the respiratory tract are relatively uncommon and many of these are utilized to examine for possible specific infectious agents, especially in immunosuppressed patients. Another reason for this discrepancy between children and adults is that it is very difficult for infants and young children to expectorate a sputum sample.

Lipid-Laden Macrophages

A relatively small number of publications have proposed the use of respiratory tract cytology to aid in the diagnosis and monitoring of nonneoplastic, noninfectious pulmonary disorders in children.[2-12] In our own experience, the assay most often requested is the evaluation of tracheal aspirates for the presence of lipid-laden macrophages. Several authors have suggested that gastroesophageal reflux with the aspiration of gastric contents contributes to the pathogeneses of chronic lung disease in neonatal infants.[2,3, 5-8]   Specimens are procured by aspirating bronchial secretions through endotracheal tubes in ventilator-dependent newborns. As described by Hewitt, the aspiration may also be performed under direct laryngoscopy.[3] The sediment so obtained is fixed with formalin vapors and stained with oil red O. The cytologist evaluates for the presence of and the relative quantities of lipid-laden macrophages and possibly extracellular lipid droplets (Image 6.1). Nearly 20 years ago Williams and Freeman described this test as being highly specific and rather sensitive for the detection of pneumonia secondary to aspiration of milk in infants.[2] They evaluated both phagocytized lipid and free fat globules, and scored their slides as either positive or negative. Negative scores included specimens with only an occasional lipid-laden macrophage or a few extracellular globules. These authors further stated, and we agree, that one of the problems with quantitating the amount of phagocytized lipid is the relatively uneven distribution of this material on the slides due to the presence of mucus.[2] 78% of the infants in their studies who suffered clinical milk inhalation had a positive specimen. They felt that this test was more sensitive for the detection of such inhalation compared to radiologic imaging. None of their control patients (infants with respiratory problems unrelated to milk inhalation) had a positive specimen. Hewitt did not include the evaluation and quantitation of extracellular fat globules as she felt that this could be possibly related to lipid entering the trachea during the aspiration procedure.[3]

Nussbaum et al studied 115 children with chronic respiratory tract diseases.[5] Nearly 2/3 of their patients also had gastroesophageal reflux disease. Each patient underwent bronchoscopic examination with bronchoalveolar lavage. The lavage fluid was cytocentrifuged onto slides and then stained with oil red O. These authors defined an alveolar macrophage as being lipid-laden if it contained 10 or more red vacuoles within its cytoplasm or if at least half of the cytoplasm stained red. A specimen was deemed positive if they could find 2 lipid-laden alveolar macrophages in at least 1 high-power microscopic field. Specimens were positive in 85% of the children with gastroesophageal reflux and in only 19% of those with lung disease but without evidence of reflux. These authors proposed that the evaluation of lavage specimens for lipid-laden macrophages should be considered in order to establish the presence of aspiration in children who may be candidates for antireflux surgery.[5] It should be noted that their patient population was not restricted to newborn infants but rather had a mean age of approximately 6 years.

A similar study was reported by Colombo and Hallberg, who evaluated 45 children with a mean age of 3 years who suffered from a variety of different respiratory disorders.[6] Their patients also underwent bronchoscopy with a bronchial washing. The obtained material was smeared on slides and stained with oil red O. These authors used a quantitation scheme very similar to that of Corwin and Irwin in which individual macrophages were scored for the amount of cytoplasmic lipid.[6,13] Their index was determined by summing the scores in 100 alveolar macrophages. 22 of their children were considered to show evidence of aspiration, while the remaining 23 did not.[6] Using their methodology, they found no overlap between the 2 groups (aspirators versus nonaspirators). All of their pediatric aspirators had an index of at least 86, whereas none of the nonaspirators had an index exceeding 72. Thus, using a cut-off value of 86, their assay was 100% specific.

However, the study of Recalde et al proved beyond doubt that the presence of intracytoplasmic lipid within alveolar macrophages is not totally specific for aspiration pneumonia.[4] They studied 74 newborn children with respiratory distress syndrome via tracheal aspiration cytology. 13 children had specimens that contained numerous macrophages with lipid-positive foamy cytoplasm. All 13 of these patients were receiving intravenous lipid administration and were not consuming milk orally, thus excluding the possibility of reflux with aspiration. Only 4 of the 61 patients who were not receiving the infusions of lipid-containing solutions had prominent numbers of lipid-laden macrophages in their tracheal aspirates. Robins and Zachariah also found a lack of specificity.[14]

Moran and colleagues also used the cellular lipid index devised by Corwin and Irwin.[7,13] Individual alveolar macrophages were evaluated for the amount of intracellular lipid droplets from grade 0 (absence of lipid) to grade 4 (numerous intracellular droplets completely occupying the cytoplasm and obscuring the nucleus). The cellular lipid index was determined by evaluating 100 consecutive macrophages and summing the score from these individual cells. They evaluated 77 newborns all of whom required mechanical ventilation for a number of different medical problems.[7] Lactose was measured biochemically in an aliquot of the tracheal aspirates. The mean lipid index for samples suggestive of aspiration (based on lactose determination) was significantly greater than the mean index for specimens thought to be negative for aspiration. Although Moran et al did not find this cytologic assay to be totally specific for aspiration pneumonia, they concluded that it was a useful test for diagnosing aspiration.[7]

It has been our own personal experience that such an elaborate quantification of phagocytized lipids is probably excessive. One of the advantages of the technique is that it produces clinically important information in a relatively rapid and effortless manner. We believe that the evaluation of individual macrophages for the amount of phagocytized lipid is too time-consuming. In our recent study, we simply counted the number of positive macrophages on each slide.[8] Scores of 0 to 3 were provided for each specimen. A score of 3 was awarded whenever a specimen contained more than 50 lipid-laden macrophages. In a blind fashion, we correlated the clinical course with the tracheal aspiration cytology specimens in 106 infants, 6 months of age or younger. 17 of the 31 patients with clinical evidence of aspiration pneumonia and/or gastroesophageal reflux had a score of 3 in their tracheal aspirate smears. Only 12 of the 75 individuals with scores less than 3 showed such clinical features. In this population of children this test had a sensitivity of 57% and specificity of 82% with an overall diagnostic efficiency of 75%.[8] Thus, by simplifying the evaluation method and apparently increasing the threshold for a positive result (that is, a score of 3), we are able to increase the diagnostic specificity (although at the expense of sensitivity). Furthermore, this methodology permits the specimen to be evaluated in a rapid manner.

We believe that the evaluation of individual macrophages for the amount of phagocytized lipid is too time-consuming

It is difficult to compare the results of different studies of lipid-laden alveolar macrophages as a marker for aspiration pneumonia. Investigations have differed on a number of important points. In some studies, only newborns have been evaluated. In others, the entire spectrum of pediatric patients have been included. Tracheal aspirates obtained through the endotracheal tube have been used to procure specimens in some, whereas bronchoscopy has been utilized in other investigations. The manner in which the cytologic specimens are evaluated has also differed from study to study, ranging from 2 positive cells in 1 microscopic field to enumerating the amount of lipid in 100 consecutive macrophages. Despite these deficiencies, the literature supports the concept that the evaluation of respiratory tract secretions for lipid-laden alveolar macrophages has clinical value in determining or confirming the etiology of chronic respiratory tract disorders.

Respiratory Distress Syndrome

A number of other acquired conditions may lead to respiratory embarrassment in neonates and older children. One of the best recognized and most common causes of respiratory difficulties in newborns is the respiratory distress syndrome of the newborn (hyaline membrane disease).[9-12] Almost always, the infant is preterm and presents with respiratory difficulty in the 1st day of life which progressively becomes more life-threatening. The basic defect in hyaline membrane disease is a relative deficiency of surfactant. Surfactant comprises a group of phospholipids that have the important role of reducing surface tension within the alveoli. Surfactant is produced by the Type II alveolar cells and immaturity of the lung in preterm infants precludes adequate production of these surface active chemicals. In general, therapy requires mechanical ventilatory assistance with the delivery of relatively high levels of oxygen to the infants. One of the major complications of this treatment is the development of bronchopulmonary dysplasia. Major pathologic alterations in the lungs associated with bronchopulmonary dysplasia include interstitial fibrosis, hypertrophy of the smooth muscle about the airways, chronic inflammatory cell infiltrates in the parenchyma, hyperplasia of the Type II pneumocytes, and variably extensive squamous metaplasia of the bronchiolar epithelium.[15]

More than a decade ago, Merritt and colleagues published their results of the use of exfoliative cytology in tracheal aspirates from infants receiving mechanical ventilation.[9,10] These authors divided their cytomorphologic findings into three classes temporally. Class I and Class II alterations occurred during the first 10 days of therapy and included the exfoliation of large numbers of bronchial epithelial cells. Early (Class I) cells showed little in the way of degeneration or regeneration. Class II features included degenerative and slight regenerative alterations in epithelial cells accompanied by infiltrates of segmented leukocytes. The Class III alterations appeared approximately at 10 days of life and included prominent regeneration among the epithelial cells, well-developed squamous metaplasia, and the presence of macrophages,

The basic defect in hyaline membrane disease is a relative deficiency of surfactant

multinucleated inflammatory giant cells, and neutrophils (Image 6.2). Their Class III alterations were found in neonates who developed radiographic features of bronchopulmonary dysplasia, but did not occur in those fortunate children who did not develop this complication. 70% of the patients who developed radiographic evidence of bronchopulmonary dysplasia had Class III cytologic alterations. Thus, using their tracheal aspiration cytology scheme, the finding of Class III cellular alterations was specific and relatively sensitive for bronchopulmonary dysplasia. Furthermore, these cytologic changes occurred earlier in the clinical course than did the diagnostic chest x-ray features of this complication. The inflammatory giant cells correlated with the clinical evidence of a pulmonary air leak (intrathoracic extraalveolar gas). The authors claimed that there was overlap between the appearances of Class I and II specimens. In an earlier report, D'Abaling et al described the cytologic features in tracheal aspirates of preterm infants with bronchopulmonary dysplasia.[12] Unlike Merritt et al, they were unable to correlate the cytologic alterations with either the concentration of oxygen or the duration of mechanical ventilation.[9,10,12]

Doshi and colleagues described the application of exfoliative cytomorphology in tracheal aspirates in the differential diagnosis of respiratory distress in newborn infants.[11] In their study, they compared the tracheal cytologic findings with the histopathologic features in 72 newborns who were autopsied. These authors utilized a battery of Papanicolaou and Gram stains, which were sometimes supplemented with other special stains. Overall, they found an agreement, either complete or partial, between the cytologic and histologic diagnoses in nearly 3/4 of the patients. At least some of the time they believed that only partial agreement was found in that the tracheal specimen had been obtained a number of days prior to death; the cytologic diagnosis rendered was hyaline membrane disease, but by the time of death, the pulmonary disease had progressed into bronchopulmonary dysplasia. Their changes were relatively similar to those of Merritt et al with the progressive appearance of metaplastic squamous cells and what they termed dysplastic cells (which may represent regenerative epithelium).[9-11] They also described the presence of detached ciliary tufts (ciliocytophthoria) early in the development of bronchopulmonary dysplasia.[11] They did not discuss the evolution of inflammatory cell infiltrates in the setting.

Cytologic alterations in idiopathic respiratory distress syndrome itself included the exfoliation of numerous respiratory columnar epithelial cells, generally in large cohesive aggregates.[11] Ciliocytophthoria was also very well developed early in the course. Also commonly seen were filamentous structures having a basophilic or yellow hue corresponding to the hyaline membranes.

Doshi et al described a single case of intraaveolar hemorrhage.[11] As expected, numerous erythrocytes were present in the tracheal aspirate. 2 infants in their series suffered massive amniotic fluid and meconium aspiration.[11] Anucleated squamous cells with basophilic cytoplasm were the predominant feature. Meconium was described as coarsely granular debris with a greenish coloration with the Papanicolaou stain. Both neutrophils and macrophages were also present. The major problem in 9 of their patients was pneumonia.[11] 7 had cytologic

Cytologic alterations in idiopathic respiratory distress syndrome itself included the exfoliation of numerous respiratory columnar epithelial cells, generally in large cohesive aggregates

evidence of such inflammation in their tracheal aspirates. The morphologic features included numerous neutrophils, fibrin, and necrotic tissue debris. With the Gram-stained smears, bacteria were recognized both extracellularly and phagocytized within macrophages.

Infections

In our experience, the major use of respiratory tract cytology in older children is to identify specific infectious agents in patients with pulmonary infiltrates. Often, but not always, these children are immunodeficient, mostly from the treatment for acute leukemia and the acquired immunodeficiency syndrome (AIDS). Although sputum and tracheal aspirates are occasionally submitted, most often specimens from bronchial washes and lavages are examined. The organism for which a specific search is most often requested is *Pneumocystis carinii*. The possibility of *Pneumocystis* infection has prompted the addition of a methenamine silver stain to one or more slides from each specimen, for it may be difficult to visualize *Pneumocystis* organisms on Papanicolaou-stained cytologic smears. In very well-developed infections, however, the alveolar cast may appear as aggregates or masses of eosinophilic material with a reticulated or honeycomb appearance (Image 6.3).[1] These alveolar casts contain numerous cysts of the organism (Image 6.4). The cysts are generally round and approximately as large as erythrocytes. Small internal structures, most often a dot less than a micron in diameter, are visualized. Some of the cysts may have a contour resembling the moon or a cup. Trophozoites of *Pneumocystis* may be visualized with the Romanowsky stain. This stage of development is either round or crescentic and generally <1 μm in diameter. The bronchial casts from children with cystic fibrosis may superficially resemble these aveolar casts (Image 6.5).

The only fungal organism that we have seen with consistency in children is *Candida albicans*. These organisms may present as pseudohyphae and/or yeast cells (Image 6.6). The pseudohypae appear as thin cylinders with points of constriction, usually with an eosinophilic staining reaction (Image 6.7). The yeast cells are oval and smaller than erythrocytes. Frequently, they will show budding. We have seen several examples of Blastomyces dermatitidis in lavage specimens in children. These organisms are much larger and the budding forms have a broad base (Image 6.8).

Exfoliative cytology provides rapid and accurate information concerning the presence of specific viral infections.[16-20] Clinically valuable information can be had demonstrating herpes simplex virus, cytomegalovirus (CMV), adenovirus, respiratory syncytial virus and measles virus. Frequently, these viruses produce histologic evidence of a necrotizing bronchitis and bronchiolitis.[15] Herpes virus can produce 2 different cytopathologic alterations.[16,17] The Cowdry Type A inclusion consists of a large basophilic intranuclear structure separated from a thickened nuclear membrane by a clear space or halo. Nuclei with such alterations may occur in cells with 1 or multiple nuclei. The

The major use of respiratory tract cytology in older children is to identify specific infectious agents in patients with pulmonary infiltrates

other characteristic change is the multinucleated giant cell in which the nuclei are molded and have a "ground-glass" appearance. That is, the nuclei have a homogeneous, basophilic appearance and are compressed against one another. With cytomegalovirus (CMV), even larger infected epithelial cells result.[1,16] However, unlike with herpes simplex, multinucleated elements are not produced. Cells have a huge basophilic nuclear inclusion surrounded by a large halo and a thickened nuclear envelope due to peripheral condensation of the chromatin (Images 6.9 and 6.10). Small basophilic inclusion bodies may also be seen within the cells' cytoplasm, they are frequently surrounded by a very small vacuole. Adenovirus may also result in intranuclear inclusions within infected epithelial cells (Image 6.11). This inclusion may be eosinophilic or basophilic and relatively small compared to those produced by CMV. As described by Bayon and Drut, thin strands of chromatin material may project from this inclusion body to the nuclear membrane resulting in rosette cells (Image 6.12).[18] Adenovirus may also produce epithelial cells with nuclei having a smudged appearance in which the chromatin appears homogeneous, structureless, and deeply basophilic (Image 6.13). Measles virus induces multinucleated giant epithelial cells that may contain more than 50 nuclei.[19] Furthermore, the nuclei may contain inclusion bodies surrounded by a thin halo. Cytoplasmic inclusion bodies may also be produced. Respiratory syncytial virus may also result in epithelial cells containing numerous nuclei. However, only intracytoplasmic and not nuclear inclusions may be seen.[20]

Alveolar Proteinosis

Alveolar proteinosis is a rare pulmonary disorder that affects adults much more frequently than children.[15] In the pediatric population this disease is almost always fatal. Cytologic descriptions of this entity are very rare.[1] We have seen a single example in an 8-year-old boy in whom the bronchial washing specimen contained abundant amorphous and acellular eosinophilic and amphophilic and somewhat flocculent material (Image 6.14 and 6.15). In conjunction with the clinical-radiographic picture, a diagnosis of alveolar proteinosis was suggested (but not definitely diagnosed). The diagnosis of alveolar proteinosis was not firmly established until autopsy. Ultrastructural study of the lavage fluid can be confirmatory when the characteristic membranous structures are present.

Allergic Disorders

Cytologic examination of nasal secretions has been proposed as a diagnostic test with allergic upper airway disorders.[21-24] Miller et al evaluated cytologic smears of nasal secretions by estimating the percentage of eosinophilic leukocytes present among all cells.[19] They considered a specimen to be positive for eosinophilia whenever the percentage of eosinophils exceeded 3% (Image 6.16). In their hands the authors found this simple assay to be highly specific, rather sensitive, and highly reproducible in separating children with seasonal allergic rhinitis from those with perennial rhinitis. Rivasi and Bergamini examined spontaneous nasal secretions from 128 children and adults with rhinorrhea, nasal obstruction and sneezing.[22] Individuals with an allergic condition were found to have increased numbers of eosinophils, goblet cells and debris in their cytologic specimens compared to those with nonatophic individuals. Pollen grains were found in greatly increased numbers in individuals with pollinosis. These authors also describe finding fungi in 5 of their patients with allergic disorders but did not further speciate the organisms.[22] Jean et al evaluated 50 children with nasal provocation tests.[23] Nasal secretions, generally obtained by nose blowing, were obtained before and after exposure to an allergen and air dried on slides. A differential cell count was performed over the entire slide. A test result was considered positive whenever the percentage of eosinophils increased by at least 10% following insufflation of the allergen. Although these authors felt that increased eosinophil counts did provide some diagnostic information, the test did not have a high level of sensitivity or specificity.[23] Bascom and colleagues reported the peak influx of eosinophils into nasal secretions occurred approximately 10 hours after exposure to allergen.[24]

Neoplasms

As mentioned earlier, primary neoplasms of the lungs are quite uncommon in children, in contrast to adults.[15] Consequently, little information exists concerning the use of exfoliative respiratory cytology to diagnose benign or malignant pulmonary tumors in the pediatric population.[1] The most common entity known to produce a solitary pulmonary nodule in a child is the inflammatory pseudotumor or plasma cell granuloma.[15,25] These proliferations may occur at any age and may be responsible for the production of cough. However, not infrequently they are found incidentally on chest x-rays in patients who are asymptomatic. These masses are well circumscribed; surgical resection is the treatment of choice and is followed by an excellent prognosis. Histologically, spindle-shaped myofibroblasts are admixed liberally with inflammatory cells.[15] The latter may include numerous lymphocytes, plasma cells and multinucleated inflammatory giant cells. Only very infrequently has the exfoliative cytopathology of the inflammatory pseudotumor been described. Occurring on a relatively clean smear background, cohesive aggregates of the myofibroblasts predominate in the brushing specimen. These cells are characterized by an oval vesicular nucleus with finely granular chromatin and small inconspicuous nucleoli. Cytoplasm is scanty and poorly stained, but overall an elongated contour may be recognized. As stated by Usuda et al, they may suggest epithelioid cells and thus granulomatous inflammation.[25] Although mitotic figures may be recognized, marked cytologic atypia is absent. Also present are neutrophils and eosinophils.

The most common entity known to produce a solitary pulmonary nodule in a child is the inflammatory pseudomotor or plasma cell granuloma

In our institutions, the most common indication for bronchoscopy in children is the presence of pulmonary infiltrates in patients who have been treated with chemotherapy and possibly bone marrow transplantation for acute leukemia or malignant lymphoma. The purpose of this examination is to look for specific infectious agents. Uncommonly, when such organisms are not identified, the washings may contain numerous neoplastic cells. A malignant lymphoreticular infiltrate may be diagnosed when a monomorphic population of mononucleated tumor cells with prominent nucleoli, irregular nuclear membranes and high N/C ratios are identified, often entrapped as noncohesive aggregates within mucus (Image 6.17). It is our experience that pediatricians are always surprised to be informed about such findings. Even in large cancer hospitals, sputum and bronchoscopic specimens are only rarely used in attempts to identify metastatic cancers (Image 6.18). As discussed in the chapter dealing with FNA of deep organs, a rare neoplasm, namely, the pulmonary blastoma is peculiar to children. Histologically and cytologically, it is composed of small undifferentiated neoplastic cells which may have rounded and plump spindle-shaped contours and high N/C ratios.

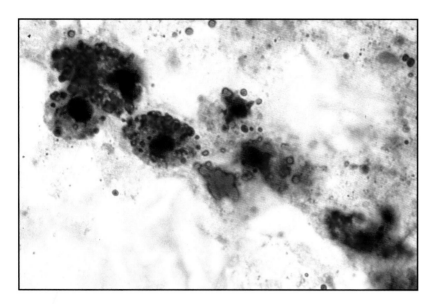

Image 6.1
Oil-red O–stained tracheal aspirate from a newborn suffering from aspiration pneumonia. The cytoplasm of these alveolar macrophages contains numerous lipid-positive droplets, which also occur in the smear background. This is from an obviously positive (heavily loaded) example.

A

B

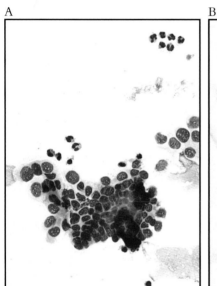
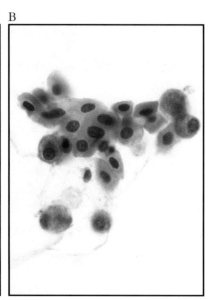

Image 6.2
A Neutrophils are admixed with degenerated epithelial cells in this tracheal aspirate of a newborn with bronchopulmonary dysplasia. (Romanowsky).
B Metaplastic squamous cells are present in this tracheal aspirate. The metaplastic nature is made evident by dense cyanophilic cytoplasm and central nuclei. (Papanicolaou).

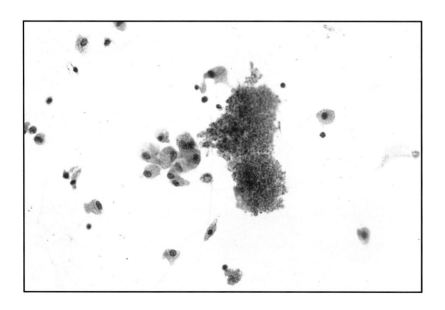

Image 6.3
Bronchial lavage (BAL) specimen from a child with AIDS and pulmonary infiltrates. Centrally, a typical 3-dimensional alveolar cast of *Pneumocystis carinii* has rather sharply defined edges and a basophilic hue with the Papanicolaou stain. It appears to be composed of small and uniform ring-like structures superimposed upon one another, creating a characteristic honeycomb appearance. Alveolar macrophages comprise the surrounding cells.

Image 6.4

BAL specimen (see Image 6.3). Gomori methenamine-silver stain reveals the readily apparent cyst form of the parasite within the alveolar cast. Cysts range from round to slightly oval to "cup-shaped," depending on their particular orientation in the plane of focus. Usually, a small dot is evident within the cyst, often applied to the inner surface of its wall. These structures are focal thickenings of the cyst wall.

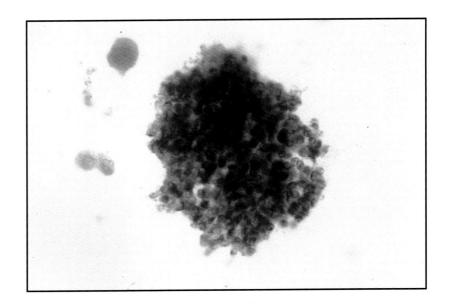

Image 6.5

Bronchial wash specimen from a young boy with cystic fibrosis and pulmonary infiltrates. This mucus cast of the bronchial lumen morphologically resembles the alveolar cast of *Pneumocystis*. On closer inspection, its internal structure has a more irregularly reticulated or stringy appearance. (Papanicolaou).

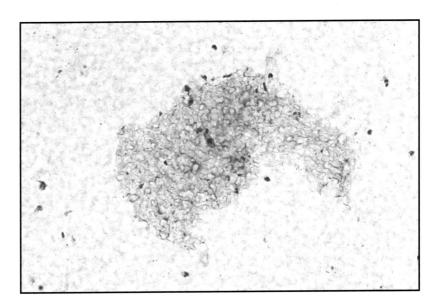

Image 6.6

Sputum from a leukemic child. Numerous small ovoid pink-staining yeast forms are present, as are a few fragments of pseudohyphae. Some yeasts show budding. It is difficult (or impossible) in many cases to determine whether the fungus is an oral contaminant or truly a pulmonary pathogen. (Papanicolaou).

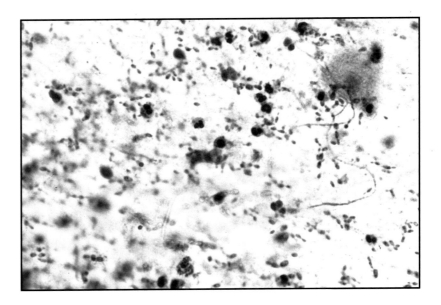

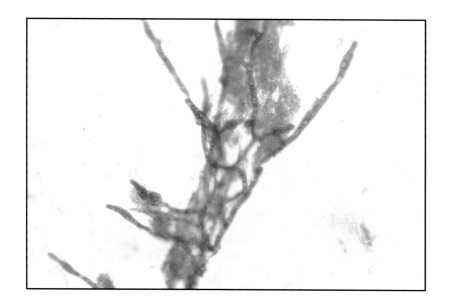

Image 6.7
Sputum from a leukemic child with pulmonary aspergillosis. The hyphae are thicker than those of *Candida*, basophilic, and demonstrate acute angle branching. Note the conidio-phore. (Papanicolaou).

A

B

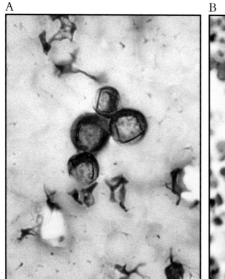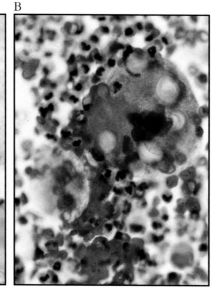

Image 6.8
A BAL specimen reveals fungal yeast forms including some showing broad-based budding consistent with *Blasto-myces*. (Romanowsky).
B BAL specimen shows multinucleat-ed giant cells containing intracytoplas-mic fungi consistent with *Blastomyces*. Also note acute inflammatory cells in the background. (Papanicolaou).

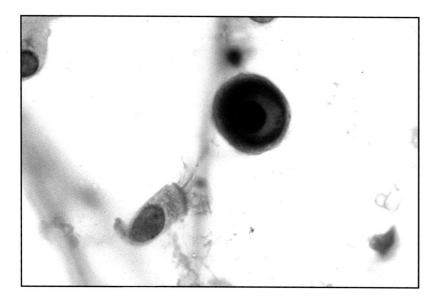

Image 6.9
BAL specimen from a girl with pul-monary infiltrates who previously had a bone marrow transplant for acute leukemia. Scattered throughout the specimen were large isolated cells with the classic picture of CMV infection. The cell (cell type not readily appar-ent) and its nucleus are huge. The nucleus creates a characteristic "owl's eye" appearance due to a large basophilic inclusion body separated from the nuclear membrane by a wide halo. (Papanicolaou).

Image 6.10
BAL specimen (see Image 6.9).
Rarely, infected cells form small cohesive aggregates. Such infected elements are generally easy to spot with the scanning lens due to their large size and overall basophilia. (Papanicolaou).

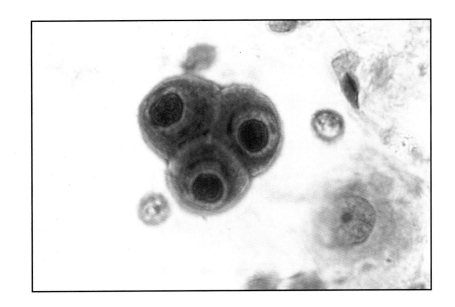

Image 6.11
Bronchial brushing from a young boy with pulmonary infiltrates. This hypertrophied bronchial epithelial cell appears to have 2 nuclei, each with a basophilic inclusion separated from the nuclear membrane by a halo due to chromatin clearing. This is an example of an adenoviral infection. (Papanicolaou).

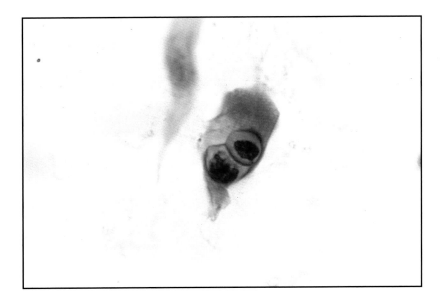

Image 6.12
Bronchial brushing (see Image 6.11). The enlarged nucleus of the intact infected bronchial cell contains an inclusion from which thin strands of chromatin extend toward the nuclear envelope, creating a rosette-cell. Compare its appearance with that of the apparently uninfected epithelial cell. (Papanicolaou).

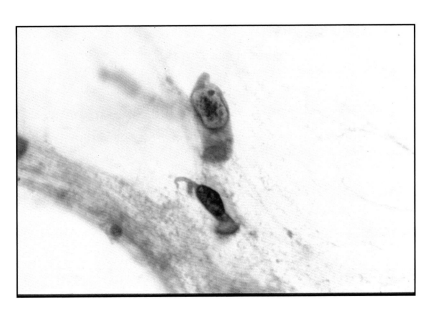

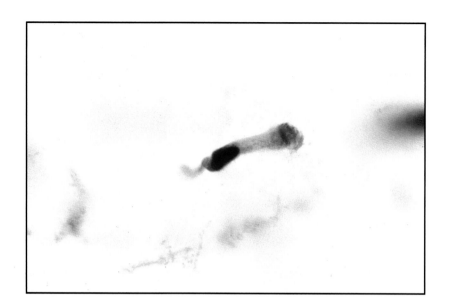

Image 6.13
Bronchial brushing (see Image 6.11). The enlarged nucleus is occupied by a structureless dark chromatin mass. Cilia persist on its luminal border. (Papanicolaou).

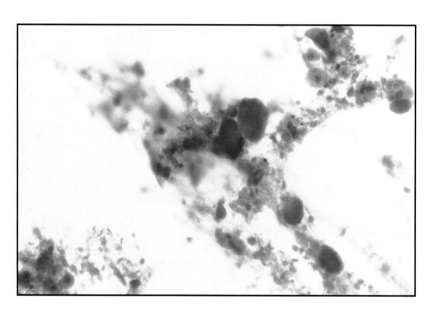

Image 6.14
Bronchial wash specimen from an 8-year-old boy who subsequently died of alveolar proteinosis. With the Papanicolaou stain, the lipoprotein material that fills the pulmonary alveoli appears blue to green and very dense. It presents in variably sized, irregularly shaped masses with well defined borders. Amyloid has a similar appearance in respiratory cytologic specimens but certainly would not be expected in a child.

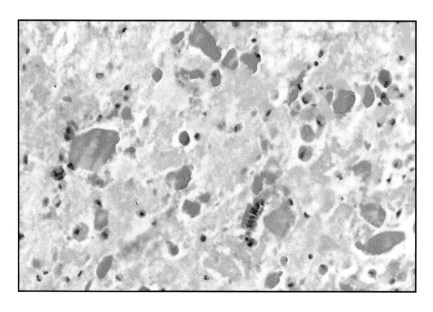

Image 6.15
Cell block preparation from the bronchial brushing specimen featured in Image 6.13. The masses of lipoprotein have a dense, almost structureless eosinophilic appearance with distinct often angulated edges. (H & E).

Image 6.16
Eosinophils form a pure "culture" in this nasal secretion specimen from a child with allergic rhinitis. (Romanowsky). (Courtesy of Dr J Georgitis).

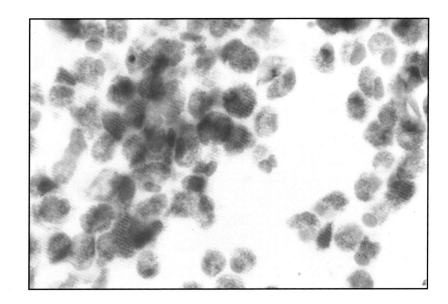

Image 6.17
Bronchial wash specimen from a 12-year-old boy with a known T-cell lymphoblastic lymphoma and bilateral pulmonary infiltrates. Concentrated within strands of mucus are numerous rather densely packed malignant cells. They have high N/C ratios and solitary nuclei. Many of the latter have complex contours including "cloverleaf" arrays. Nucleoli are small and indistinct. Infectious agents were not identified. (Papanicolaou).

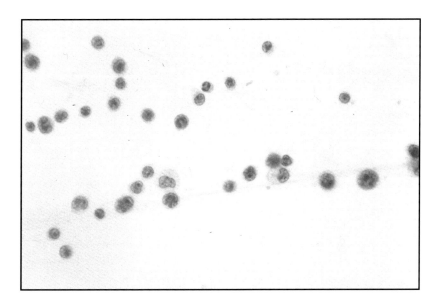

Image 6.18
Bronchial wash specimen from a 15-year-old boy with a previously treated femoral osteosarcoma who later developed pulmonary infiltrates (no mass was detected radiologically). Dispersed individually were obviously malignant cells characterized by large hyperchromatic nuclei and variable N/C ratios. Without a history of osteosarcoma, it would not be possible to characterize this beyond the large cell tumor category. (Papanicolaou).

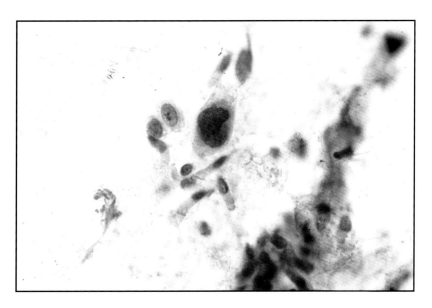

References

1. Johnston WW, Elson CE. Respiratory Tract in Comprehensive Cytopathology. M. Bibbo, ed. WB Saunders, Philadelphia, 1991.

2. Williams HE, Freeman M. Milk inhalation pneumonia. The significance of fat filled macrophages in tracheal secretions. *Aust Paediat J* 9:286-288,1973.

3. Hewitt VM. Effect of posture on the presence of fat in tracheal aspirate in neonates. *Aust Paediat J* 12:267-271,1976.

4. Recalde AL, Nickerson BG, Vegas M, Scott CB, Landing BH, Warburton D. Lipid-laden macrophages in tracheal aspirates of newborn infants receiving intravenous lipid infusions: a cytologic study. *Pediat Pathol* 2:25-34,1984.

5. Nussbaum E, Maggi JC, Mathis R, Galant SP. Association of lipid-laden alveolar macrophages and gastroesophageal reflux in children. *J Pediat* 110:190-194,1987.

6. Colombo JL, Hallberg TK. Recurrent aspiration in children: lipid-laden alveolar macrophage quantitation. *Pediat Pulmonol* 3:86-89,1987.

7. Moran Jr, Block SM, Lyerly AD, Brooks LE, Dillard RG. Lipid-laden alveolar macrophage and lactose assay as markers of aspiration in neonates with lung disease. *J Pediat* 112:643-645,1988.

8. Collins Orris KA, Geisinger KR, Block SM, Wagner PH. The cytologic evaluation of lipid-laden alveolar macrophages as an indicator of aspiration pneumonia in young children. *Acta Cytol* 36:598,1992.

9. Merritt TA, Stuard ID, Puccia J, Wood B, Edwards DK, Finkelstein J, Shapiro DL. Newborn tracheal aspirate cytology: classification during respiratory distress syndrome and bronchopulmonary dysplasia. *J Pediat* 98:949-956,1981.

10. Merritt TA, Puccia JM, Stuard ID. Cytologic evaluation of pulmonary effluent in neonates with respiratory distress syndrome and bronchopulmonary dysplasia. *Acta Cytol* 25:631-639,1981.

11. Doshi N, Kanbour A, Fujikura T, Klionsky B. Tracheal aspiration cytology in neonates with respiratory distress. Histopathologic correlation. *Acta Cytol* 26:15-21,1982.

12. D'Ablang G III, Bernard B, Zaharov I, Barton L, Kaplan B, Schwinn CP. Neonatal pulmonary cytology and bronchopulmonary dysplasia. *Acta Cytol* 19:21-27, 1975.

13. Corwin RW, Irwin RS. The lipid-laden alveolar macrophage as a marker of aspiration in parenchymal lung disease. *Am Rev Respir Dis* 132:576-581,1985.

14. Robins D, Zachariah S. Lipid-laden macrophages in adult and pediatric bronchoalveolar lavage specimens. Utility of quantitative scoring as a diagnostic aid. *Mod Pathol* 7:40A, 1994.

15. Dehner LP. Lungs in Pediatric Surgical Pathology. 2nd ed. Williams and Wilkins, Baltimore, 1987.

16. Coleman DV. Cytological diagnosis of virus-infected cells in Papanicolaou smears and its application in clinical practice. *J Clin Pathol* 32:1075-1098,1979.

17. Drut RM, Drut R. Congenital herpes simplex virus infection diagnosed by cytology of aspirated tracheo-bronchial material. *Acta Cytol* 29:712-713,1985.

18. Bayon MN, Drut R. Cytologic diagnosis of adenovirus bronchopneumonia. *Acta Cytol* 35:181-182,1991.

19. Siegel C, Johnston S, Adair S. Isolation of measles virus in primary Rhesus monkey cells from a child with acute interstial pneumonia who cytologically had giant-cell pneumonia without a rash. *Am J Clin Pathol* 94:464-469,1990.

20. Parham DM, Bozeman P, Killian C, Murti G, Brenner M, Hanif I. Cytologic diagnosis of respiratory syncytial virus infection in a bronchoalveolar specimen from a bone marrow transplant recipient. *Am J Clin Pathol* 99:588-592, 1993.

21. Miller RE, Paradise JL, Friday GA, Fireman P, Voith D. The nasal smear for eosinophils. Its value in children with seasonal allergic rhinitis. *Am J Dis Child* 136:1009-1011,1982.

22. Rivasi F Bergamini G. Nasal cytology in allergic processes and other syndromes caused by hyperactivity. *Diagn Cytopathol* 4:99-105,1988.

23. Jean R, Lellouch-Tubiana A, Bruent-Langot D, Scheinmann P, Pfister A. Nasal eosinophilia in children: its use in the nasal allergen provocation test. *Diagn Cytopathol* 4:23-27,1988.

24. Bascom R, Pipkorn U, Lichtenstein LM, Naclerio RM. The influx of inflammatory cells into nasal washings during the late response to antigen challenge. Effect of systemic steroid pretreatment. *Am Rev Res Dis* 138:406-412,1988.

25. Usuda K, Saito Y, Imai T, Ota S, Sato M, Fujimura S, Tamahashi N. Inflammatory pseudotumor of the lung diagnosed as granulomatous lesion by preoperative brushing cytology. A case report. *Acta Cytol* 34:685-689,1990.

○ CHAPTER SEVEN

Additional Applications of Exfoliative Cytology

Gastrointestinal Cytology

Very little information exists concerning the use of brushing cytology of the gastrointestinal mucosa in children.[1] In large part this is due to the rarity of primary malignant neoplasms involving these hollow viscera. However, there are some specific applications which will be discussed briefly here.

By far, brushings of the esophagus are the most common type of specimen seen in our laboratories.[1,2] The number 1 indication for this procedure is to look for specific infectious agents in children with the symptoms of esophagitis and a history of cancer. Often patients have been treated for acute leukemia or malignant lymphoma and are variably immunosuppressed. The most frequent organism identified is *Candida albicans*.[2] In smears, this fungus is often readily recognized with its eosinophilic pseudohyphae and budding yeast cells aggregated into relatively large masses (Image 7.1). When the organisms are not associated with large numbers of neutrophilic leukocytes, it may be that the fungus is simply a contaminant and not responsible for clinical symptoms such as dysphagia. A potential diagnostic pitfall occurs when the fungal organisms are entrapped within inflammatory necrotic debris. In this setting, we routinely perform methenamine silver stains to bring out the presence of the fungus. Cytologic preparations, in our hands, are more sensitive than a histologic examination by endoscopic biopsy.[3] The other major organism responsible for esophagitis is Herpes simplex, which is diagnosed when the characteristic cytopathologic alterations within squamous epithelial cells, namely, prominent intranuclear inclusion bodies surrounded by halo and multinucleated cells with molded nuclei with homogeneous chromatin are found (Image 7.2). Usually these altered cells are quite numerous and easily recognized. However, we have seen examples in which only a very few squamous cells with the diagnostic changes were present.[2] This is in sharp contrast to the situation with cytomegalovirus (CMV) esophagitis. Only very rare infected cells with characteristic cytopathologic changes will be found in esophageal brushings with this condition.[4] This is due to the fact that CMV does not infect squamous epithelial cells. Rather, this virus attacks glandular cells, endothelial cells and fibroblasts in the ulcer bed. Thus, the base of an ulcer needs to be sampled with the endoscopic brush in order to procure infected cells.

In all types of esophagitis including those secondary to radiation and chemotherapy, the squamous epithelial cells may show prominent but benign atypia.[1,2] Whenever there is an ulcer, regardless of its etiology, reparative changes may be seen within the epithelium. The cells have enlarged nuclei with very finely granular or vesicular chromatin, distinct but thin and smooth nuclear membranes and a solitary prominent round nucleolus. Importantly, these cells will be present within cohesive sheets in which there may be a whorled or flowing appearance. Characteristic morphologic changes include marked but relatively proportionate nucleomegaly and cytomegaly, vacuolization of the cytoplasm and possibly the nucleus and multinucleation. Degenerative changes in the nucleus may also be expected in some of these cells. Fortunately from a diagnostic standpoint, such benign alterations pose little difficulty in distinguishing them from pediatric malignancies.

Although it is certainly much more frequent in adults, glandular metaplasia of the distal esophageal mucosa may occur as a consequence of chronic gastroesophageal reflux disease.[5] Also known as Barrett's esophagus, it is important to recognize this change as it is a morphologic marker of reflux. In brushings, the most characteristic appearance of Barrett's epithelium is the presence of large, flat cohesive sheets of epithelial cells with sharp, smooth margins.[1,2,6,7] Within the aggregates the epithelial nuclei are uniformly distributed and have uniform appearances with round or slightly ovoid contours, finely granular chromatin and generally inconspicuous nucleoli. In order to render a cytologic diagnosis of Barrett's esophagus, one must have total confidence in the fact that the brushings were obtained proximal to the gastroesophageal junction. It is now widely recognized that Barrett's esophagus is a premalignant condition and is the overwhelming precursor to esophageal adenocarcinoma. The intermediate morphologic stage between benign Barrett's epithelium and adenocarcinoma is glandular dysplasia. Recently, several groups have described the cytologic features of glandular dysplasia in endoscopically obtained brushing specimens.[1,6,7] Fortunately, however, although Barrett's metaplasia does occur with some frequency in children with reflux disease, it is exceedingly rare for a pediatric patient to develop dysplasia or adenocarcinoma.

Very uncommonly, patients with known leukemia may develop a clinical picture of severe erosive esophagitis which is not due to known infectious agents, acid reflux, or chemotherapy but rather due to extensive infiltration of the esophageal mucosa by the leukemic elements. Although we have seen several examples of this in esophageal brushings

In all types of esophagitis including those secondary to radiation and chemotherapy, the squamous epithelial cells may show prominent but benign atypia

from adult leukemics, we are unaware of a single example diagnosed in such a specimen in a pediatric patient.[8]

In the stomach the most common microbial pathogen is *Helicobacter pylori* which is associated with peptic ulcer disease. Although several very recent studies have shown brushing cytology of the stomach to be comparable to biopsies in the detection of this bacterium in adults, we are unaware of any such investigation that involves pediatric patients.[9] Cytologic specimens may be used to enhance the diagnostic armamentarium for the identification of *Helicobacter*. Davenport described the morphologic features of *H pylori* organisms in Papanicolaou-stained gastric brushing specimens.[9] This bacterial rod was described as having a curved or spiral contour, a basophilic staining reaction and a length of approximately 1 μm. The organisms were typically present within gastric mucus or in association with the surface of gastric epithelial cells. Davenport compared the brushings with concurrently obtained gastric biopsies and their abilities to provide a morphologic diagnosis.[9] 10 of the 49 brushing specimens and 11 of the biopsy specimens contained this bacterium. In 3 of the 10 specimen pairs in which smears contained *Helicobactor*, the biopsy finding was negative. Davenport thus claimed, and we agree, that gastric brushings may increase the diagnostic sensitivity for the identification of this organism.[9] We are unaware of any significant experience with this clinical situation in children. Other authors have recently described the use of cytologic smears of the gastric biopsy specimens in order to facilitate identification of this organism.[10] This type of preparation also appears to increase diagnostic sensitivity. We favor a Diff-Quik stained, air-dried smear because the organism is well visualized (Image 7.3).

Until recently, gastric stromal tumors (smooth muscle neoplasms) were almost unheard of in children. Within the last few years, an association between AIDS and the development of malignant gastric stromal tumors (leiomyosarcomas) has emerged among children.[11,12] These neoplasms arise beneath the mucosa and thus present as bulging nodules in which the overlying mucosa may remain intact or be ulcerated. When stromal tumors are sampled cytologically, characteristic spindle-shaped tumor cells may appear in the smears.[1] This is especially likely with the advent of transmucosal needle aspirates.[13,14] In any case, it is probably impossible to distinguish between benign and malignant stromal tumors. Furthermore, it may be quite difficult to separate these neoplastic elements from fibroblasts associated with the granulation tissue of an ulcer.[1]

In the pediatric population, the most common primary cancer of the entire gastrointestinal tract is malignant lymphoma. In contrast, in adults lymphomas occur more frequently in the intestines than in the stomach. The most frequent histologic type in children is the diffuse small noncleaved-cell form of non-Hodgkin's lymphoma. In brushings one would expect to see moderately sized mononuclear elements with very high N/C ratios with thick nuclear membranes, which may be smooth or irregular, and multiple prominent nucleoli. Cytoplasmic vacuoles due to neutral lipid may also be seen. Typically, the lymphomatous elements would be concentrated in a noncohesive grouping within mucus. The monomorphic appearance of these cells is important in distinguishing the neoplastic elements from reactive lymphocytes as may occur in nodular lymphoid hyperplasia.[1,15] In the latter

In the pediatric population, the most common primary cancer of the entire gastrointestinal tract is malignant lymphoma

entity, one sees a variety of sizes and appearances of the lymphoid elements. Most of the cells are small and mature-appearing, but large lymphocytes with prominent nucleoli as well as intermediate forms with more irregular nuclear contours can also be detected. It is this polymorphic or heterogeneous appearance of the lymphoid cells in hyperplasia that allows one to feel comfortable that one is dealing with a benign process. Tingible-body macrophages are typically present in hyperplasia as well. However, such elements may also be present in the malignant lymphomas. Another potential pitfall in the cytologic diagnosis of lymphoma is the presence of numerous benign glandular nuclei which have been stripped of their cytoplasm. In the latter, the chromatin is very finely granular and evenly distributed rather than clumped as in lymphomatous cells, and nucleoli will be very inconspicuous.

Giardia lamblia is a protozoan parasite sometimes associated with nodular lymphoid hyperplasia in the small intestine. *Giardia* may be seen in brushings of the duodenum which may or may not contain such hyperplasia. The trophozoites measure 12 μm and 15 μm and are pear-shaped when seen in full profile. They characteristically have two "mirror image" nuclei with prominent karyosomes displaced to one pole of the organism. With the Papanicolaou stain, flagella are not readily visualized.

Another intestinal parasite that may be diagnosed in cytologic brushings is *Cryptosporidium*. This organism has become a common cause of diarrhea in immunosuppressed children, especially those with AIDS. In cytologic brushings, these organisms appear as round to pyramidal structures that measure 2 μm to 4 μm and that characteristically appear attached to the luminal borders of unremarkable columnar epithelial cells.[16]   Thus, they are most easily recognized when the epithelium is arranged in a "picket-fence" manner.   is more easily vizualized in Diff-Quick–stained smears.

There appears to be very little diagnostic utility for cytologic brushings of the large intestine of children. As elsewhere in the gastrointestinal tract, immunosuppressed patients may develop prominent clinical symptoms and signs due to mucosal infection by CMV. The morphologic features are similar to those described earlier in this section.

Chronic inflammatory bowel disease can certainly affect pediatric patients. However, in contrast to adults, the development of glandular dysplasia and subsequent adenocarcinoma is not a major concern in children. In part, this is due to the fact that it generally takes many years for patients to develop colitis-associated dysplasia. Melville et al have, in a large study, demonstrated the distinct utility of brushing cytology of the colon in the evaluation of these premalignant changes in patients with ulcerative colitis.[17]

Mucocutaneous Cytology

Diagnostic exfoliative cytology plays a small role in the evaluation of cutaneous lesions in the pediatric population. However, scrapings from skin lesions may provide a rapid and inexpensive diagnosis (considered by many to be only a presumptive interpretation) for selected dermatologic conditions. Buchino has provided an excellent review of the use of exfoliative cytology in the diagnosis of cutaneous infections.[18] In varicella zoster (chicken pox) and cutaneous Herpes simplex infections (Image 7.4), one may find the characteristic multinucleated epithelial giant cells in which the nuclei are molded and have a homogeneous or "ground glass" appearance (so-called Tzanck test). In children, especially newborn infants, pyogenic bacteria may produce bullae and pustules. Scrapings from the base of these lesions may demonstrate neutrophils and Gram-positive cocci in large numbers. As expected, scrapings of *Candida* infection sites will yield an admixture of yeast, pseudohyphae and mixed inflammatory cell infiltrates. A transient benign dermatologic condition that occurs in newborns is erythema toxicum. Eosinophils are present in abundance in specimens obtained from this idiopathic condition (Image 7.5). Another transient condition is neonatal pustular melanosis, which occurs predominantly in black newborns. Clinically this will mimic erythema toxicum but scrapings of the vesicle will yield a predominance of neutrophils rather than eosinophils and an absence of bacterial organisms. Rarely, cutaneous lesions in children with acute leukemia are related to infiltrates of the leukemic elements (Image 7.6).

The majority of instances of inflammatory conditions of the conjunctiva and cornea have either an infectious or allergic etiology.[19] A relatively common form of conjunctivitis in newborn infants is due to chylamydial infections acquired during passage through an infected birth canal. In combination with the patient's history and the clinical appearance of the patient, exfoliative ocular cytology may provide useful diagnostic information.[20-24] Basically, the conjunctiva or cornea are locally anesthetized and then scraped in order to obtain cellular material. Some authors prefer air-dried, Romanowsky-stained preparations, others prefer alcohol-fixed, Papanicolaou-stained smears. The classic publications of Naib describe in detail the cytomorphologic features of this condition.[20-22] The diagnostic finding is the presence of intracytoplasmic inclusions (Image 7.7). These typically have a perinuclear location and vary in appearance with the stage of infection. The inclusions may occur as small (≤ 1 μm) granular structures typically surrounded by small individual vacuoles. The staining reaction of the inclusion bodies is usually basophilic. With maturation there is a coalescence of these small granules into a much larger body also surrounded by a halo or vacuole. Infected epithelial cells themselves may be enlarged and show degenerative cytoplasmic and nuclear alterations. According to Thelmo et al, in addition to the distinctive inclusion bodies, the cytologic picture is distinctive.[23] The predominant inflammatory cell is mononuclear and lymphocytic. In fact, some of the lymphocytes may be aggregated into follicular structures. They described these follicles as being heterogeneous with the inclusion of neutrophils, histiocytes and necrotic debris within their centers. In addition, these authors noted the number of goblet cells to be increased in this condition. Duggan and colleagues compared the diagnostic utility of the Papanicolaou and Giemsa stains, and favored the Giemsa stain as they believed it permitted the recognition of the inclusion bodies with greater ease.[24] In part, this was felt to be due to the large number of artifacts that could simulate inclusions with the Papanicolaou stain. Although the

A relatively common form of conjunctivitis in newborn infants is due to chlamydial infections acquired during passage through an infected birth canal

diagnostic sensitivity of the Geimsa stain was only marginally better than that of the Papanicolaou stain, diagnostic specificity was certainly much higher with the Romanowsky preparation. Duggan et al also evaluated an immunoperoxidase reaction using a monoclonal antibody with these two stains and found it to be diagnostically helpful.[24]

Another condition that may include lymphoid follicles in the smears is adenoviral conjunctivitis. These follicular structures are cytologically more homogeneous than those in inclusion conjunctivitis and are composed largely of relatively large lymphoid elements. According to Thelmo et al, neutrophils, histiocytes and necrotic debris are absent. Epithelial cells may be present in large numbers and show degenerative changes.[23] In addition, some of these cells will contain the diagnostic nuclear inclusions.[22,23] Early in the infection, these inclusion structures are very small, multiple and eosinophilic. With progression, these inclusions fuse to form a single large basophilic inclusion placed centrally within the nucleus and surrounded by a halo due to chromatin condensation. One will not find an increased number of goblet cells.[23]

Rare viral infections producing conjunctivitis include measles and vaccinia. In measles, one may find giant epithelial cells that contain numerous small round distinct nuclei and eosinophilic inclusions surrounded by a vacuole within the cytoplasm.[20] A solitary huge "brick-like" inclusion may be found adjacent to nuclei of epithelial cells in vaccinial infections.[20] Herpes simplex virus may infect the conjunctiva and/or cornea, leading to their characteristic cytopathic alterations.[25,26]

Acute bacterial conjunctivitis is most often related to an infection by *Staphylococcus*. The neutrophilic leukocyte will be the major cellular element in conjunctival scraping specimens (Image 7.8). Although many of these may appear intact and viable, degenerative changes will also be well developed. The smear background will contain cellular debris and fibrin, but only a few epithelial elements, typically degenerated, will be present.[23]

Several distinct clinical forms of allergic conjunctivitis and keratitis exist.[19,27] Exfoliative cytology can be useful in the separation of these allergic conditions from infectious disease. Of course, viral inclusions and bacteria are not seen in smears from the allergic processes. The characteristic cellular element is the eosinophilic leukocyte, which may degranulate, yielding its characteristic eosinophilic cytoplasmic granules within the smear background. According to Naib et al, basophils are present in prominent numbers in vernal conjunctivitis.[22] Goblet cells may be well represented in these specimens as well. The smear background will be clean. Very recently, Rivasi and colleagues provided a quantitative analysis of conjunctival cytology in patients with allergic inflammatory states.[27] Their 65 patients included both children and adults and were divided into atopic and nonatopic groups. Eosinophils, neutrophils and lymphocytes were present in relatively equal proportions in the two groups. In addition, noncellular material, including pollen grains, fungal organisms, and other foreign material were also present in relatively equal distributions. Goblet cells were found more frequently in patients with the atopic form of disease, but according to the authors' data, this would not be very helpful in the distinction for a given individual patient.[27]

Natadisastra et al have described the application of conjunctival

Exfoliative cytology can be useful in the separation of allergic conditions from infectious disease

impression cytology to aid in the diagnosis of vitamin A deficiency in young children.[28] The exfoliative specimens were stained with a combined periodic acid-Schiff and Papanicolaou stain. Specimens were considered positive if goblet cells and/or extracellular masses of mucin were present in the specimens. 93% of the children with clinical evidence of vitamin A deficiency and a low serum vitamin level had an abnormal specimen. Conversely, 94% of the children with a normal ocular examination and serum levels had a normal cytologic specimen. Of note was the fact that nearly half of the children who were clinically normal but who had depressed serum vitamin A levels also lacked goblet cells. Thus, it would appear that this impression cytologic test could be applied as a screening procedure in certain parts of the world.[28]

Urinary Cytology

In distinct contrast to adults, conventional cytopathologic examination of the urine (as distinct from routine urinalysis) plays a relatively small diagnostic role in children. In large part, this reflects the rarity of urinary tract neoplasms in the pediatric population. Urinary cytology, however, does have a place in selected situations.

The most common cause of an inflammatory cytologic picture in the urine is an acute bacterial infection of the urinary bladder. Such infections may occur throughout the entire range of the pediatric population. Bacterial infections in young children often reflect a congenital abnormality causing varying degrees of obstruction to the flow of urine. Almost always the cytologic smears show a nonspecific picture that includes large numbers of inflammatory cells, predominantly neutrophils, which may show well-developed degenerative alterations.[29] Degenerative changes are also frequently seen in rare urothelial cells. Pyknosis and karyorrhexis may be seen, as may a peculiar but nonspecific cytoplasmic inclusion. The latter consists of one or more perfectly round eosinophilic and almost refractile structures within the cell's cytoplasm. Although latter inclusions are thought by some to be characteristic of specific entities (such as Kawasaki disease), we believe that usually they are nonspecific and reflect simply degeneration.[29,30] At times bacterial organisms may be visualized within the smears of the sediment.

Several viral infections are recognized as producing characteristic cytopathologic alterations within exfoliated cells in the urine. The best known of these is CMV.[29] The characteristic large intranuclear inclusion and the uncommon cytoplasmic inclusions are seen in exfoliated renal tubular epithelial cells (Image 7.9). Most often, these are seen as solitary cellular elements but may be seen in small cohesive aggregates as well. The number of infected cells in a given specimen is usually quite low. In addition to congenital CMV inclusion disease, this infection may appear in children who are immunosuppressed.

Immunosuppression also may lead to the presence of cells within the urine showing characteristic changes induced by human polyomavirus.[29,31,32] It appears as if immunosuppression of various etiologies (and at times no apparent cause) may cause an activation of a previously

Bacterial infections in young children often reflect a congenital abnormality causing varying degrees of obstruction to the flow of urine

acquired infection by this virus. This clinical recrudescence manifests as bizarre cytologic changes, but apparently the infection has no long-term adverse effects on patients. The major diagnostic problem is that the cells may be confused with neoplastic urothelial elements. In children, fortunately, this is not a major diagnostic dilemma in that carcinoma of the lower urinary tract is most uncommon. The altered cells, which have been referred to as decoy cells, are often prominently enlarged, although size is variable within a given patient's specimen.[29] The most typical alteration is the transformation of the nucleus into a solitary deeply basophilic inclusion which appears structureless (Image 7.10). That is, chromatin granules are not recognized within the confines of this altered nucleus. In some cells, a very thin clear ring separates this homogenous inclusion from the relatively delicate nuclear membrane. Cytoplasmic inclusion bodies are not produced. Koss has described what he calls the postinclusion stage.[29] The dark homogenous appearance of the enlarged nucleus is replaced by one with a pale, washed-out look. Delicate skeins of chromatin may be seen within these nuclei. These alterations are reversible. The presence of polyomavirus can be confirmed by the use of immunocytochemistry and electron microscopy, although this is usually clinically unnecessary.[31, 32]

In addition to nonspecific degenerative changes and viral cytopathic alterations, cellular inclusion bodies may be seen in exfoliated cells in the urine from other causes. Due to significantly improved public health measures, lead poisoning in children is much less frequent than it was several decades ago. However, occasional cases may be seen and the cytologic picture within a urine specimen may call attention to the problem or provide an early preliminary confirmation. The characteristic inclusion occurs within the nucleus of exfoliated renal tubular cells.[32] These inclusions are basophilic and do not appear to greatly enlarge the nucleus. These bodies are acid-fast, apparently due to the high content of protein with sulfhydryl groups. As demonstrated in the study of Landing and Nakai, this finding is not common among affected children (low sensitivity).[33]

A number of congenital lipid storage disorders affect the renal parenchyma and may shed morphologically altered cells into the urine. As discussed by Sane, most of these disorders will produce a nonspecific cellular change, namely the presence of numerous small clear vacuoles within an abundant volume of cytoplasm.[34] Only the cells found in the urinary sediment of patients with Gaucher's disease may be distinguishable in that they may have a "wrinkled tissue paper" appearance in contrast to the small round vacuoles in the other lipidosis.[34] Sane described the cytoplasm of cells from a patient with Nieman-Pick disease as showing red birefringence with polarized light and autofluorescence.[34] She felt that this was due to the relative abundance of sphingomyelin in the cytoplasm of the storage cells.

The optimal therapy for children with many different types of malignant neoplasms include the administration of one or more cytotoxic pharmacologic agents. Such drugs, especially the alkylating agents, may also be given to children in preparation for bone marrow transplantation. Several of these toxic drugs may produce clinical problems referable to the urinary tract and marked cytologic alterations within urothelium.[29,35] The most notorious is cyclophosphamide,

The optimal therapy for children with many different types of malignant neoplasms include the administration of one or more cytotoxic pharmacologic agents

which may incite a mild to severe hemorrhagic cystitis. Koss has elegantly and extensively described the morphologic features of the altered epithelial cells.[29] The most prominent change is a marked enlargement of these cells involving both the nucleus and the cytoplasm. According to Koss, nucleomegaly may precede cytomegaly.[29] The enlarged nuclei are generally very darkly stained and may have irregular contours. Nucleoli may also be prominently enlarged and irregular. Usually, the nuclear membrane remains delicate and the chromatin is uniformly distributed throughout the nucleus. Cytoplasm may become very opaque but typically shows one or more vacuoles. Some of these altered benign cellular elements may be impossible to distinguish from transitional cell carcinoma. Fortunately, such neoplasms are very infrequent in children and thus do not pose a frequent diagnostic challenge. However, their presence does serve as a marker of cytotoxic damage to the urinary bladder.

Urine is a very low-yield specimen for neoplastic cells, reflecting the low frequencies with which both carcinomas arise within the urinary bladder and nonurothelial tumors metastasize to the lower genitourinary tract. Kmetz and Newton did not find a single urine sample to contain malignant cells in a total of 61 specimens over a 4-year period in a children's hospital.[36] From a different perspective, namely a large cancer hospital, Helson and Hajdu reviewed urine samples from 112 children with known cancers.[36] 56 patients had nonlymphoreticular malignancies and urine samples were positive in 4: 2 for Wilms' tumor, and 2 for rhabdomyosarcoma. Only 2 of the children with lymphoreticular tumors had positive urine samples, both of whom had non-Hodgkin's lymphoma. Therefore, no child with leukemia or Hodgkin's disease had a positive urine specimen. Radiographic evidence of distortion of the wall of the urinary bladder or of renal alterations were present in all 6 patients with positive urine samples. Geisinger et al found rhabdomyosarcoma to be the most common tumor cell type in urine; in all patients with positive urine samples, this sarcoma arose in the pelvic organs and soft tissues (Image 7.11).[38] Other relatively frequent cancers that yielded positive urine specimens included Wilms' tumor and Ewing's sarcoma.[38,39] With this latter neoplasm, the primary site for those with positive urine samples was usually the bones of the pelvis. In this last series, almost all of the positive urine specimens contained only scanty numbers of neoplastic cells.[38]

Finally, it has been proposed that the pattern of maturation of the epithelium derived from the trigone of the urinary bladder may be a simple, rapid and inexpensive test of the gestational age of newborn infants. Robine et al found that the maturation index could be used to distinguish premature from term newborn boys, whereas the estrogen and pyknotic indices made this separation possible in neonatal girls.[40]

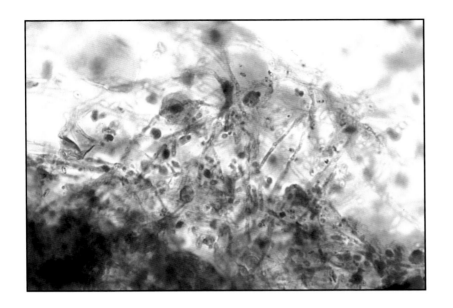

Image 7.1
Esophageal brushing specimen from a young child with acute leukemia and odynophagia. A tangle of pseudohyphae and yeast forms of *Candida* are admixed with squamous epithelial cells. The narrow pseudohyphae show points of constriction simulating septation. (Papanicolaou).

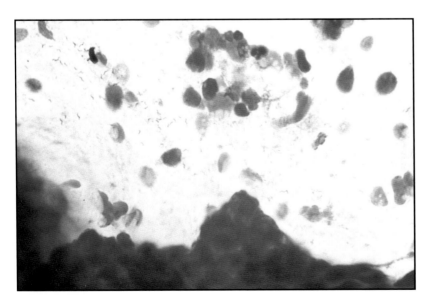

Image 7.2
Esophageal brushing specimen from a 12-year-old boy who presented with odynophagia, but no known predisposing conditions. The features are diagnostic of herpes esophagitis. The essential finding in this field is two multinucleated giant squamous epithelial cells. In one of these, each of the nuclei contains the classic Cowdry type A inclusion body separated from the thick nuclear membrane by a halo. In the other, the molded nuclei show the characteristic homogenization of their chromatin. (Papanicolaou).

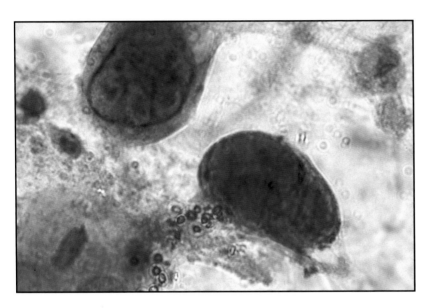

Image 7.3
In this gastric brushing, numerous *Helicobacter* are evident as spiral or twisted rods adjacent to glandular epithelial cells. (Papanicolaou).

Image 7.4
Skin scraping specimen from a child with leukemia and cutaneous vesicles. Changes similar to those seen in Image 7.2 include the multinucleated squamous cells with molded "ground glass" nuclei. (Papanicolaou).

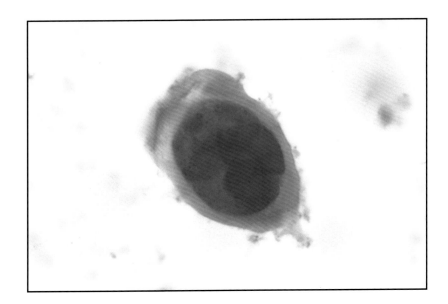

Image 7.5
Skin scraping specimen from buttocks of 2-day-old boy showing numerous eosinophils, including many that are degranulated. Note the numerous eosinophilic granules in the background. Differential diagnosis in this age group includes incontinentia pigmenti, allergic contact dermatitis, and erythema toxicum neonatorum. Based on the clinical findings, the latter diagnosis is most likely in this patient. (Romanowsky).

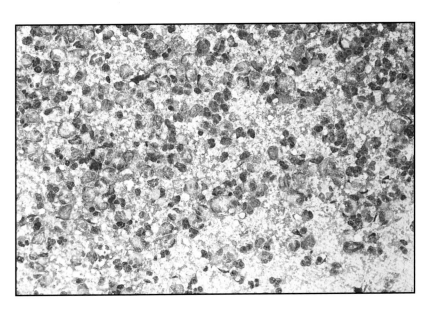

Image 7.6
Skin scraping specimen from another child with ALL. The key finding is the presence of leukemic blasts, which are admixed with a smaller number of neutrophils. Although cutaneous infiltrates of leukemic cells are relatively uncommon, the inflammatory cell infiltrate should not be ignored. The blasts are characterized by a single round to irregular nucleus, a conspicuous nucleolus, and only a scanty rim of cytoplasm. (Papanicolaou).

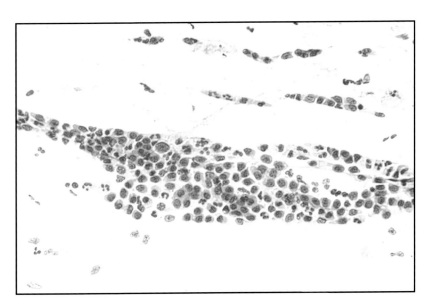

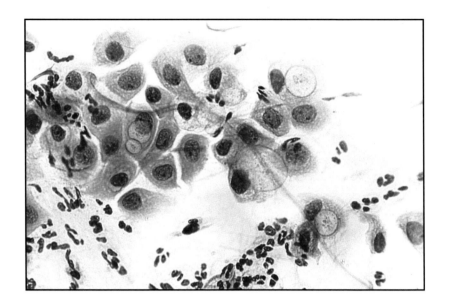

Image 7.7
Chylamydial conjunctivitis. Several of the epithelial cells show the characteristic intracytoplasmic inclusion bodies. These consist of vacuoles that contain finely granular material that may coalesce to form a larger body. (Papanicolaou).

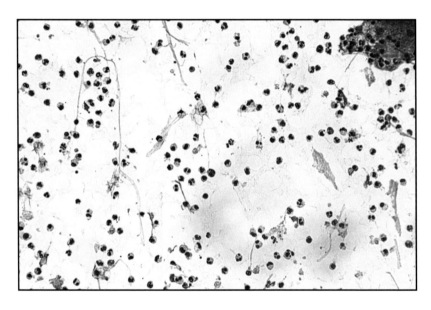

Image 7.8
Neutrophils predominate in this conjunctival specimen associated with a bacterial infection. (Papanicolaou).

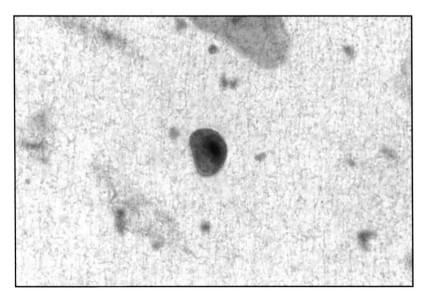

Image 7.9
Urine specimen from an infant with CMV infection. Scattered about in small numbers were isolated altered epithelial cells. The nucleus in this cell was expanded and occupied, for the most part, by a large basophilic inclusion body which is separated from the nuclear membrane by a halo due to chromatin clearing. (Papanicolaou).

Image 7.10
Urine specimen from a child who had previously undergone a renal transplantation. Both of the epithelial cells have nuclei that are altered by a polyomavirus infection. Enlarged nuclei have been replaced by very homogenous deeply basophilic masses. Such cells have been called decoy cells as they may morphologically imitate cells from a transitional cell carcinoma, although such a problem would be most unusual in a child. (Papanicolaou).

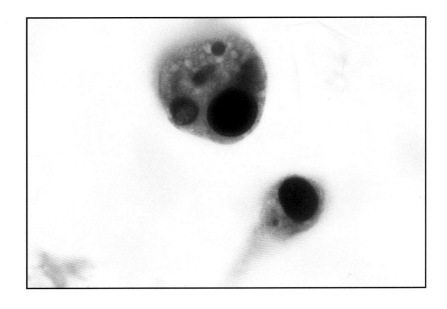

Image 7.11
A This rhabdomyosarcoma of the urinary bladder of a pediatric patient contains elongated neoplastic cells with abundant eosinophilic cytoplasm with obvious cross-striations (H & E). **B** Some of the malignant "strap" cells seen in A exfoliated into the urine. (Papanicolaou). (Courtesy of Dr B Naylor).

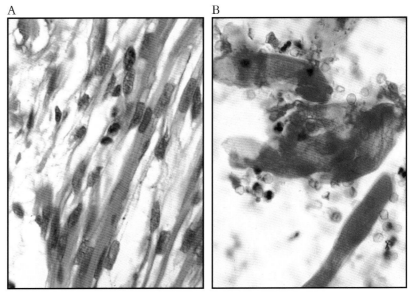

References

1. Geisinger KR, Wang HH, Ducatman BS, Teot LA. Gastrointestinal cytology. *Clinics Lab Med* 11:403-441, 1991.
2. Teot LA, Geisinger KR. Diagnostic esophageal cytology: an overview. In: Cytopathology Annual. WA Schmidt, ed. Williams and Wilkins, Baltimore, 1993, p 89-114.
3. Geisinger KR. Endoscopic biopsies and cytologic brushings of the esophagus are diagnostically complementary. *Am J Clin Pathol.* In press.
4. Teot LA, Ducatman BS, Geisinger KR. The cytologic diagnosis of cytomegaloviral esophagitis: a report of three AIDS-related cases. *Acta Cytol* 37:93-96, 1993.
5. Dahms BB, Rothstein FC. Barrett's esophagus in children: a consequence of chronic gastroesophageal reflux. *Gastroenterology* 86:318-323, 1984.
6. Robey SS, Hamilton SR, Gupta PK, Erozan YS. Diagnostic value of cytopathology in Barrett's esophagus and associated adenocarcinoma. *Am J Clin Pathol* 89:493-498, 1988.
7. Geisinger KR, Teot LA, Richter JE. A comparative cytopathologic and histologic study of atypia, dysplasia, and adenocarcinoma in Barrett's esophagus. *Cancer* 69:8-16, 1992.
8. Fulp SR, Nestock BR, Powell BL, Evans JK, Geisinger KR, Gilliam JH III. Leukemic infiltration of the esophagus. *Cancer* 71:112-116, 1993.
9. Davenport RD. Cytologic diagnosis of *Campylobacter pylori*-associated gastritis. *Acta Cytol* 34:211-213, 1990.
10. Faverly D, Fameree D, Lamy V, Fievez M, Gompel C. Identification of *Campylobacter pylori* in gastric brush smears. *Acta Cytol* 34:205-210, 1990.
11. Chadwick EG, Connor EJ, Hanson CG, Joshi VV, Abu-Farsakh H, Yogev R, McSherry G, McClain K, Murphy SB. Tumors of smooth-muscle origin in HIV-infected children. *JAMA* 263:3182-3184, 1990.
12. McLoughlin LC, Nord KS, Joshi VV, DiCarlo FJ, Kane MJ. Disseminated leiyomyosarcoma in a child with acquired immune deficiency syndrome. *Cancer* 67:2618-2621, 1991.
13. Layfield LJ, Reichman A, Weinstein WM. Endoscopically directed fine needle aspiration biopsy of gastric and esophageal lesions. *Acta Cytol* 35:69-74, 1991.
14. Abdul-Karim FW, O'Mailia JJ, Wang KP, Deeds DA, Yang P. Transmucosal endoscopic needle aspiration: utility in diagnosis of extrinsic malignant masses of the gastrointestinal tract. *Diagn Cytopathol* 7:92-94, 1991.
15. Rilke F, Pilotti S, Clemente C. Cytology of non-Hodgkin's malignant lymphomas involving the stomach. *Acta Cytol* 22:71-79, 1978.
16. Silverman, JF, Levine J, Finely JL, Larkin EW, Norris HT. Small-intestinal brushing cytology in the diagnosis of *Cryptosporidium* in AIDS. *Diagn Cytopathol* 6:193-196, 1990.
17. Melville DM, Richman PI, Shepherd NA, Williams CB, Lennard-Jones LE. Brush cytology of the colon and rectum in ulcerative colitis: an aid to cancer diagnosis. *J Clin Pathol* 41:1180-1186, 1988.
18. Bucchino JJ. Cytopathology in Pediatrics. Karger, Basel, 1991, p 8-20.

19. Friedlaender MH. Immunologic aspects of diseases of the eye. *JAMA* 26:2869-2873, 1992.

20. Naib ZM, Clepper AS, Elliott SR. Exfoliative cytology as an aid in the diagnosis of ophthalmic lesions. *Acta Cytol* 11:295-303, 1967.

21. Naib ZM. Cytology of TRIC agent infection of the eye of newborn infants and their mothers' genital tracts. *Acta Cytol* 14:390-395, 1970.

22. Naib ZM. Cytology of ocular lesions. *Acta Cytol* 16:178-185, 1972.

23. Thelmo W, Csordas J, Davis P, Marshall KG. The cytology of acute bacterial and follicular conjunctivitis. *Acta Cytol* 16:172-177, 1972.

24. Duggan MA, Pomponi C, Kay D, Robboy SJ. Infantile chlamydial conjunctivitis. A comparison of Papanicolaou, Giemsa, and immunoperoxidase staining methods. *Acta Cytol* 30:341-346, 1986.

25. Kobayashi TK, Umezawa Y, Uemura M, Kurosaka F, Matsunaga Y, Tinaka B, Chiba S. Cytodiagnosis of herpes simplex virus infection in the newborn infant. Report of a case. *Acta Cytol* 26:65-68, 1982.

26. Kobayashi TK, Mizuhara S, Sawaragi I. Cytodiagnosis of herpes simplex keratitis by means of an immunoperoxidase technique. A case report. *Acta Cytol* 29:708-711, 1985.

27. Rivasi F, Cavallini GM, Longanesi L. Cytology of allergic conjunctivitis. Presence of airborne, nonhuman elements. *Acta Cytol* 36:492-498, 1992.

28. Natadisastra G, Wittpenn JR, Muhilal, West KP Jr., Mele L, Sommer A. Impression cytology: a practical index of vitamin A status. *Am J Clin Nutr* 48:695-701, 1988.

29. Koss LG. Diagnostic Cytology and Its Histopathologic Bases. 4th ed. JB Lippincott, Philadelphia, 1992, p 890-1017.

30. Kobayashi TK, Sugimoto T, Nishida K, Sawaragi I. Intracytoplasmic inclusions in urinary sediment cells from a patient with mucocutaneous lymph node syndrome (Kawasaki disease). A case report. *Acta Cytol* 28:687-690, 1984.

31. Akura K, Hatakenaka M, Kawai K, Takenaka M, Kato K. Use of immunochemistry on urinary sediments for the rapid identification of human polyomavirus infection. A case report. *Acta Cytol* 32:247-251, 1988.

32. Braza F, Johnson KA, Grigg LM, Lopez VF, Kavirajan V. Human papovavirus in a routine urine specimen of a four-year-old boy. *Diagn Cytopathol* 5:286-288, 1989.

33. Landing BH, Nakai H. Histochemical properties of renal lead-inclusions and their demonstration in urinary sediment. *Am J Clin Pathol* 31:499-503, 1959.

34. Sane SY. Urinary sediment in storage diseases: differential diagnosis of Neiman-Pick disease by cytologic means. *Diagn Cytopathol* 6:122-123, 1990.

35. Stella F, Battistelli S, Marcheggiani F, DeSantis M, Giardini C, Baronciani D, Mattioli S, Troccoli R. Urothelial cell changes due to busulfan and cyclophosphamide treatment in bone marrow transplantation. *Acta Cytol* 34:885-890, 1990.

36. Kmetz DR, Newton WA Jr. The role of clinical cytology in a pediatric institution. *Acta Cytol* 7:207-210, 1963.

37. Helson L, Hajdu SI. The cytology of urine of pediatric cancer patients. *J Urol* 108:660-662, 1972.

38. Geisinger KR, Hajdu SI, Helson L. Exfoliative cytology of non-lymphoreticular neoplasms in children. *Acta Cytol* 28:16-28, 1984.
39. Helson L, Krochmal P, Hajdu SI. Diagnostic value of cytologic specimens obtained from children with cancer. *Ann Clin Lab Sci* 5:294-297, 1975.
40. Robine N, Relier JP, Le Bars S. Urocytogram, an index of maturity in premature infants. *Biol Neonate* 54:93-99, 1988.

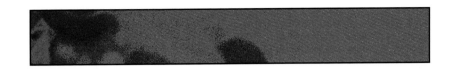

CHAPTER EIGHT

Radiologic Imaging in Children

Percutaneous fine needle aspiration (FNA) biopsy of deep-seated mass lesions in infants and children has become possible due to the advent of the cross-sectional imaging techniques of ultrasonography (US) and computed tomography (CT). The imaging modality used to identify the presence of a mass lesion will depend in part upon the anatomic site under clinical suspicion. As it is not invasive and requires no ionizing radiation, we believe that US is the initial imaging procedure of choice in the abdomen and pelvis.[1(p39-43)] Often US is the only modality necessary to localize a mass in its organ of origin, and it provides a means for performing biopsy under real-time guidance. CT may be necessary to stage completely the extent, or in cases where the lesion is not well seen, to both identify the mass and provide localization for biopsy guidance. This has been our experience with deep pelvic masses of musculoskeletal origin and, occasionally, with small nodal masses, which can be obscured by bowel gas on an US examination. Magnetic resonance imaging (MRI) is primarily used to answer questions not clarified by US or CT.

In the case of mass lesions involving the lung or mediastinum, the initial imaging modality for diagnosis remains the standard chest radiograph.[2] CT is almost always used to characterize better thoracic lesions prior to biopsy. The cross-sectional imaging display of CT precisely localizes masses, whether in the lung or mediastinum, without confusing overlying shadows and allows planning of the safest approach to the lesion.

Lesions of the extracranial head and neck can be imaged well with US. However, CT more precisely localizes mass lesions in the

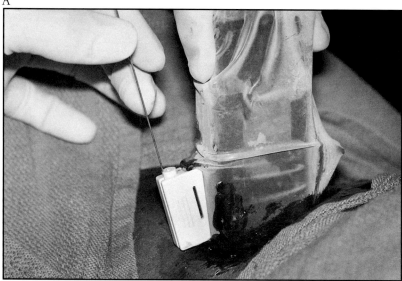

Figure 8.1

A The transducer is covered with a sterile drape. The plastic needle guide is attached to the transducer and the appropriate needle is placed in a groove in the guide.

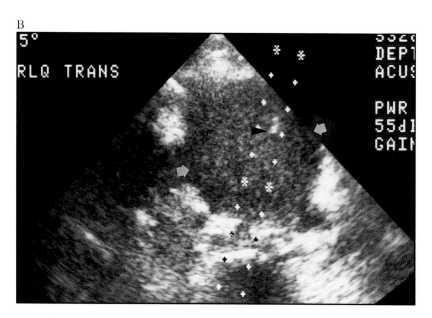

B A nodal mass (arrows) is positioned within the electronically generated lines on a CRT screen. When the needle is passed through the guide, it will follow the path between the lines. The bright echo (arrowhead) is the needle tip, the position of which is monitored during the specimen acquisition in real time.

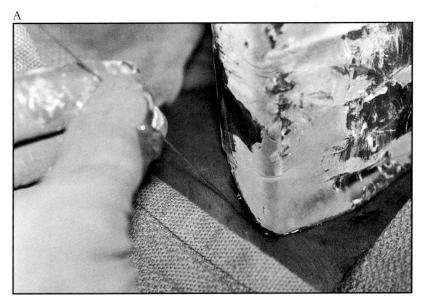

Figure 8.2

A With the free-hand technique, the needle is placed at the end of the transducer and angled toward the target. The target and the needle are positioned within the ultrasound beam and monitored as the needle is advanced toward the target.

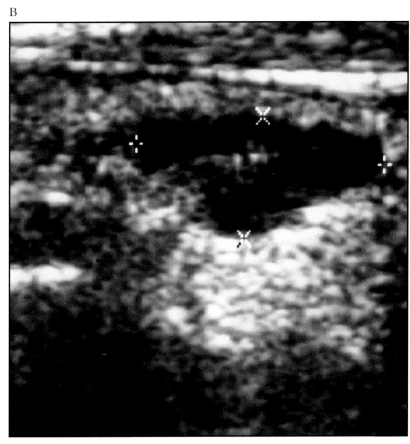

B Papillary cancer of the thyroid. Long-axis image of the right lobe containing a necrotic mass (cursors) which was biopsied using the free-hand technique. Note the proximity of the mass to the skin surface.

compartment of origin, which is helpful in the initial diagnosis and aids in determining the extent of the disease, particularly nodal involvement in lymphoma. The biopsy can be performed with US when the lesion is well seen, but may require CT guidance, particularly with lesions in the deeper compartments of the neck.

Biopsy Technique

Patient Preparation

With infants and young children, sedation is usually required for the performance of the biopsy. We have found intravenous Nembutal in a dose of 5 mg/kg (maximum) with continuous monitoring of PO_2 with a pulse oxymeter to be a safe and effective regimen. With older children, local anesthesia will usually suffice. Midazolam and phentonyl may be used in addition to local anesthesia.

Three major techniques are used for biopsy guidance: CT, US and fluoroscopy. Whenever possible, we prefer US guidance as this technique allows real-time monitoring of the needle pass and sample acquisition, particularly when the child is not completely cooperative. Two methods of US guidance are used, one is a "free hand" technique where the target is localized and the needle is either angled under the transducer or placed perpendicular to the target and directed toward the lesion with real-time correction of the needle trajectory. This technique is generally used for very superficial lesions such as thyroid nodules. The second technique involves the use of a guide attached to the transducer through which the needle passes (Figure 8.1). The computer generates lines on the US monitor that depict the potential needle course. The target is positioned within the electronically generated lines and the needle pass is made with real-time guidance (Figure 8.1). We prefer the guided technique because of its accuracy and speed. Very superficial lesions, however, may require a free-hand technique because the type of transducer needed to visualize the lesion (linear configuration) does not permit the use of a guide (Figure 8.2).

With CT guidance, the image slice that best depicts the lesion is identified and the safest approach is determined. The skin is marked at the appropriate site and the degree of angulation of the needle and the depth of the target are estimated. Usually the needle will be placed part way to the target and repeat scans made to evaluate the trajectory and to confirm that the tip is within the target. A coaxial needle system can be used to facilitate repeated sampling (Images 8.1 and 8.2). The technique is time consuming, particularly when compared with US or fluoroscopy.

Fluoroscopic guidance is used primarily for pulmonary and mediastinal lesions not in contact with the chest wall. When thoracic lesions are in contact with the chest wall, ultrasound guidance is possible as there is no intervening air-containing lung to obscure the sound beam.

We prefer the guided technique because of its accuracy and speed

Imaging Characteristics of Common Pediatric Tumors

Abdomen

The majority of abdominal masses (57%) detected by physical exam in the pediatric age group are due to organomegaly, the remaining 43% represent developmental anomalies or neoplasms. 90% are retroperitoneal and 50% are of urinary tract origin, equally divided between benign and malignant lesions.[3-5] Sonography is ideally suited to confirm organomegaly and to characterize renal masses into solid or cystic lesions. Solid renal lesions are usually malignant while cystic lesions are usually benign. Usually the retroperitoneal location of a mass can be readily determined by the multiplanar capability of ultrasonography.

Neuroblastoma

As neuroblastomas arise from neural crest epithelium, they may be found anywhere along the sympathetic chain from the base of the skull to the pelvis. 75% of neuroblastomas are from the retroperitonium, 50% from the adrenal medulla and 25% from the paraspinal ganglia.[3] Plain radiography of the abdomen precedes CT imaging techniques to identify calcifications (Image 8.3), present in approximately 60% of patients with neuroblastoma.[6] The calcifications are often punctate or stippled. Sonographically, neuroblastomas present as uniformly echogenic masses, which on the right side are suprarenal in location, and extrinsic to both the liver and kidney. On the left side, the mass is often both above and anterior to the kidney. Bright echoes with acoustic shadowing may be seen secondary to calcification (Images 8.4 and 8.5). Occasionally, hypoechoic foci can be seen within the mass secondary to tumor necrosis. Neuroblastomas often cross the midline with a lobular contour.[7(p243)] A meticulous search must be made to identify regional adenopathy, liver metastases and vascular encasement. Occasionally, venous invasion (inferior vena cava and renal vein) is identified. Neuroblastomas may directly invade the kidney mimicking Wilms' tumor.[6,7(p243)] Once the mass is identified and staged with sonography, the safest route for a percutaneous biopsy is chosen. Preferably, a posterior approach is used in an attempt not to violate the peritoneal cavity. With knowledge of the cytologic diagnosis, additional appropriate staging studies can then be planned, which usually include CT, nuclear bone scans and a plain radiographic skeletal survey. MRI will be used if there is a question of spinal cord involvement, vascular encasement or invasion not adequately demonstrated with sonography or CT (Images 8.6 and 8.7). With CT exam, the mass is usually a lobulated, soft tissue density mass often crossing the midline. Calcifications are seen with a much higher frequency (approaching 90%) than with plain radiography (Image 8.8). There is usually variable contrast enhancement and often central areas of necrosis can be identified. A careful evaluation of the liver is made for metastases, as well as the node-bearing areas for regional and distant lymphadenopathy.[8]

> *Sonographically, neuroblastomas present as uniformly echogenic masses, which on the right side are suprarenal in location, and extrinsic to both the liver and kidney*

Wilms' Tumor

Children with Wilms' tumor are more likely to present with an asymptomatic mass than those with neuroblastoma. Imaging begins with plain radiographs to confirm the presence of a mass and to look for calcification, which is present in approximately 10% of children with Wilms' tumors and is often wavy, linear or curvilinear (Image 8.9), unlike the punctate calcifications of neuroblastoma.[9] We then proceed with ultrasonography for the reasons discussed above.[10] Wilms' tumors typically are well-circumscribed masses with mixed echogenicity, often containing foci of necrosis. However, the radiologic hallmark of Wilms' tumor is its renal origin. While this finding is usually easily confirmed sonographically, when the mass is large, the site of origin becomes more difficult to ascertain. It is less likely than neuroblastomas to cross the midline or encase vessels. Venous invasion, however, is quite common and a meticulous exam must be made of the renal veins and inferior vena cava, as well as the right atrium. A search is made for regional lymphadenopathy and liver metastases. The contralateral kidney must be carefully evaluated to exclude bilaterality as well as signs of nephroblastomatosis. Chest radiographs should be made as pulmonary metastases in the face of an abdominal mass is highly suggestive of Wilms' tumor. As with neuroblastoma, CT is performed to stage the tumor in the abdomen and chest. The CT appearance of Wilms' tumor is that of an intrarenal mass, which enhances in an inhomogeneous fashion after intravenous contrast, often with a rim of residual kidney at the periphery. With meticulous technique, bolus enhancement and dynamic scanning, vascular involvement can be evaluated. Invasion of the renal vein and inferior vena cava is well seen. Unlike neuroblastoma, adjacent organs and vessels are usually displaced rather than invaded or encased (Image 8.10).[11] CT is more sensitive than US in identifying subtle bilateral tumors as well as nephroblastomatosis. As with neuroblastoma, we invariably use ultrasound guidance in suspected Wilms' tumor biopsies. When possible, we use a posterior approach, so as not to violate the peritoneal cavity.

Sonography in Wilms' tumors demonstrates either a predominantly exophytic mass with preservation of a portion of the kidney or replacement and distortion of most of the kidney (Images 8.11 and 8.12). Due to the presence of a pseudocapsule, the mass is often well defined. Occasionally, it may be difficult to differentiate a neuroblastoma invading the kidney from an infiltrating Wilms' tumor. The echo texture of the latter is variable, reflecting the heterogeneous tissue components found. Usually the mass is solid, but cystic areas due to necrosis and hemorrhage are common. Rarely, a Wilms' tumor will be predominantly cystic with internal septations. This pattern may be impossible to differentiate from a multilocular cystic nephroma.

Other primary renal tumors of childhood have similar imaging characteristics, with the exception of rhabdoid tumor which tends to infiltrate the renal parenchyma and is poorly defined. The presence of a renal mass and bony metastases suggests a clear cell sarcoma of the kidney.

The radiologic hallmark of Wilms' tumor is its renal origin

Primary Liver Lesions

Most benign masses commonly found in the liver of infants and children have imaging and clinical characteristics that preclude the need for a percutaneous biopsy. Cavernous hemangiomas and capillary endotheliomas, when symptomatic, produce the combination of high output congestive failure with single or multiple liver masses. The abdominal aorta proximal to the celiac axis is often large with abrupt tapering distal to the celiac axis. The hepatic veins and inferior vena cava may be dilated from arteriovenous shunting within the mass. The hepatic artery is enlarged with either lesion. The combination of the US, CT and radionuclide studies is often quite specific.

Focal nodular hyperplasia produces well-defined hypo- to isoechoic liver masses with US and accumulates sulphur colloid on technetium sulphur colloid scintigraphy. Although quite characteristic, this finding, however, is not pathognomonic as occasionally liver adenomas and hepatomas will be avid for sulphur colloid (Images 8.13 and 8.14).[12,13]

Mesenchymal hamartomas are typically cystic intrahepatic masses with multiple septations but may be solid and thus mimic hepatoma or hepatoblastoma. They may be quite large projecting into the peritoneal cavity so that their origin in the liver may be difficult to ascertain by any imaging technique (Image 8.15 and 8.16). The uncommon predominantly solid mesenchymal hamartoma may also mimic a hemangioma being hyperechoic with a large hepatic artery, dilated proximal aorta with large draining veins.[14]

Cysts are quite characteristic on US and require no additional studies. Solitary cavernous hemangiomas are hyperechoic on US and rarely >3 cm in diameter.

Liver masses that generally are amenable to percutaneous biopsy are either inflammatory lesions or neoplastic lesions

Liver masses that generally are amenable to percutaneous biopsy are either inflammatory lesions or neoplastic lesions. Abscesses most commonly present as cystic or complex masses with US or hypodense masses on CT, often with rim enhancement with intravenous contrast. Percutaneous aspiration will serve to confirm the diagnosis of abscess and provide access for percutaneous drainage for treatment and microbiologic studies.

In both hepatoma and hepatoblastoma, plain radiographs confirm the presence of the mass and its general location, as well as identify calcification present in up to 55% of hepatoblastomas and hepatomas.[15] Sonography is usually the next imaging procedure. Most hepatoblastomas and hepatomas are hypoechoic solid masses, either localized with a well defined pseudocapsule or multicentric with involvement of more than one lobe. A careful search of the inferior vena cava and portal vein is necessary, as these tumors have a propensity for vascular invasion (Images 8.17 and 8.18).

Prior to surgical resection radiologic exam allows a careful anatomic "dissection" of the liver to identify which liver segments are involved. MRI promises to be a useful technique here because of its multiplanar capability and excellent demonstration of vascular structures without the need for intravenous contrast.[16] Currently, we use MRI to answer specific questions raised by US and/or CT.

Hepatic adenomas are uncommon in children, but when present, produce hypoechoic solitary or multiple masses with US. Hepatic echogenicity is often increased as these lesions are common in children with glycogen storage disease or Fanconi's anemia treated with androgenic steroids. On CT scans these lesions are typically hypodense before intravenous contrast and enhance in a homogeneous fashion.[17] Radionuclide angiograms reveal hypervascular lesions in 50% of cases, similar to hepatomas. With MRI, the adenomas are usually isointense to liver on T1-weighted images and hyperintense to liver on T2-weighted images. However, occasionally they may be isointense on both T1- and T2-weighted images, mimicking focal nodular hyperplasia.[16]

Cavernous hemangiomas, when peripheral in the liver, are well-defined homogeneous hyperechoic masses on ultrasonography. When central, they tend to be larger and inhomogeneous in echo texture. Symptomatic cavernous hemangiomas are usually large, solitary masses with well-defined borders. Hypo- or anaechoic spaces are common secondary to vascular channels. Doppler studies typically show no or little signal as the flow is extremely slow. On dynamic CT, the enhancement pattern may be characteristic with peripheral enhancement early followed by gradual centripetal opacification; delayed scans show isodense total opacification. This typical pattern, however, can be seen with other hepatic lesions and does not occur with all hemangiomas. Technetium-tagged red blood cell studies are specific with decreased activity during the radionuclide angiogram phase and increased activity relative to the liver on delayed images (Images 8.19 and 8.20).[18,19] MRI typically reveals cavernous hemangiomas to be low intensity on T1-weighted images and high intensity on heavily T2-weighted images. Although characteristic, this finding is not always present and may be mimicked occasionally by metastatic disease.[20]

Hemangioendotheliomas are typically multiple or demonstrate diffuse hepatic infiltration. Sonographically, these usually produce well-defined, hypoechoic nodules similar to metastatic disease. The presence of a dilated hepatic artery, hepatic veins, inferior vena cava and upper abdominal aorta together with the clinical picture of congestive heart failure separates lesions from metastases.

Hepatic Metastases

Neuroblastoma is the most common childhood tumor to spread to the liver. In the 1st year of life, neuroblastoma in the liver may be diffuse with massive enlargement, and irregular echo texture, but without discrete lesions, particularly with stage IV S disease. Older children with neuroblastoma are more likely to have discrete lesions (Image 8.21).[7(p261)] Lymphoma and leukemia usually diffusely infiltrate the liver and spleen and are difficult to identify on any imaging study. Burkitt's lymphoma may produce discrete, often very hypoechoic masses within the liver.

Pelvis

Imaging usually begins with US, particularly in young girls. The goal of imaging is first to identify the organ of origin and the organ systems involved. Most ovarian masses are cystic or complex. Purely cystic masses are benign and do not require biopsy. Teratomas characteristically are complex, often with very ectogenic foci due to calcification or fat. Signs of malignancy include ascites and nodal or liver metastases. In the absence of these, one cannot differentiate benign from malignant ovarian tumors by imaging techniques.[21] After ovarian masses, rhabdomyosarcomas are the most common tumor of the pelvis in the pediatric population. When botryoid rhabdomyosarcoma occurs in the vagina, uterus or bladder, the US appearance is often characterized by multiple fluid filled spaces. On CT, the mass will be low in density and the septations are best shown with contrast enhancement.[22] CT is best suited to evaluate the full extent of rhabdomyosarcomas of the pelvic floor (Images 8.22 and 8.23).

Retroperitoneum

In addition to the retroperitoneal tumors discussed above, masses due to enlarged lymph nodes are encountered in children as metastatic disease or malignant lymphoma. With US, lymph nodes are typically well defined hypoechoic masses which follow the retroperitoneal and abdominal vasculature (Image 8.24). The major vessels are traced for enlarged lymph nodes. With non-Hodgkin's lymphoma, the nodal masses are often bulky and, in addition to a paravascular location, may be within the root of the mesentery as well as the retrocrural spaces.

A more complete nodal search can be made with CT as portions of the retroperitoneum are often obscured by gas. Meticulous technique with complete opacification of the gastrointestinal tract with contrast is essential to avoid confusing opaque bowel with large lymph nodes. Bolus intravenous contrast, preferably with a power injector, is also essential to separate vascular structures from nodal masses. This is especially true in the pelvis. With CT, enlarged lymph nodes are seen as soft tissue density masses adjacent to vascular structures or in the retrocrural space or the root of the mesentery. Lymph nodes may enhance with contrast and may occasionally demonstrate central necrosis (Images 8.25 and 8.26).[23]

The percutaneous FNA biopsy of nodal masses may be accomplished either with CT or US guidance. We prefer US guidance when feasible and resort to CT guidance in those cases when either a safe route cannot be found with ultrasound or when a nodal mass cannot be seen.

Bone and Soft Tissue

The primary imaging modality to identify and characterize primary and metastatic lesions of bone remains the plain radiograph

The primary imaging modality to identify and characterize primary and metastatic lesions of bone remains the plain radiograph. The pattern of bone destruction and repair, as well as the presence and type of matrix formation, and the type of periosteal new bone formation are well shown with good quality radiographs. The above features coupled with the age of the child and the location of the lesion are the most helpful features in determining the aggressiveness of a lesion and the probability of its being benign or malignant (Image 8.27).[24]

Bone scintigraphy is the procedure of choice to survey the skeletal system for metastatic disease. In cases of neuroblastoma and histiocytosis X, the plain film skeletal survey is complementary.

MRI is now used routinely to determine the true extent of primary bone tumors, both within the medullary cavity, and for the extent of soft tissue involvement. On T1-weighted images, the normally high signal from marrow will be replaced by low-signal tumor. On T2-weighted sequences, most tumors will be high signal, both within the marrow and the adjacent soft tissues. While MRI is very sensitive to the presence of tumor and edema, the findings are not entirely specific (Images 8.28 through 8.30).[25]

Biopsy guidance for bone tumors is determined by the location and characteristics of the lesion. Bone tumors with a significant soft tissue mass can be sampled with US guidance as the soft tissue component is clearly depicted. CT guidance is generally used when either there is no soft tissue mass or the location precludes visualization with US (Image 8.31). Various needle types can be used for FNA of bone tumors. When a significant soft tissue mass is associated with a lytic or blastic lesion, 20 and 21 gauge Chiba needles can be used. When there is considerable destruction of cortical bone, these same needles can still be used as destroyed cortex can be penetrated with little effort. In those cases where the marrow space must be entered through intact cortical bone, either a Craig needle must be used, or one of the newer, relatively small-gauge bone cutting needles.

Extracranial Head and Neck

Masses localized in the extracranial head and neck are most commonly congenital anomalies, enlarged lymph nodes or primary neoplasms. Imaging of the extracranial head and neck is best accomplished with contrast-enhanced CT, which best localizes the mass to the compartment of origin. The location of the mass and its morphologic appearance and enhancement pattern often provide either a specific diagnosis or a short differential diagnosis. For example, a cyst along the anterior border of the sternocleidomastoid muscle is typical for a branchial cleft cyst and a multiloculated cyst in the posterior cervical triangle is typical for cystic hygroma. Lymph nodes are most commonly located in the carotid space along the common carotid artery and internal jugular vein, the spinal accessory space, the retropharyngeal space and the submandibular and submental spaces. Lymph node size and enhancement patterns aid in differentiating benign from malignant nodes. Lymph nodes > 1 cm with ring enhancement are generally malignant (Image 8.32).[26]

Imaging of the extracranial head and neck is best accomplished with contrast-enhanced CT, which best localizes the mass to the compartment of origin

Central Nervous System

Tumors of the brain and spinal cord are identified and characterized by CT and MRI. MRI, with its multiplanar capability and exquisite sensitivity, characterizes most brain tumors, even when initially diagnosed with CT, and is the imaging modality of choice for examining the spinal cord.[27] The use of intravenous gadolinium has increased the sensitivity of MRI in identifying and localizing central nervous system (CNS) neoplasms (Images 8.33 and 8.34). Biopsy of

CNS masses can be accomplished either intraoperatively with real-time ultrasound guidance or stereotactically through a burr hole. The intra-operative technique requires turning a bone flap in preparation for both biopsy and resection. Preferably, scanning is accomplished through the intact dura. The ultrasound transducer is draped with a sterile cover and saline is placed in the operative defect to provide an acoustic window. Brain tissue provides an excellent medium for sound transmission hence, relatively high-frequency transducers can be used, allowing excellent resolution. Most brain tumors are hyperechoic, relative to normal brain tissue.[28] In addition, many tumors have cystic components that are well seen with ultrasound. The ventricles of the brain, as well as the ectogenic midline falx, provide anatomic landmarks that aid in localizing masses. FNA can be performed under real-time guidance with the same guidance system described for percutaneous biopsies elsewhere in the body (Images 8.35 and 8.36).

The stereotactic system is a CT-guided technique in which a specially designed head ring is attached to the patient's calvarium via burr holes and the patient is scanned in the CT gantry with the head ring in place. A CT-generated trajector and distance is calculated from the scan and the patient returned to the operating room where the neurosurgeon performs the biopsy using a guidance system attached to the head ring and the information gained from the CT scan. This technique has the advantage of using a small burr hole rather than a bone flap.

Chest

Most thoracic lesions which come to percutaneous biopsy are identified initially on standard frontal and lateral radiographs of the chest. Mediastinal masses are best evaluated according to the compartment of the mediastinum from which they arise. The location of the mass, together with imaging characteristics, the age of the child and the clinical picture allows for a short differential diagnostic list. Masses such as the normal large infant thymus are characteristic and require no further imaging studies or biopsy. Others such as bronchogenic cysts are diagnostic based on their middle mediastinal location and cystic imaging characteristics on CT, US or MRI; therefore, biopsy is not necessary. The plain radiographic findings of mediastinal masses are uniform water-density masses that can usually be localized to a given compartment. Calcifications are frequent in germ cell tumors, thymic cysts and neurogenic tumors. The margins (lobulated or smooth) of masses are helpful in narrowing the differential diagnosis. CT is the next imaging step, both to localize precisely the mass and better characterize the type of tissue present. The greater tissue specificity of CT and MRI allows identification of subtle calcification, fat and hemorrhage.

In the anterior mediastinum, solid masses are candidates for FNA biopsy. Most solid anterior mediastinal masses will usually be thymomas, teratomas or lymphomas.[1(p200),29] Benign thymomas have well-defined borders, calcify in an eggshell pattern in 25% and arise from the surface of the thymus or may replace the gland. Extension to the pleura, lung or pericardium is usually indicative of malignancy. A mul-

The location of the mass, together with imaging characteristics, the age of the child and the clinical picture, allows for a short differential diagnostic list

ticystic appearance on contrast-enhanced CT strongly suggests malignancy. Teratomas often have specific imaging characteristics including the presence of fat, calcium or fat-fluid levels. Both CT and MRI are effective in demonstrating these characteristics. Invasion of adjacent tissues implies a malignant teratoma or cyst, whereas fat-fluid levels implies benignity.

The most common middle mediastinal mass in children is adenopathy due to lymphoma. Non-Hodgkin's lymphoma often presents with bulky multilobulated middle mediastinal masses, often with associated pleural effusions. Airway and vena caval compression are not uncommon and may produce symptoms leading to diagnosis by chest radiography. Hodgkin's lymphoma most commonly manifests as both hilar and mediastinal lymphadenopathy, often with concomitant cervical node enlargement. The thymus may be infiltrated with Hodgkin's disease which may be difficult to differentiate from nodal disease on chest radiographs; however, CT can usually separate these two sites of involvement.[30]

Most posterior mediastinal masses in children are neurogenic. On chest radiographs, neurogenic tumors present as a unilateral homogeneous mass in the posterior mediastinum. Calcification occurs in approximately 25%. CT is essential for staging and to confirm the posterior mediastinal origin. MRI is valuable to identify intraspinal extension as well as marrow infiltration.[31]

Parenchymal mass lesions are uncommon and fall into two broad categories: solitary and multiple. Multiple nodular opacities are most commonly metastases from Wilms' tumor, osteosarcoma, rhabdomyosarcoma, germ cell tumors, hepatoblastoma, thyroid carcinoma and neuroblastoma, and are typically peripheral in location. The etiology usually is obvious due to a known primary malignancy. Solitary mass lesions are less common and are nonspecific on imaging studies with the exception of characteristic calcifications found in several benign lesions. Hamartomas may have a "popcorn"-type calcification, and granulomas may have a central nidus or concentric rings. Pulmonary blastomas may have amorphous calcification and are typically located in the upper lobes. Bronchial adenomas tend to be central in location, related to the main stem bronchi and may produce bronchial obstruction with peripheral collapse or partial obstruction with air trapping. Finally, among the most common solitary mass lesions are pseudotumors. These lesions are usually quite large and often calcify in an amorphous pattern.[32]

The imaging modality used for percutaneous biopsy of lung lesions is chosen by the location of the lesion. Our preference is to use US guidance when the lesion is in contact with the chest wall (Images 8.37 through 8.39). Air-containing lung between the lesion and the transducer will obscure the target; however, if even a small portion of the mass is in contact with the chest wall, the lesion can usually be seen well and a biopsy safely performed. The needle path will not traverse air-containing lung, reducing the risk of pneumothorax.

If the lesion is completely surrounded by air-containing lung, either fluoroscopic or CT guidance must be used. We prefer fluoroscopic guidance due to the rapidity of the procedure. CT guidance is reserved for lesions that are difficult to see on chest radiographs and fluoroscopy.

We prefer fluoroscopic guidance due to the rapidity of the procedure

Image 8.1

CT guidance was used with the child prone to perform a biopsy on eosinophilic granuloma involving a vertebral body. The line labeled (2) identified the distance from the spinous process where the puncture will be made. The line labeled (1) provides the depth to the target as well as the angle which will be used.

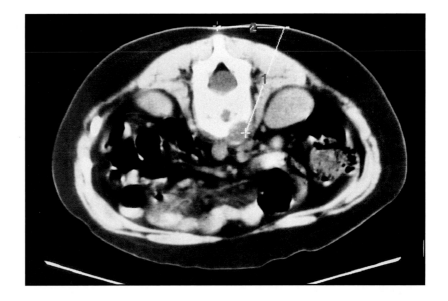

Image 8.2

CT image made with the needle in place with the tip at the surface of the mass (arrow). The actual sample was obtained immediately following confirmation of the position of the biopsy needle.

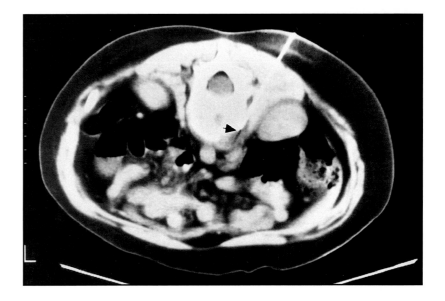

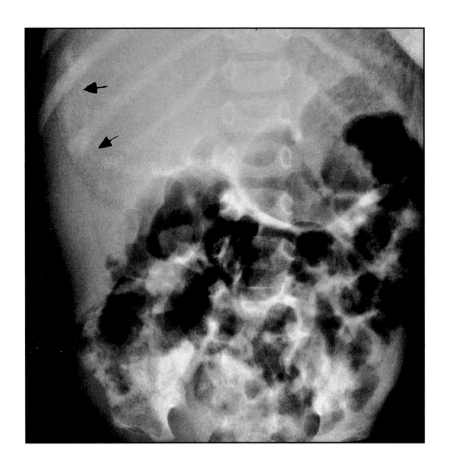

Image 8.3
2-year-old child with right adrenal neuroblastoma. Note the coarse foci of calcification in the right upper quadrant mass (arrows).

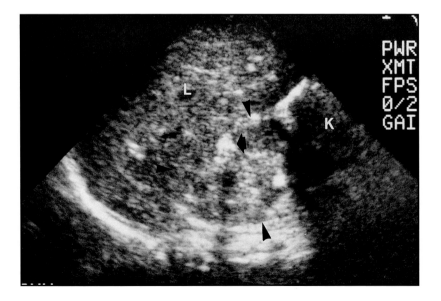

Image 8.4
Longitudinal ultrasound image of a right adrenal neuroblastoma demonstrating a slightly hyperechoic mass (arrowheads) containing bright ectogenic foci with acoustic shadowing due to calcifications (arrow). The kidney (K) and the liver (L) are below and above the mass, respectively.

Image 8.5
Large left neuroblastoma flattening the left kidney producing a lateral beak (black arrow). This appearance may mimic a tumor rising from the kidney. Note the coarse calcifications within the mass typical of neuroblastoma (red arrow).

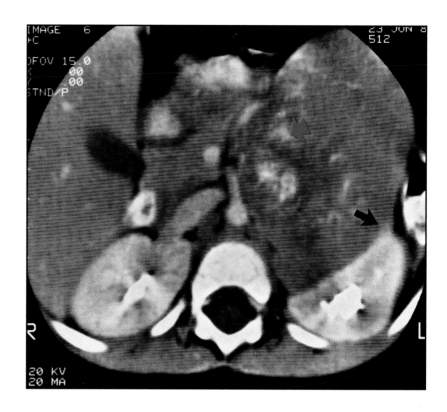

Image 8.6
6-year-old with neuroblastoma with back pain. Plain radiographs and a nuclear bone scan were not conclusive for bony involvement (not shown). Axial T1-weighted MR image shows abnormal low signal replacing fatty marrow in the left pedicle with extension into the vertebral body (black arrows). The intraspinal contents are not involved (red arrows).

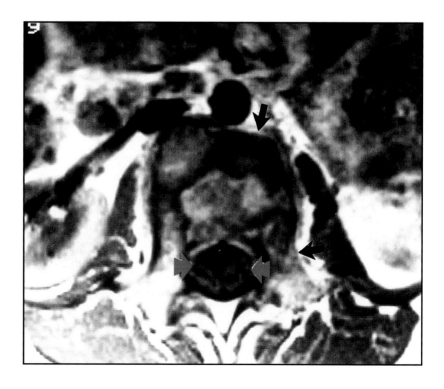

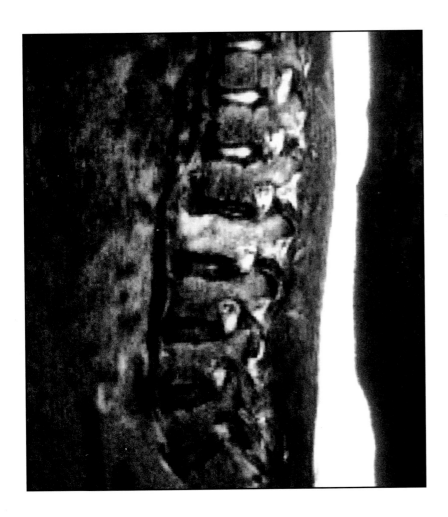

Image 8.7
Sagittal T2-weighted MR image of neuroblastoma shows abnormally high signal replacing the marrow of the vertebral body with extension into the pedicle. The lack of intraspinal involvement was confirmed on midline sections (not shown).

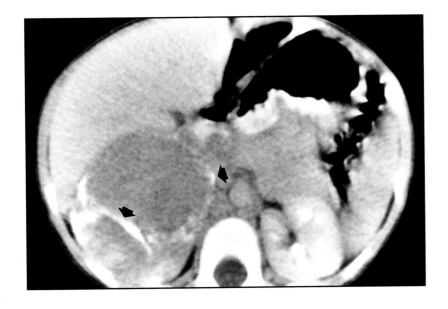

Image 8.8
Right upper quadrant neuroblastoma with characteristic calcification within the mass (arrows).

Image 8.9
Plain radiograph of the abdomen in an infant with a large left upper quadrant mass demonstrating wavy, linear calcifications which are very suggestive of Wilms' tumor (arrow).

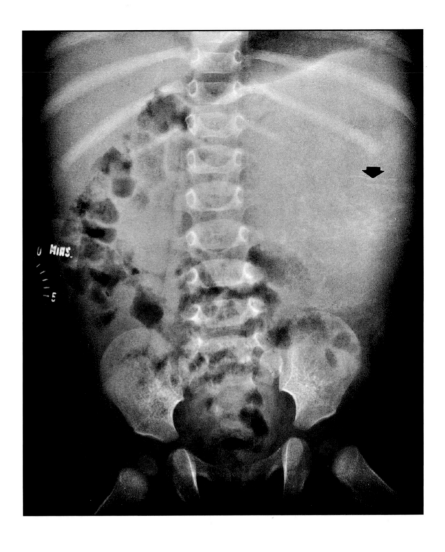

Image 8.10
CT scan of a large mass arising from and displacing the left kidney anteriorly due to a necrotic Wilms' tumor (K=kidney).

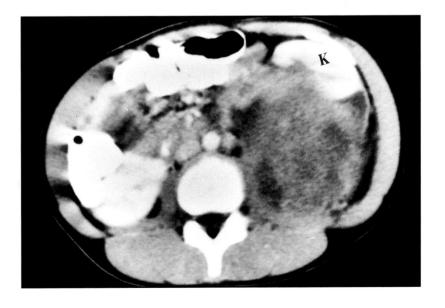

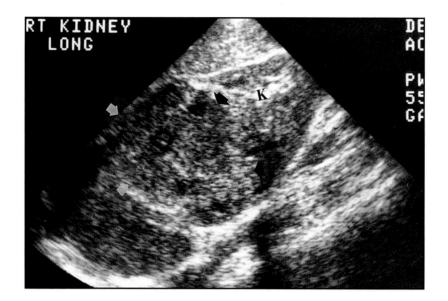

Image 8.11
Wilms' tumor arising from the upper pole of the right kidney. The mass (white arrows) splays the upper pole of the kidney (K; black arrows) and is of mixed echogenicity containing small foci of necrosis (arrowhead).

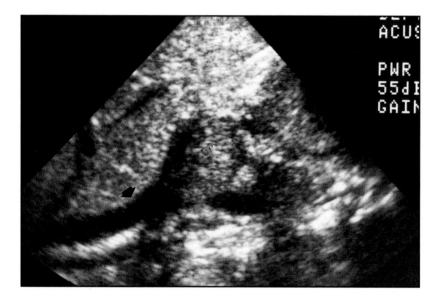

Image 8.12
Ultrasound is well suited to identify vascular invasion commonly seen with Wilms' tumor. A longitudinal image of the inferior vena cava (arrow) contains tumor mass (T) extending from the right renal vein into the inferior vena cava secondary to a right-sided Wilms' tumor.

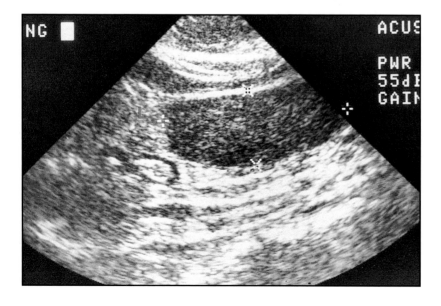

Image 8.13
Long axis view of a large homogenous hypoechoic mass (outlined by cursors) arising from the inferior aspect of the left lobe of the liver (L), which proved to be due to focal nodular hyperplasia.

Image 8.14

Technetium sulfur colloid scan of another patient with focal nodular hyperplasia in which there is uniform uptake indicating the presence of Kupffer cells which is characteristic of focal nodular hyperplasia.

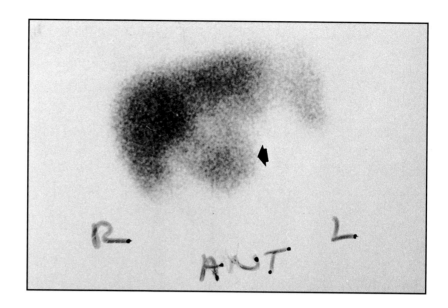

Image 8.15

Transverse ultrasound image of a large right upper quadrant mass containing both cystic (white arrow) and solid elements (black arrow). The size of the lesion made it difficult to be certain of the organ of origin.

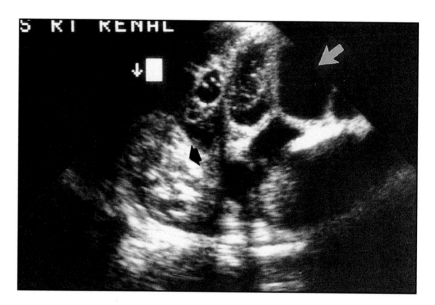

Image 8.16

A CT scan of the same patient as in Image 8.15 more clearly identified the liver as the site of the mass. The combination of the liver origin and the mixed solid and cystic nature of the mass are characteristic of mesenchymal hamartoma of the liver.

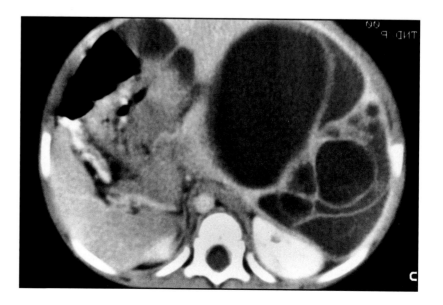

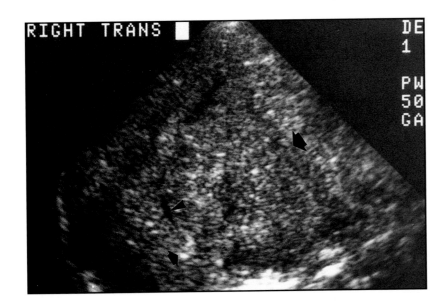

Image 8.17
Transverse ultrasound image of the right lobe of the liver demonstrating a slightly hyperechoic mass (arrows). Note the displacement of the right hepatic vein by mass (arrowhead).

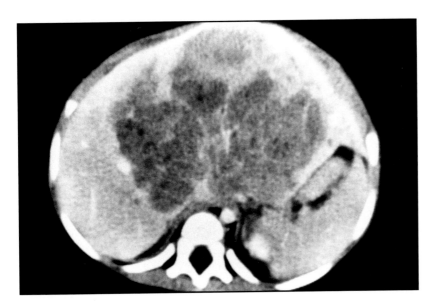

Image 8.18
Transverse CT image of the same patient demonstrates a hypodense mass with peripheral contrast enhancement replacing much of the right lobe of the liver with an extension into the left lobe.

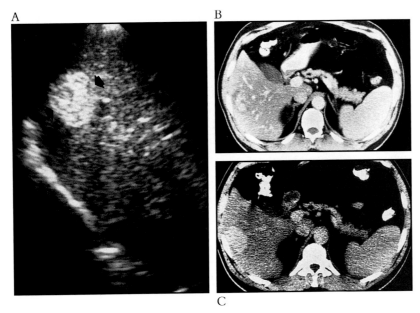

Image 8.19
A Long axis ultrasound view of the right lobe of the liver demonstrating the well-circumscribed hyperechoic mass (arrows) with acoustic enhancement posterior to the mass. The enhancement is due to the fluid nature of a hepatic hemangioma which absorbs less acoustic energy than the liver parenchyma.
B and **C** Early and late CT images, respectively, demonstrating peripheral enhancement early, followed by total opacification on delayed scans.

Image 8.20
Delayed image from a tagged erythrocyte study demonstrating the characteristic intense activity within a hemangioma (arrow).

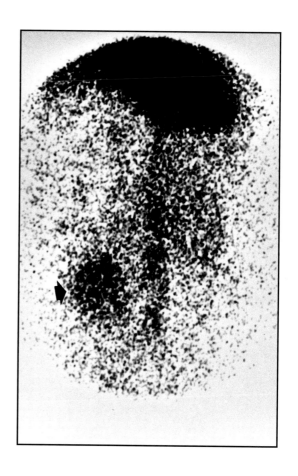

Image 8.21
Long axis view of the right lobe of the liver in a child with a left adrenal neuroblastoma. A solitary metastatic deposit with focal hyperechoic foci due to calcification is outlined by cursors.

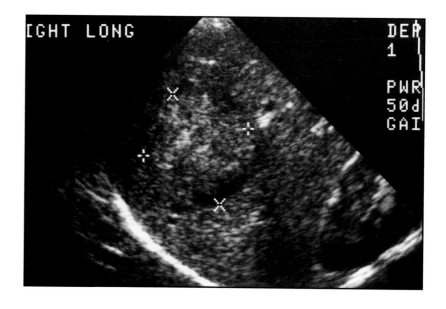

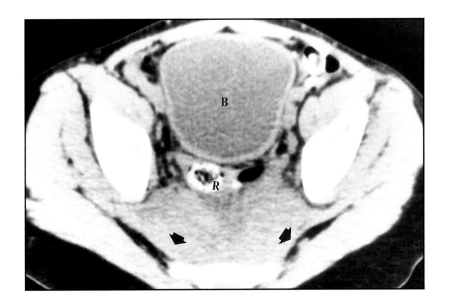

Image 8.22
Pelvic rhabdomyosarcoma.
Transverse CT image of a soft tissue mass posterior to the rectum (R) and bladder (B). The mass is inseparable from the pyriformis muscles (arrows).

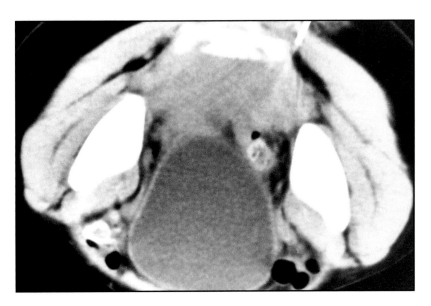

Image 8.23
CT guidance was used to perform a biopsy on the mass. The needle is entering the sciatic notch with the patient in a prone position.

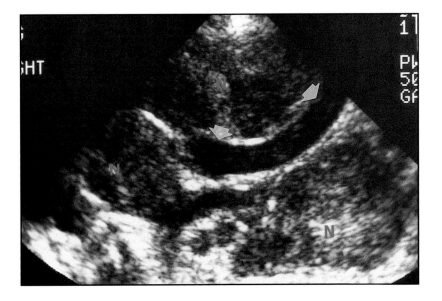

Image 8.24
Pelvic lymph nodes. Long axis ultrasound image of the left common iliac artery (arrowheads) in a child with Hodgkin's disease. There are three well defined common iliac nodes (N) contiguous with long axis of the artery.

Image 8.25

Retroperitoneal lymphadenopathy. Transverse image of the mid-abdomen with a mantel of soft tissue surrounding the aorta secondary to lymphadenopathy in this teenager with non-Hodgkin's lymphoma (arrows) is visible in this CT scan.

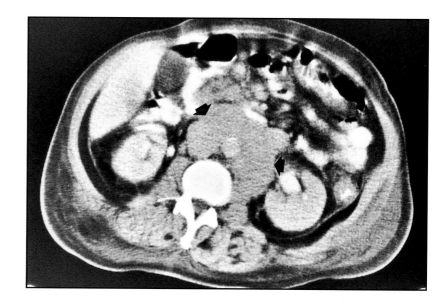

Image 8.26

Extensive bilateral external iliac nodes can be seen with this transverse image through the pelvis (arrows).

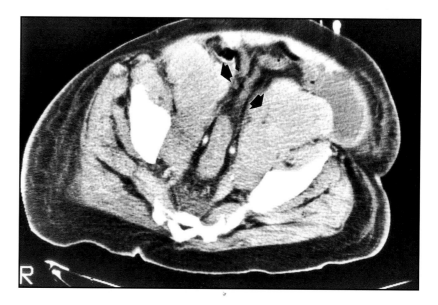

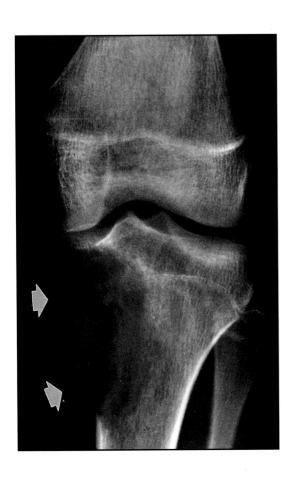

Image 8.27
Osteosarcoma. AP radiograph of a 12-year-old girl demonstrating an aggressive lytic lesion of the metaphysis of the tibia with a large soft tissue mass (arrows). An eccentric metaphyseal aggressive tumor in a child of this age is typical of osteosarcoma. The only characteristic feature not present is neoplastic bone formation within the soft tissue mass.

A
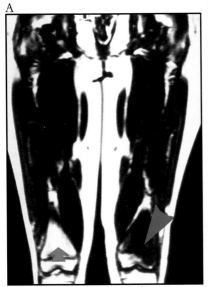

B
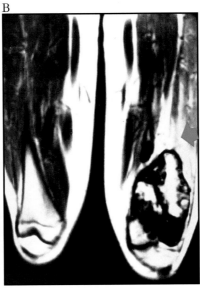

Image 8.28
A Osteosarcoma. T1-weighted MR image of a distal femoral osteosarcoma. Note the replacement of the normal high intensity marrow on the right side by low signal tumor (blue arrowhead). The tumor can be seen extending to the joint surface. On the left side normal high signal fatty marrow is preserved (red arrow).
B Longitudinal proton density weighted image of the same patient demonstrates mixed signal within the primary tumor mass. The extent of the tumor as well as edema in adjacent muscles (red arrow) are clearly shown.

Image 8.29

Osteosarcoma. Transverse ultrasound image of the soft tissue component of a tibial osteosarcoma (arrows) prior to biopsy. Note the bright linear reflectors at the interface with bone.

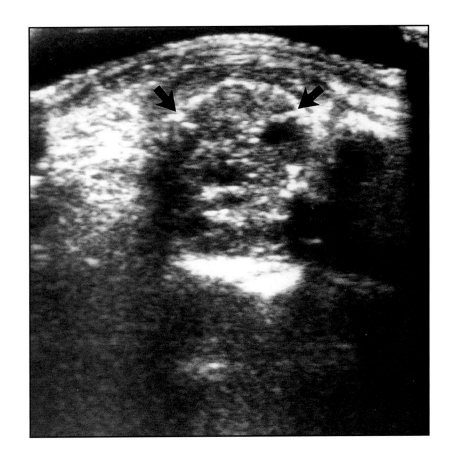

Image 8.30

Aneurysmal bone cyst. Transverse CT scan in a child with a sacral bone cyst on which a biopsy was performed under CT guidance. The soft tissue mass is completely encased within the expanded posterior elements of the sacrum (arrow).

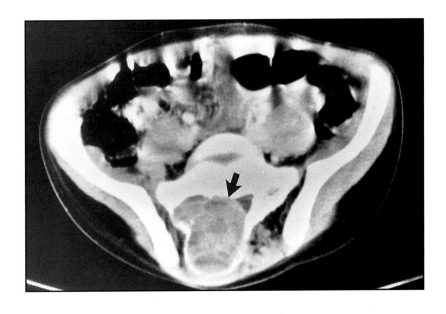

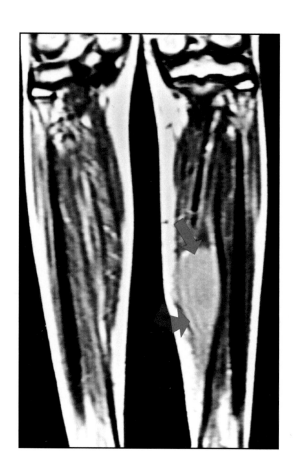

Image 8.31
Soft tissue involvement by myelogenous leukemia is well shown on this proton density weighted MR image of a child with a painful lower extremity (arrows). Plain radiographs (not shown) were entirely normal.

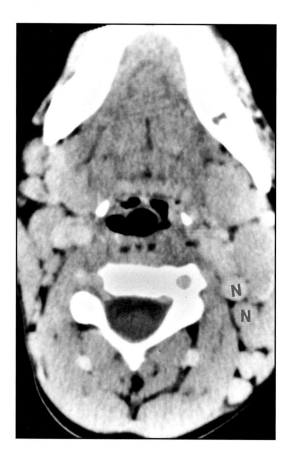

Image 8.32
Lymphoma. Transverse CT image of a child with non-Hodgkin's lymphoma. Extensive nodal masses are demonstrated in the spinal accessory space (N).

Image 8.33
Child with a medulloblastoma.
A Axial CT scan demonstrating a homogeneously enhancing mass involving the cerebellar vermis.
B Axial T2 weighted MR image demonstrating mixed signal within the mass (arrows) as well as edema in the adjacent part of the brain.

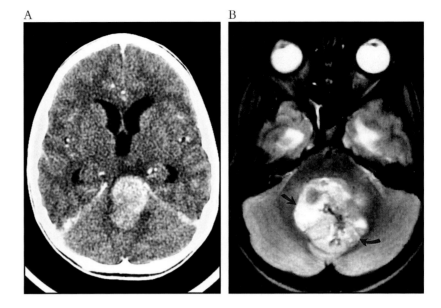

Image 8.34
The sagittal plane clearly depicts the origin of the mass in the vermis (arrows).

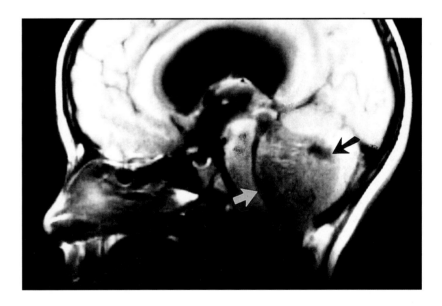

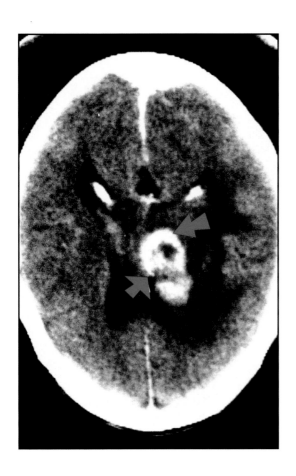

Image 8.35
Metastatic brain tumor. Enhanced CT scan of a mass involving the head of the caudate nucleus with extension into the thalamus (arrows).

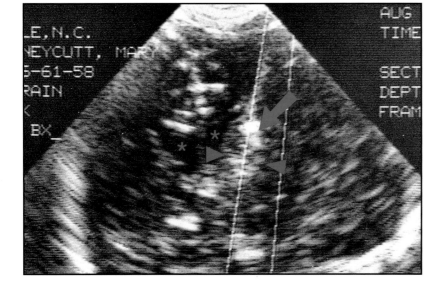

Image 8.36
A biopsy of the same mass as in Image 8.35 under real-time ultrasound guidance through the intact dura following turning of a bone flap (ultrasound image reversed left-right). Note the electronic guidelines generated by the ultrasound computer (dotted lines). The bright echo (arrow) is the needle tip within the ectogenic mass (arrowheads). The echo-free lateral ventricle (asterisk) is displaced to the left.

Image 8.37
Immunologically compromised child due to chemotherapy for leukemia with two nodular opacities on a chest radiograph.

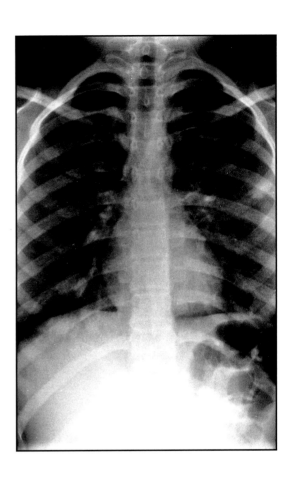

Image 8.38
CT scan demonstrating the lesion on the left in contact with the chest wall, (arrow) whereas the lesion on the right is almost completely surrounded by air-containing lung.

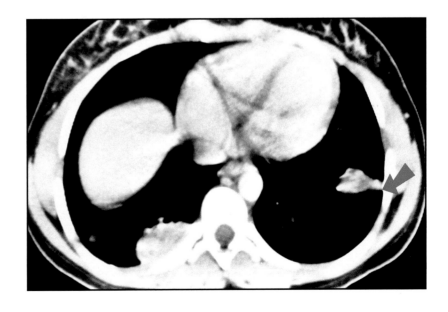

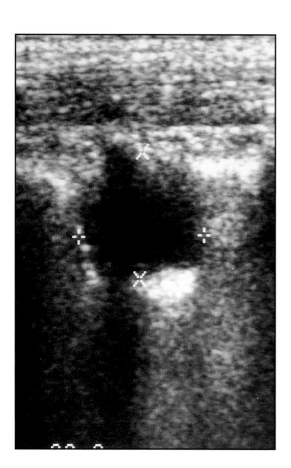

Image 8.39
Ultrasound of the left-sided lesion which is well seen as contact with the chest wall provided an acoustic window. FNA under ultrasound guidance proved the mass to be a fungal lesion.

References

1. Sty JR, Wells RG, Starshek RJ, Gregg DC. Diagnostic Imaging of Infants and Children. Aspin, Gaithersburg, Md, 1992.
2. Kirks D. Practical Pediatric Imaging: Diagnostic Radiology of Infants and Children. Little Brown, Boston, 1984, p 401-403.
3. Mahaffey SM, Ryckman FC, Martin LW. Clinical aspects of abdominal masses in children. *Sem Roentgenol* 23(3):161-174, 1988.
4. Mellicou MM, Uson AC. Palpable abdominal masses in infants and children: A report based on a review of 653 cases. *J Urol* 81:705-710, 1959.
5. Stevenson RJ. Abdominal masses. *Surg Clin North Am.* 65:1481-1504;1985.
6. Daneman A. Adrenal neoplasms in children. *Sem Roentgenol* 23(3):205-215, 1988.
7. Teele RL, Share JC. Ultrasonography of Infants and Children. WB Saunders Co, Philadelphia, 1991.
8. Stark DD, Mass AA, Brasch RC, et al. Neuroblastoma: Diagnostic imaging and staging. *Radiology* 148:101, 1983.
9. Donaldson JS, Shkolnik A. Pediatric renal masses. *Sem Roentgenol* 23(3):194, 1988.
10. Jaffee MH, White SJ, Silver JM, Heidolberger KP. Wilms' tumor: Ultrasound features pathologic correlation and diagnostic pitfalls. *Radiology* 140:147, 1981.
11. Relman AJ, Siegel MJ, Shackelford GD. Wilms' tumor in children: Abdominal US and CT evaluation. *Radiology* 160:501, 1986.
12. Lipman JC, Tumeh SS. The radiology of cavernous hemangioma of the liver. *Current Review Diagnostic Imaging* 1:30, 1990.
13. Dachman AA, Lichtenstein JE, Friedman AC, Hartman DS. Infantile hemangioendothelioma of the liver: a Radiologic-Pathologic Clinical Correlation. *AJR* 140:1049, 1983.
14. Stanley P, Hall TR, Woolley M, Diament MJ, Gilsanz V, Miller JH. Mesenchymal hamartoma of the liver in childhood: Sonographic and CT findings. *AJR* 147:1035-1039, 1986.
15. Dachman AH, Pakter R, Ros PR, et al. Hepatoblastoma: Radiologic-pathologic correlation in 50 cases. *Radiology* 164:15-19, 1987.
16. Cohen MD, Edwards MIC. Magnetic Resonance Imaging of Children. BC Decker, Inc, Philadelphia, 1990, p 639-642.
17. Grossman H, Ram PC, Coleman RA, et al. Hepatic US in type I glycogen storage disease (von Gierke's disease): Detection of hepatic adenoma and carcinoma. *Radiology* 141:753-756, 1981.
18. Brodsky RI, Friedman AC, Maurer AH, Radecki PD, Caroline DF. Hepatic cavernous hemangioma: Diagnoses with 99m TC labeled red cells and single photon emission CT. *AJR* 148:125-129, 1987.
19. Boechat MI, Kangerloo H, Gilsaz SV. Hepatic masses in children. *Sem Roentgenology* 23:185-193, 1988.
20. Lik C, Glaser GM, Quint LE, et al. Distinction of cavernous hemangioma from hepatic metastases with MR Imaging. *Radiology* 169:409-415, 1988.
21. Haller JO, Bass IS, Friedman AP. Pelvic masses in girls: An 8-year analysis stressing US as the prime imaging modality. *Ped Radiol* 14:363-368, 1984.

22. Geoffrey A, Coevanent D, Montague JP, et al. US and CT for diagnosis and follow-up of pelvic rhabdomyosarcoma in children. *Ped Radiol* 17:132-136, 1987.

23. Jing BS. Diagnostic imaging of abdominal and pelvic lymph nodes in lymphoma. *RCNA* 28(4):801-829, 1990.

24. Dalinka MA, Zlatkin MB, Chao P, Dvicun M, Kvessel HY. The use of magnetic resonance imaging in the evaluation of bone and soft-tissue tumors. *RCNA* 28(2):461, 1990.

25. Seeger LL, Eckavolt JL, Bassett JW. Cross-sectional imaging in the evaluation of osteogenic sarcoma: MRI and CT. *Sem Roentgenol* 23(3):174, 1989.

26. Som PM, Bergeon RI. Head and Neck Imaging. Mosby Year Book, 1991, p 566.

27. Stark DD, Bradley WG. Magnetic Resonance Imaging. Mosby Year Book, Vol. II. 1991, p. 1271.

28. Rumack CM, Wilson SR, Charboneau JW. Diagnostic Ultrasound. Mosby Year Book. 1991, p 461.

29. Levitt RG, Husband JE, Glazer HS. CT of primary germ cell tumors of the mediastinum. *AJR* 142:73-78;1984.

30. Heron CU, Husband JE, Williams MP. Hodgkins Disease: CT of the thymus. *Radiology* 167:647-651;1988.

31. Siegel MJ, Jamroz GA, Glazer HS, Abramson CL. MR imaging of intraspinal extension of neuroblastoma. *J Comput Assist Tomogr* 10:593-595;1986.

32. Schwartz EE, Katz SM, Mandell GA. Post inflammatory pseudo-tumors of the lung: Fibrous histiocytoma and related lesions. *Radiology* 136:609-613;1980.

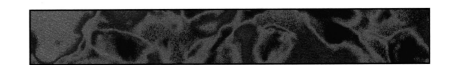

CHAPTER NINE

Lymph Nodes

Lymph nodes are among the most frequent sites of fine needle aspiration (FNA) biopsy in children.[1,2] While the great mjority of palpable lymph nodes in children occur in the head and neck and represent reactive hyperplasia, the presence of an enlarged lymph node remains a worrisome feature to parents and pediatricians alike. Lymphnode enlargement in a child may be watched for a period of a few weeks and event treated empirically with antibiotics. If a adenopathy persists, however, the pediatrician is faced with the clinical dilemma of either continuing observation with the risk that treatment for a serious illness may be delayed, or subjecting the child to open (and possibly unnecessary) biopsy with the risks and cost associated with that procedure. Although a model using a combination of chest x-ray findings, lymph node size and clinical symptomatology had claimed high specificity and sensitivity for predicting lymphoid pathology[3] other pediatricians have argued that there is no single clinical feature that can preselect for those nodes which will show treatable pathology at biopsy.[4] Selective use of FNA biopsy has many advantages for management of these children (Table 9.1).

The utility of lymph node FNA biopsy in children and young adults has been demonstrated in a study by Kardos et al.[5] They found a sensitivity and specificity of 93% and 95%, respectively, from lymph node FNA biopsy of 126 patients in the first 3 decades of life. In the 3 patients with a false negative FNA biopsy diagnosis, the delay in follow-up surgical biopsy was only 0, 5 and 14 days.

Not all masses presenting in the neck are lymph nodes (Table 9.2[6]), although many are clinically misdiagnosed as such. FNA biopsy can fre-

Table 9.1
Advantages of Pediatric Lymph Node FNA Biopsy

Ability To Triage Children With Lymphadenopathy:

    a. Can avoid open surgical biopsy in benign conditions that will regress, eg FNA can select those patients who could be followed with conservative management versus those who should undergo excisional biopsy.

    b. Helps to determine the nature of primary site of origin in malignant states for the first time patient.

    c. Helps the pediatrician to focus on an informed workup in various disease states potentially limiting extraneous and costly laboratory tests.

    d. Information from a less than optimal aspirate may still provide information that is of use to the pediatrician.

Capable Of Rapid, Effective Diagnosis:

    a. Confirmed diagnostic sensitivity and specificity in experienced centers.

    b. Minimal trauma and morbidity (if any) to the child (wide parental acceptance).

    c. Rapid turnaround time.

    d. Readily repeatable and applicable to multiple lesions.

Confirms That Mass in Question Is Indeed a Lymph Node.

Helps Select the Best Site for Biopsy in the Patient with Multiple Nodes or Nodes in Multiple Sites, if Biopsy Becomes Necessary.

Provides Material for Culture of Infectious Lesions.

Helps in Tumor Staging of a Patient with a Known Cancer.

Documents Metastatic or Recurrent Tumor in a Known Cancer Patient.

Preserves a Neoplastic Mass as a Marker for Response to Treatment.

Preserves Tissue Architecture if Subsequent Open Biopsy is Undertaken.

May Substitute for Open Biopsy in Selected Situations:

    a. Patients who are high risk or unacceptable surgical candidates.

    b. Patients (the child's parents) who refuse surgery.

    c. Where surgery is contraindicated or conservative management is more appropriate.

    d. Neoplasms where chemotherapy rather than surgery is the optimal treatment (eg lymphoblastic lymphoma).

May Alleviate Anxiety of both Parent and Pediatrician in a Benign yet Clinically Worrisome Condition.

Economical (applicable to both outpatient and inpatient settings).

Capacity to Obtain Cells for all Known Special Techniques in Pathology with Ease and Little Trauma to the Child, eg: cell culture, lymphocyte surface markers, immunocytochemistry, flow cytometry, electron microscopy, morphometry, karyotyping, diagnostic molecular methods including fluorescent in situ hybridization and polymerase chain reaction.

Table 9.2
Neck Masses Potentially Mistaken for Lymph Nodes in Children

Branchial Cleft Lesions
Thyroid Lesions
Inflammatory Masses: Subcutaneous Fat Necrosis, Abscess
Lymphangioma/Hemangioma
Other Benign Soft Tissue Neoplasms: Fibromatosis, Neural Tumor
Salivary Gland Lesions: Inflammation, Cyst, Neoplasm
Cervical Teratoma
Soft Tissue Sarcoma
Undescended/Aberrant Thymus
Skeletal Muscle and Bone[6]

quently explain the nature of a mass in the head and neck region, and not infrequently offer a difinitive diagnosis.

Children who are old enough to understand the procedure are generally quite cooperative in our experience; only rarely have we not attempted FNA because of a noncompliant child. Infants, of course, need to be restrained as do younger children. Some have advocated sedation prior to FNA. Local anesthesia is administered to the periphery of the lesion prior to FNA in some centers.

FNA is operator dependent. Expertise is necessary for representative sampling of the node, and in preparation and interpretation of smears. FNA biopsy has certain limitations, and, of course, is not the solution to all problems related to childhood lymphadenopathy. False-negative diagnoses occur on occasion for various reasons (Table 9.3). Further, severe coagulation disorder may be a contradiction to FNA biopsy of an enlarged superficial lymph node. Hematoma formation is the only complication we have experienced from lymph node FNA. Occasional reports of hemorrhage, fibrosis and partial or total infarction of lymph nodes have appeared.[7]

FNA biopsy of lymph nodes is not meant to replace clinical judgment. A nonmalignant interpretation requires clinical follow-up, and clinically suspicious lymphadenopathy should undergo either reaspiration or biopsy. Nevertheless, it is our belief that the advantages out-weigh the disadvantages, that the technique far outperforms the clinical indicators listed in the aforementioned series, and when combined with meaningful communication between pediatrician and pathologist enhances the care of the pediatric patient (Tables 9.1 and 9.3).

Table 9.3
Limitations and Causes of False-Negative Diagnoses of Pediatric Lymph Node FNA Biopsy

Inadequate Sampling. Cytologic Material May Not Be Representative of the Lesion, or May Miss the Lesion Entirely:

   a.   This is particularly important when a benign diagnosis is issued, and the question of adequacy is raised.

   b.   Fibrosis and/or necrosis within the node limits the amount of diagnostic material obtained.

   c.   Dilution of specimen from a bloody aspiration may obscure or limit the amount of diagnostic cellular material.

   d.   Aspiration smears are misleading if the node is only partially involved by a lesion and this area is not sampled.

Small or Deep Seated Lymph Node.

Subtyping of Certain Diseases Not Possible with Cytology Alone (eg Hodgkin's Disease).

Definitive Diagnosis of Certain Non-Neoplastic Conditions Requiring Knowledge of Histologic Architecture Not Possible (eg angiofollicular hyperplasia, progressive transformation of germinal centers).

Incorrect Interpretation by Pathologist.

Requires Expertise in Interpretation and Technique:

   a.   Although experience and training are required before consistently reliable results can be expected, this is not an insurmountable task. Faulty technique leads to an inability to obtain sufficient numbers of cells during the aspirate. Cells may be damaged beyond recognition due to improper aspiration or subsequent smearing of material onto slides.

   b.   Limited FNA biopsy experience exists in the U.S.

General Features

Although we perform both air-dried modified Romanowsky [May-Grunwald-Giemsa (MGG) or Diff-Quik] and alcohol-fixed, Papanicolaou-stained smears, we believe the former is particularly helpful for lymph node aspirates.

Methodical assessment of smear cellularity, cell pattern, predominant cell type and background material will ensure optimal evaluation of lymph node aspirates.[8] FNA biopsy smears from children with enlarged lymph nodes typically show intermediate to high cellularity. Low cellularity usually indicates that something other than a lymph node was aspirated or that a fibrotic process (eg, Hodgkin's disease, nodular sclerosis type) exists within the node.

Primary lymphoid lesions show individually scattered cells on the slide. There are exceptions to this pattern. Lymphohistiocytic aggregates are irregular, syncytial clusters of intermixed lymphocytes and histiocytes. They are considered derived from the germinal centers of secondary follicles, and generally indicate a benign process. Clusters of epithelioid histiocytes can be loosely or tightly arranged in granulomatous inflammation. Their nuclei are generally boomerang-shaped, which distinguishes them from dendritic histiocytes. Epithelioid histiocytes also do not exhibit the phagocytosis typical of tingible-body macrophages. Artificial clustering of lymphoid cells may occur in thick preparations: at the edge of an otherwise well-made smear, and in some lymphomas that exhibit extremely high cellularity from which a cell monolayer cannot be easily obtained. Unlike hematopoietic lesions, metastatic neoplasms (including many of the primitive small cell tumors of children) typically are distributed in both clusters and single cells.

Documenting the predominant cell type is helpful in distinguishing benign from malignant lesions. The small mature lymphocyte is ubiquitous in benign lymphoid proliferations of children. Although no one feature differentiates benign hyperplasia from malignant lymphoma, awareness of a heterogeneous rather than monotonous lymphoid cell population combined with the predominance of mature lymphocytes are keys to recognizing a benign process.

"Lymphoglandular bodies," a term coined by Söderstrom, are thought to represent cytoplasmic fragments of lymphoid cells sheared from the cells during the procedure.[9] They are a consistent background element of both benign and malignant lymph node aspirates, and appear as globular or flakelike structures, which may be vacuolated. Their presence in conspicuous numbers indicates, with some exceptions, that many cells (if not all) are lymphoid in nature.[10] Lymphoglandular bodies are better appreciated in Romanowsky-stained smears, in which they stain a light blue or blue-gray color, though they may be visualized with the Papanicolaou stain also. Other background elements of note include necrotic debris and foreign material.

Reactive Lymph Node Hyperplasia

In general, lymphoid tissue develops a much more florid proliferative response to antigenic stimuli in children than adults. Usually, a sin-

Table 9.4
Reactive Hyperplasia-Cytomorphology

Moderately to markedly cellular smears.

Admixture of large and small lymphocytes with a range of intermediate forms. Mature small lymphoid cells predominate.

Tingible-body macrophages.

Plasmacytoid cells ranging in size from mature plasma cells to plasmacytoid immunoblasts.

Lymphohistiocytic aggregates (follicular center fragments). These are sparse to absent in paracortical hyperplasia.

Variable number of histiocytes.

"Lymphoglandular bodies" in background.

gle node is involved, and the etiology is unknown. Clinical presentation is variable with most lymphadenopathy occurring in the cervical region, and usually <3 cm in greatest dimension.

Follicular hyperplasia is the most common histologic pattern. Sharply demarcated germinal centers within secondary follicles are usually prominent and contain readily apparent tingible-body macrophages. A variably heterogeneous population of plasma cells, histiocytes and plasmacytoid lymphocytes occupy an expanded interfollicular region in cases of marked hyperplasia. The sinus pattern shows prominent, distended sinuses with numerous histiocytes.

Smears are moderately to markedly cellular (Table 9.4). The key cytologic feature to recognizing a reactive lymph node in a child is the heterogeneous nature of the lymphoid cells.[11,12] A mixture of large and small lymphocytes exists with a range of intermediate forms, but it is the mature, small lymphocyte that predominates (Image 9.1). Tingible-body macrophages are common when hyperplasia is secondary to follicle proliferation rather than paracortical expansion of nonneoplastic lymph nodes (Image 9.2). Tingible-body macrophages in and of themselves are not, however, diagnostic of a binign process as they are commonly seen in high-grade lymphomas such as lymphoblastic or small non-cleaved cell lymphoma. Plasmacytoid cells ranging in size from mature plasma cells to plasmacytoid immunoblasts are common. Lymphocytes are ordinarily spread as single cells on the smear without nuclear overlapping or molding. Clusters of lymphohistiocytic aggregates, presumably representing follicular (germinal) center fragments, are also generally present (Image 9.3). The number of individual histiocytes depends on the amount of medullary sinus histiocytosis in the node.

Potential Problems in Diagnosis: As mentioned, a major clue to differentiating a benign form malignant lymphoid proliferation lies in recognizing the heterogeneous (po;ymorphous) nature of lymphoid cells on the smear. None of the major childhood non-Hodgkin's lymphomas (NHLs) demonstrate this range of various lymphoid elements. One should be careful not to overlook the mononuclear Reed-Sternberg cells of Hodgkin's disease in smears that otherwise appear to show reactive lyperplasia.

A major clue to differentiating a benign from malignant lymphoid proliferation lies in recognizing the heterogeneous (polymorphous) nature of lymphoid cells on the smear

Since lymphohistiocytic aggregates are common in benign pediatric lymph node aspirates, they should not be confused with deposits of metastatic tumor. Their presence, however, does not preclude a lymph node metastasis. Several such aggregates on smears have a positive correlation with the follicular form of hyperplasia. They are sparse to absent in those enlarged nodes with few or no secondary follicles such as sinus histiocytes or paracortical hyperplasia.

Ancillary studies demonstrate immunoreactivity for both T and B cell lymphocyte surface markers. B cells predominate in florid follicular hyperplasia and demonstrate both kappa and lambda light chains. Flow cytometry for lymphocyte surface markers can be performed readily directly from FNA biopsy material, and may be helpful in difficult cases. Electron microscopy has a limited role in diagnosis.

Acute Lymphadenitis

Clinical presentation is variable. Infections of the scalp, mouth, pharynx, and in children particularly, the middle ear may cause localized lymphadenopathy in the head and neck. An isolated enlarged lymph node or group of nodes may be involved. Fever and tenderness to palpation are common, but not universal findings. Skin overlying the nodes may be erythematous. Histologically, a diffuse infiltration of the node by neutrophils is seen with or without microabscess formation. Alternatively, the node may be entirely destroyed by acute suppurative inflammation.

Smears of an aspirated abscess are hypercellular and contain sheets of neutrophils with varying degrees of cell necrosis (Image 9.4). In acute lymphadenitis without overt abscess formation, the cellular elements of reactive hyperplasia may also be present (Table 9.5). Occasionally, bacteria and fungi may be seen directly with Romanowsky-stained smears (Image 9.5). Nonetheless, stains for bacteria, fungi, and acid-fast bacilli should and can be performed directly on aspirate smears. A portion of the aspirate also should be sent for direct microbiologic culture.

Table 9.5
Lymphadenitis-Cytomorphology

Suppurative lymphadenitis: sheets of neutrophils with varying degrees of individual cell necrosis; bacteria may be present.

Granuloma: loosely or tightly clustered epithelioid histiocytes [cells with eccentric oval or elongated nuclei and moderate amount of cytoplasm].

Granulomatous lymphadenitis:

a.   Epithelioid histiocytes, necrosis, inflammation, (suggests mycobacteria, cat-scratch disease, fungal infections), "negative image" bacilli (mycobacteria).

b.   Low cellularity with groups of epithelioid histiocytes, multinucleate giant cells and few lymphoid cells (suggests sarcoid, foreign body granuloma, early mycobacteria infection).

Cell elements described for reactive hyperplasia may be seen.

Granulomatous Lymphadenitis

Clinical presentation and anatomic site are variable, but the head and neck region are most commonly involved. Either an isolated enlarged lymph node or matted group of nodes may be involved. There may be tenderness and firmness of the node upon palpation. The node may suppurate and form a draining sinus, but this is unusual. One should ask about recent scratches by a cat.

In necrotizing granulomatous lymphadenitis, the fully developed lesion is characterized by necrotizing granulomas. Granulomas contain either bland necrosis, or central microabscesses with numerous neutrophils. They are lined by palisading epithelioid cells and occasional multinucleated giant cells.

Nonnecrotizing granulomatous lymphadenitis shows partial or complete replacement of the node by discrete noncaseating granulomas (eg, sarcoid). Multinucleated giant cells are often present. In some cases, clusters of epithelioid histiocytes are present in the paracortex, at the edge or within germinal centers without necrosis or giant cells (toxoplasmosis). Follicular hyperplasia is a common component.

Smears of necrotizing granulomatous lymphadenitis unveil a moderate to highly cellular population of neutrophils, a variable degree of background cell necrosis, and occasional multinucleated giant cells (Table 9.5). Granulomas are found in varying numbers. They appear as loose or tightly clustered epithelioid histiocytes. The latter are recognized as cells with eccentrically placed oval to elongated nuclei simulating a "footprint" or boomerang shape and a moderate amount of cytoplasm, which may be vacuolated (Image 9.6).

Causes include cat-scratch disease, and infections due to mycobacteria, *Yersinia*, tularemia, brucellosis, fungi, and lymphogranuloma venereum. Mycobacterial (tuberculosis and atypical mycobacteria) infection more commonly displays necrosis without a large component of neutrophils. Some of the granulomas on the FNA biopsy smears of cat-scratch disease may have a stellate configuration and a central scattering of neutrophils, which closely echos characteristic tissue histopathology findings (Image 9.7).[13]

In nonnecrotizing granulomatous lymphadenitis, smears are more likely to be hypocellular or have only moderate cellularity (Table 9.5). Granulomas (loosely or tightly clustered), and multinucleated giant cells are found. Usually, lesser numbers of histiocytes are incorporated into granuloma formation in the nonnecrotizing than in necrotizing form. The cellular elements described for reactive hyperplasia may be present in both necrotizing and nonnecrotizing processes.

Potential causes include toxoplasmosis, sarcoid, foreign body granuloma, Hodgkin's disease, lymphangiogram effect, and early mycobacterial infection. In the presumptive case of toxoplasmosis that we have encountered, epithelioid histiocytes were only very loosely assembled, and widely scattered on smears. This is similar to previous descriptions of *Toxoplasma* lymphadenitis.[14] It is very rare for cysts of *T gondii* to be found. Serologic testing is necessary to confirm the diagnosis.

Children with AIDS or who are otherwise severely immunocompromised do not mount an effective granulomatous response to certain infectious organisms. Mycobacterial or fungal infection may elicit only

Potential causes include toxoplasmosis, sarcoid, foreign body granuloma, Hodgkin's disease, lymphangiogram effect and early mycobacterial infection

a simple acute or chronic inflammatory response. Stains for organisms are mandatory in these patients. Attention has been called to the "negative image" phenomenon of both intra- and extracellular acid-fast bacilli, which are readily discerned in Romanowsky-stained smears of these individuals, but not with the Papanicolaou stain (Image 9.8).[15,16] Silverman et al have made us aware that crystals of the antimycobacterial drug clofazimine may be ingested by macrophages and thus closely mimic the appearance created by acid-fast bacilli.[17] Both appear as multiple needle-shaped and rhomboid structures within macrophage cytoplasm producing a "pseudo-Gaucher" cell. Unlike acid-fast bacilli, clofazimine crystals are polarizable, are readily seen with the Papanicolaou stain, do not occur extracellularly and are not positive with stains for acid-fast bacilli.

Definitive diagnosis for the infectious causes of granulomatous lymphadenitis requires culture of the organism. If one is clinically suspicious for such a lesion at the time of FNA biopsy, a portion of the aspirate may be directly submitted for culture, or the patient may be immediately reaspirated to obtain such material. One of the advantages of immediate interpretation of the aspirate is to recognize this inflammation, and reaspirate the mass for culture (if it was not done initially) while the child is still on the premises. Special stains for acid-fast bacilli and fungi made directly on aspirate smears are useful and easily performed.

Infectious Mononucleosis

Infectious Mononucleosis (IM) is a self-limited disorder caused by infection with the Epstein-Barr virus (EBV). The IM syndrome of fever, pharyngitis, peripheral blood atypical lymphocytosis, and splenomegaly usually affects adolescents and young adults. Lymphadenopathy is typically cervical, but may be generalized, and affected nodes may be tender to palpation. Lymph node enlargement usually regresses within 2 to 3 weeks. Tests for heterophil IgM antibody are positive in a majority of patients. Serologic profiles for antibodies specific to EBV are also confirmatory.[18]

Lymph nodes demonstrate follicular and interfollicular hyperplasia with a marked proliferation of immunoblasts. Individual cell necrosis and mitoses are common. Occasionally, Reed-Sternberg–like cells with prominent nucleoli are seen. The lymph node capsule is frequently infiltrated by immunoblasts, plasma cells, and plasmacytoid lymphocytes.

Aspiration smears are extremely cellular (Table 9.6). A heterogeneous lymphoid cell population occurs with obviously increased numbers of plasmacytoid lymphocytes. Immunoblasts, which appear as large cells with fine nuclear chromatin, prominent nucleoli, and ample pale-to-dark blue cytoplasm either predominate or constitute a large percentage of lymphoid cells (Image 9.9).[19,20] Rarely, pleomorphic cells simulating Reed-Sternberg cells may be found.

Potential Problems in Diagnosis: The role of FNA biopsy in IM is to suggest this as a presumptive diagnosis, which should be followed up by confirmatory serologic testing, thus avoiding an unnecessary excisional biopsy in a child. Cytologic differentiation from reactive hyperplasia lies in recognizing the quantitative increase in immunoblasts and plas-

Cytologic differentiation from reactive hyperplasia lies in recognizing the quantitative increase in immunoblasts and plasmacytoid lymphocytes

Table 9.6
Infectious Mononucleosis-Cytomorphology

Smears usually quite cellular.

Immunoblasts [large cells with fine nuclear chromatin and prominent nucleoli, and deep blue or grey cytoplasm in Romanowsky smears] predominate with a mixture of small and large lymphocytes.

Plasmacytoid lymphocytes easily found.

Tingible-body macrophages.

Pleomorphic cells rare to absent.

"Lymphoglandular bodies" in background.

---

macytoid lymphocytes. Hodgkin's disease with plasmacytoid cells is another possible source of confusion.

Aspirates of Hodgkin's disease, however, are not usually as cellular, and the immunoblasts are cytologically different from Reed-Sternberg cells. Immunoblasts have abundant cytoplasm that varies from a pale shade to dark blue, and round nuclei with fine chromatin and regular nucleoli, while Reed-Sternberg cells and their variants tend to have gray cytoplasm, with nuclei that are irregular in contour, irregular nucleoli, and coarse chromatin.[19]

Definitive diagnosis requires confirmatory serologic studies for heterophile antibody or specific Epstein-Barr virus antibodies.

Immunostaining or flow cytometry shows a heterogeneous immunologic phenotype with a predominance of CD8 (suppressor) T cells.

Rosai-Dorfman disease (Sinus Histiocytosis with Massive Lymphadenopathy)

This disorder of unknown etiology characteristically involves the cervical lymph nodes of young children, especially blacks. Lymph node enlargement not uncommonly is massive, bilateral, and painless. This disorder often includes fever, leukocytosis, and hypergammaglobulinemia. Transformation to malignant lymphoma has not been reported.

Histologic examination reveals marked distention and hyperplasia of medullary sinuses within lymph nodes with few, if any, residual follicular centers. A mixed lymphoid population exists, but the most obvious cell is a phagocytic histiocyte. Phagocytosis of red blood cells and viable lymphocytes (emperipolesis) is common.

Smears reveal characteristic features of reactive hyperplasia (Table 9.4). In addition, scattered throughout the smear are histiocytes which have engulfed cytologically intact small, mature lymphocytes within their cytoplasm (Image 9.10).[21,22]

Potential Problems in Diagnosis: Collections of engulfed cytoplasmic lymphocytes may be so numerous as to obscure the underlying histiocytic nucleus, and thus miss the diagnosis. The aspirate may also be dismissed as reactive hyperplasia if only a few such phagocytic histiocytes are found. One should make sure that mature lymphocytes are actually intracytoplasmic, otherwise typical lymphohistiocytic aggregates of a nonspecific reactive lymph node could be confused with this entity. Sometimes bacterial, viral, or fungal infections will demonstrate an occasional histiocyte with lymphocytic phagocytosis, but not in the quantity characteristic of Rosai-Dorfman disease. Finally, S-100 positive immunostaining of phagocytic histiocytes (which can be performed directly on the smear) combined with the proper clinical presentation confirms the diagnosis.

Hodgkin's Disease

Hodgkin's Disease occurs principally in late adolescence and young adults; it is rare before 5 years of age. Cervical and supraclavicular lymph nodes are most commonly involved, but axillary, mediastinal and inguinal lymph nodes are sometimes affected.

Hepatomegaly/splenomegaly, fever, night sweats, and weight loss may coexist with lymphadenopathy. With the nodular sclerosis subtype, the node may be very firm to palpation. The aspirator may experience a gritty sensation during the aspiration procedure, and a meager amount of cells may be procured. If multiple nodes are involved, smaller nodes may contain connective tissue and thus yield a greater amount of diagnostic material (Dr M Glant, personal communication).

Histologic classification has subdivided Hodgkin's Disease into four subtypes. The nodular sclerosis subtype is the most common. The lymph node is partially or completely effaced by a diverse cell population, collagen bands, and Reed-Sternberg cells of lacunar type. The mixed cellularity subtype is second in incidence, and includes a similar diverse cell mixture (eosinophils, mature lymphocytes, plasma cells, histiocytes) without the fibrosis, more numerous Reed-Sternberg cells, and mononuclear variants. The other forms are distinctly uncommon in children.

Cellularity of smears may range from low to intermediate depending on the amount of sclerosis within the node (Table 9.7). With extensive fibrosis, diagnostic cells may not be obtained at all. Partial involvement of the node will yield increased smear cellularity. The smear picture described for reactive hyperplasia is found. In addition, a concentrated search for classic Reed-Sternberg cells and variants is required (Image 9.11). Classic Reed-Sternberg cells are large cells with two or more mirror-image nuclei and prominent, irregularly shaped macronucleoli (Images 9.12, 9.13). Reed-Sternberg variants are large mononuclear cells with irregular (frequently lobated) nuclear contours, coarse chromatin, and grayish cytoplasm (Romanowsky stain) (Images 9.14, 9.15, 9.16). Nucleoli may be prominent, but in the so-called polyploid variants, nucleoli are absent or indistinct, and cytoplasm is often stripped from nuclei.[23] Background fibrous stoma (anucleate metachromatic staining material in Romanowsky stain), eosinophils, necrosis, plasma cells, and neutrophils are present in varying amounts. Granulomas (usually cellular) may occasionally be found.

Potential Problems in Diagnosis: Identifying Reed-Sternberg variants combined with the proper polymorphous cell background is key to sug-

Table 9.7
Hodgkin's Disease-Cytomorphology

Moderately or sparsely cellular smears.

Polymorphous lymphoid cell population similar to reactive hyperplasia.

Reed-Sternberg cells (classic binucleate, multinucleate and mononuclear forms); mirror-image nuclei with prominent, large nucleoli.

Polyploid cells very common (large cells with densely hyperchromatic single or multinucleate and often lobulated nuclei. Bytoplasm often striooed from cell nuclei).

Fragments of collagen, eosinophils, epithelioid histiocytes (granuloma formation), necrosis, plasma cells and neutrophils variable in amount.

"Lymphoglandular bodies" in background.

---

gesting the cytologic diagnosis because classic binucleated Reed-Sternberg cells may not exist on smears. One should diligently search for such cells particularly in a node which is clinically suspicious for lymphoma, but at first appears merely reactive. Reed-Sternberg variants may be few in number, but ordinarily are more readily found than classic Reed-Sternberg cells. Their size usually makes them discernible from the surrounding reactive lymphoid population. If one requires classic Reed-Sternberg cells to suggest the cytologic diagnosis of Hodgkin's Disease and discounts these Reed-Sternberg variants, the node may be mistakenly dismissed as reactive hyperplasia.

A suspicion of Hodgkin's Disease arising from a lymph node FNA biopsy in a new patient, in our view, should be confirmed with surgical biopsy. We have not been able to subtype confidently Hodgkin's Disease by cytology alone, although others have had mixed results doing so using differential cell counts.[24,25]

Immunoperoxidase staining of smears or cell blocks from aspirates can occasionally be helpful in differentiating Hodgkin's disease from other lymphomas. Classic Reed-Sternberg cells and variants express both CD15 (Leu M1) and CD30 (Ki-1), and are negative for CD45 (leukocyte common antigen) (Image 9.17). The lymphocyte-predominant subtype of Hodgkin's Disease stains just the opposite, and is both CD15- and CD30- negative, while showing immunoreactivity for CD45. Large cell anaplastic (Ki-1) lymphoma may have cells indistinguishable from Reed-Sternberg cells. Generally, atypical cells stain positively with CD30 and CD45 and do not stain with CD15.

A suspicion of Hodgkin's disease arising from a lymph node FNA biopsy in a new patient, in our view, should be confirmed with surgical biopsy

Childhood NHL

Childhood NHL incorporates three major histopathologic classes: Lymphoblastic lymphoma, Small Non-Cleaved Cell lymphoma (Burkitt and non-Burkitt types), and Large Cell lymphoma. Unlike lymphomas of adults, those of children are commonly extranodal, almost always high grade, and only rarely demonstrate a follicular pattern.[26] Knowledge of both morphologic and immunophenotypic characteristics are necessary for definitive diagnosis (Table 9.8).

Table 9.8

Comparative Cytology Of Pediatric Non-Hodgkin's Lymphomas

Feature	Lymphoblastic	Small Non-Cleaved Cell	Large Cell
Cell Size	monomorphic; about 1.5-2 x larger than a mature lymphocyte	monomorphic; about 1.5 x larger than a mature lymphocyte	variable; greater than 2-3 x larger than a mature lymphocyte
Nuclear chromatin	finely granular	coarsely granular	variable; finely granular to clumped
Nucleoli	indistinct, small	prominent; 1 to 5	variable; single to multiple; indistinct to prominent
Mitotic index	high	high	variable
Cytoplasm	meager	moderate	variable; may be ample
Cytoplasmic vacuoles	inconspicuous	common	inconspicuous
Tingible-body macrophages	common	common	variable
Surface markers (+)	Tdt, CD10, T-cell antigens, Ki-67	B-cell antigens, kappa, lambda, CD10, Ki-67	variable; most type as B-cells

Modified from Kjeldsberg et al.

Lymphoblastic Lymphoma

In the International Working Formulation (IWF) classification of non-Hodgkin's lymphoma, lymphoblastic lymphoma is categorized as a high-grade, rapidly progressive neoplasm. It comprises anywhere from 30% to 50% of pediatric non-Hodgkin's lymphomas, in contrast to the situation in adults where it comprises less than 5% of all lymphomas. Lymphoblastic lymphoma occurs principally in adolescence and young adults; it affects males four times more frequently than females. It is nearly always supradiaphragmatic, and the patient routinely presents with an anterior mediastinal mass. As a rule, some degree of respiratory compromise secondary to tracheal compression exists at the time of clinical presentation (Image 9.17). As these patients are high-risk surgical candidates due to tracheal compression (which is exacerbated by tracheal relaxation under general anesthesia), FNA biopsy is a perfect alternative to surgical biopsy in this setting.[27]

Peripheral lymphadenopathy is likely to be cervical, supraclavicular, or axillary. Bone marrow involvement at the time of diagnosis is not uncommon. Only a small percentage of patients have a leukemic presentation with anemia, and thrombocytopenia, but transformation to a leukemic phase commonly occurs during the course of disease. Gonadal and central nervous system involvement is not unusual during relapse.

Diffuse effacement of the lymph node occurs in tissue sections by lymphoblasts that are morphologically identical to those of acute lymphoblastic leukemia.[28,29] A starry-sky pattern (presence of tingible body macrophages diffusely scattered throughout the patternless population of lymphoblasts) occurs in about one-third of cases. Lymphoblasts are small with a meager amount of cytoplasm, powdery chromatin, and indistinct nucleoli. Their nuclei are smaller than those of the benign histiocytes.

The aspirate will produce highly cellular smears containing noncohesive, monotonous lymphoblasts (Table 9.9). Lymphoblasts are about twice the size of mature lymphocytes. Their nuclei incorporate the features of L1 and L2 morphology of the French-American-British classification for acute lymphoblastic leukemia. Nuclei are commonly round, but may be irregularly shaped with nuclear clefts and convolutions.[30] Nuclear chromatin is fine and delicate with imperceptible nucleoli (Image 9.18). Mitotic figures are frequent. Cytoplasm is sparse with either obscure or absent vacuoles. Plasma cells and plasmacytoid lymphocytes are typically absent. Tingible-body macrophages and necrosis vary in extent.

Most cases are immature T-cell lymphomas with a small percentage being of pre-B cell lineage.[27] TdT (terminal deoxynucleotidyl transferase) is immunoreactive in greater than 80% of cases (Image 9.19); CALLA (CD10) is immunoreactive in greater than 40%. Other T-cell antibodies (CD 5, 8, 4, 3, 1, and 7) may be immunoreactive. Because of the high mitotic rate in lymphoblastic lymphoma, Ki-67 proliferation antigen almost always yeilds a positive reaction. Punctate cytoplasmic staining occurs with acid phosphatase. PAS stain shows coarse granular cytoplasmic staining ("block positivity") in some cases. Cytogenetic abnormalities are variable.

In our experience, the presence of the aforementioned cytopathology and confirmatory immunophenotype in a patient with the typical clinical setting is sufficient for a difinitive diagnosis of lymphoblastic NHL. We have treated several patients on protocol with a turnaround time of <24 hours using FNA solely to establish the diagnosis.

Small Non-Cleaved Cell NHL (Burkitt type)

Small non-cleaved cell lymphoma (SNCL) is a high-grade, prognostically unfavorable neoplasm in the IWF classification. Highest incidence is

Table 9.9
Lymphoblastic Lymphoma-Cytomorphology

Highly cellular smears with non-cohesive, uniform cell population.

Blasts about twice the size of mature lymphocytes.

Nuclei: delicate fine chromatin, imperceptible nucleoli, variable nuclear shape-convolutions may be present (L1/L2 morphology).

Frequent mitotic figures.

Cytoplasm: very sparse with absent or obscure vacuoles.

Plasmacytoid cells absent.

Tingible-body macrophages and necrosis may be present.

"Lymphoglandular bodies" in background.

---

in the first 2 decades of life. In contrast to lymphoblastic lymphoma, small non-cleaved cell lymphoma is primarily a subdiaphragmatic, extranodal neoplasm in North America, most often affecting the terminal ileum, appendix, cecum, ovaries, and colon. Presenting clinical symptoms include abdominal pain, ascites, nausea and vomiting, intussusception, and gastrointestinal bleeding. Other sites of involvement may include Waldeyer's ring. Involvement of the mandible and maxilla, a common mode of presentation in Africa, is unusual in developed Western countries. Peripheral lymphadenopathy, if present, is most likely to be inguinal.

Histologically, there is diffuse effacement of lymph nodes by a monotonous lymphoid cell population. A starry-sky pattern with a very high mitotic index exists in the majority of cases.[31] The morphologic distinction between Burkitt and non–Burkitt subtypes is somewhat subjective with the latter demonstrating greater cell heterogeneity, and differences in number of nucleoli.[32] It has questionable clinical relevance in children, and we do not attempt to make this distinction cytologically.

Aspirate smears are highly cellular and consist of dyshesive, monotonous lymphoid cells which are $1^1/_2$ to 3 times the size of a mature lymphocyte (Table 9.10). Most nuclei are round with coarsely clumped chromatin and one to several discrete nucleoli (Image 9.20). Cell cytoplasm is deeply basophilic, moderate in amount, and typically laden with lipid vacuoles (Image 9.21). Background lymphoglandular bodies are also not uncommonly vacuolated. Tingible-body macrophages and individual cell necrosis are common. There are innumerable mitoses throughout the smear.

These are lymphomas of B cell lineage (Image 9.22).[34] Staining for TdT is negative with rare exceptions, but cell immunoreactivity occurs in most cases for monoclonal kappa or lambda light chain, CD19, CD20, and CD10 (CALLA). Ki-67 proliferation antigen is almost always positive. Cytogenetics shows a translocation of the *c-myc* oncogene between chromosomes 8;14 in 80% of cases; t(8;22), and t(2;8) translocations are the other chromosomal derangements that can occur.

Large Cell NHL

The age at presentation for large cell NHL is variable. Anatomic sites of involvement are frequently extranodal and include the abdomi-

Table 9.10
Small Non-Cleaved Cell Lymphoma-Cytomorphology

Highly cellular smears with non-cohesive, uniform cell population.

Blasts about 2 - 3 times the size of mature lymphocytes.

Nuclei: variable shape (although most are round), coarsely clumped with one to several nucleoli.

Cytoplasm: moderate, frequently vacuolated (lipid).

Innumerable mitoses.

Tingible-body macrophages and necrosis common.

"Lymphoglandular bodies" in background.

Table 9.11
Large Cell Lymphoma-Cytomorphology

Usually highly cellular smears with non-cohesive uniform or variable sized population of larger cells, usually greater than 3 times size of mature lymphocyte.

Nuclei: variable in shape and number of nucleoli. Immunoblasts defined as large cells with single, strikingly obvious nucleoli.

Cytoplasm: moderate to abundant.

Tingible-body macrophages and necrosis may be present.

"Lymphoglandular bodies" in background.

---

nal cavity, mediastinum, skin, and tonsils. Large cell anaplastic (polymorphous immunoblastic) lymphoma with the CD 30 (Ki-1) antigen phenotype may occur in older children and young adults.[35] Peripheral T-cell lymphomas are uncommon in children, but when they occur are typically of the large cell type. A recent series of 22 children with peripheral T-cell lymphomas\ revealed 10 as morphologically diffuse large cell lymphoma, and 5 as large cell anaplastic type.[36] Skin was the most common site of extranodal involvement.

Diffuse effacement of lymph nodes with immunoblastic, large non-cleaved and large cleaved cell types occurs in histologic sections. Nuclei are large with prominent and, commonly, multiple nucleoli. Large cell anaplastic lymphoma has a paracortical and sinusoidal pattern of involvement mimicking metastatic carcinoma and Hodgkin's disease.

There is a greater degree of variability in cellular morphology in this type of childhood lymphoma than in the prior two entities (Table 9.11).[37] Highly cellular smears of non-cohesive, uniform or variably sized lymphoid cells are the rule. Cells are generally greater than 3 times the size of a mature lymphocyte. Nuclei are larger than those of tissue macrophages, are more variable in shape and in the number of nucleoli they contain (Image 9.23). Cell cytoplasm is moderate to abundant. Immunoblasts, large cells with a single, strikingly obvious nucleolus and deeply basophilic cytoplasm, may be present on smears. Tingible-body macrophages and necrosis are not uncommon.

Immunologic phenotyping is inconsistent, although B-cell neoplasms are somewhat more common than T-cell types. Large cell anaplastic lymphoma is usually a T-cell neoplasm, but may be B-cell or null cell.[38]

Metastatic Neoplasms

In contrast to adults, lymph node metastases are not frequent in children. In children, papillary carcinoma of the thyroid may metastasize early in the course of the disease, and present as primary lymphadenopathy. Among the malignant small round cell tumors of childhood, neuroblastoma, and rhabdomyosarcoma are more likely to metastasize to lymph nodes, and, only infrequently is, lymph node metastasis is the initial clinical manifestation of disease.

The cytologic diagnosis of a metastatic neoplasm in a lymph node is usually much less difficult than that of malignant lymphoma. In papillary carcinoma and most examples of nonlymphoreticular malignant small round cell tumors of childhood, discrete cell aggregates or some loose clustering of cells usually helps differentiate these neoplasms from malignant lymphoma. Depending on the degree of involvement in the node there may be no lymphoid elements on the smear. As previously stated, the absence of numerous "lymphoglandular bodies" in the smear background is good evidence that lymphoid cells have not been aspirated.

Undifferentiated Nasopharyngeal Carcinoma (Lymphoepithelioma)

This neoplasm is common in adolescents and young adults. The primary tumor is located in the roof and lateral walls of the nasopharynx, but it is most frequently detected as an enlarged unilateral or bilateral cervical lymph node harboring metastatic carcinoma. Epstein-Barr virus has been implicated as a causative agent in nasopharyngeal carcinoma.

Lymph nodes histologically show a variable degree of replacement of tumor deposits. Carcinoma may be distributed either as large or small cohesive islands of obvious epithelial cells or may be scattered as few or single cells admixed with and obscured by the lymphoid cell background.

The cytologic findings of a reactive lymph node are generally present. Individual as well as small syncytial groups of poorly differentiated epithelial cells occur, sometimes in very small numbers (Image 9.24). These epithelial cells are somewhat larger cells with crowded, sometimes overlapping oval and spindled nuclei with fine chromatin, single prominent nucleoli, and moderate amounts of cytoplasm with indistinct cell borders.[39,40] Bare nuclei are common. Individual cell necrosis may occur; however, cytoplasmic keratinization is largely absent.

Potential Problems in Diagnosis: Aspiration smears of lymphoepithelioma may be troublesome because the overwhelming population of lymphoid elements can obscure individual and small clusters of undifferentiated malignant cells. A diligent effort must be made to examine all cell clusters in a lymph node aspirate.

Cytokeratin is expressed by malignant epithelial cells, which are, conversely, CD45-negative. Electron microscopy will reveal cytoplasmic tonofilaments and desmosomes. Cells obtained by FNA biopsy have been used in the polymerase chain reaction to test for Epstein-Barr virus genomes.[41]

Epstein-Barr virus has been implicated as a causative agent in nasopharyngeal carcinoma

Image 9.1

Reactive hyperplasia.

A There is a range in cell sizes with small mature lymphocytes predominating. Note the numerous lymphoglandular bodies in the background indicative of the lymphoid nature of these cells. (Romanowsky).

B The heterogeneity of lymphoid cells is somewhat more difficult to appreciate in alcohol-fixed smears. Tingible-body macrophages are at the center and far right. (Papanicolaou).

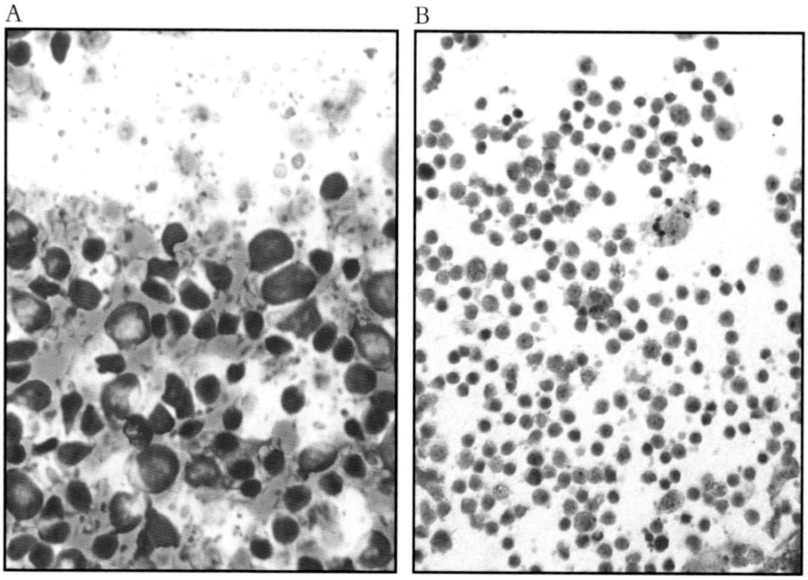

Image 9.2

Reactive hyperplasia.

A Tingible-body macrophages. (Romanowsky).

B (Papanicolaou).

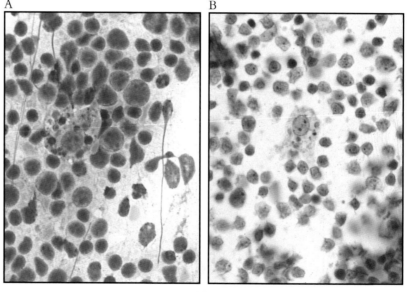

Image 9.3

Reactive hyperplasia.

A and **B**, Lymphohistiocytic aggregates. A delicate capillary can be seen traversing through the cluster in **A**. (Romanowsky).

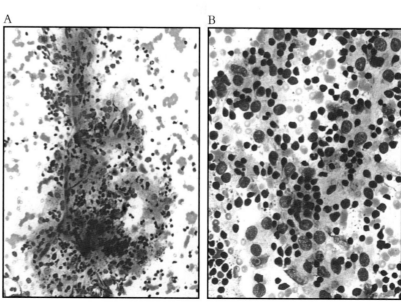

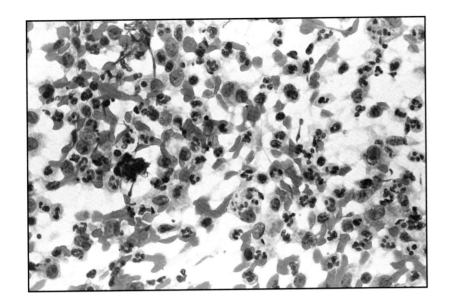

Image 9.4
Acute lymphadenitis. Neutrophils have obscured most of the remaining lymphoid cells. (Papanicolaou).

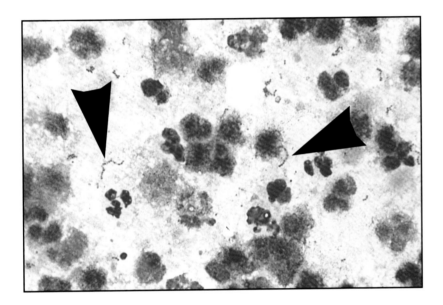

Image 9.5
Acute lymphadenitis. Bacterial cocci (arrowheads) can be found among the degenerating neutrophils. Culture from the aspirate grew *Staphylococcus*. (Romanowsky).

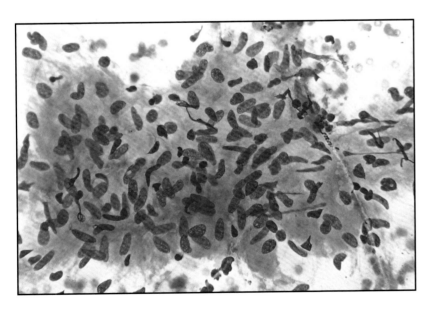

Image 9.6
Granuloma formation. A tight cluster of epithelioid histiocytes with abundant cytoplasm and elongated sometimes comma-shaped nuclei. (Romanowsky).

Image 9.7
Nectotizing granulomatous lymphadenitis.
A Central granuloma amidst a myriad of neutrophils. (Romanowsky).
B Loosely formed granuloma. (Papanicolaou).

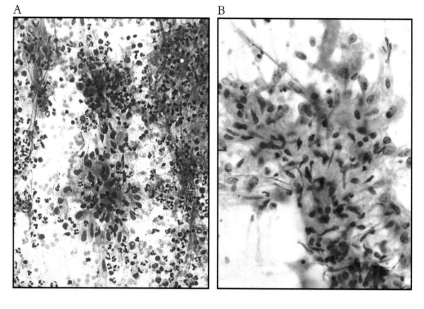

Image 9.8
Mycobacterium avium-intracellulare lymphadenitis, HIV-positive child.
A Numerous linear striations ("negative images") caused by acid-fast bacilli both extracellularly (arrowhead), and within a histiocyte simulating the appearance of a Gaucher cell. (Romanowsky).
B Intra–and extracellular acid-fast bacilli. (Ziehl-Neelsen).

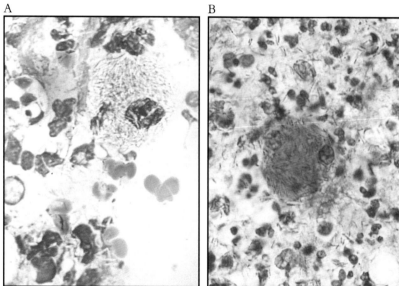

Image 9.9
Infectious mononucleosis. Numerous immunoblasts are scattered amongst mature lymphocytes and plasmacytoid cells (arrowhead). (Romanowsky).

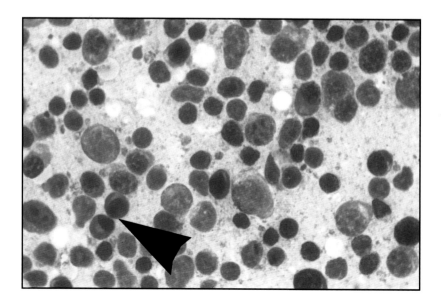

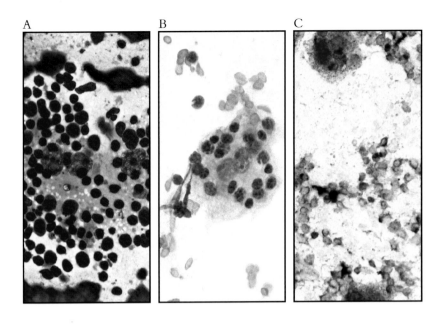

Image 9.10
Rosai-Dorfman disease. Histiocytes with numerous engulfed mature lymphocytes.
A Romanowsky.
B Papanicolaou.
C Positive S-100 immunocytochemistry.

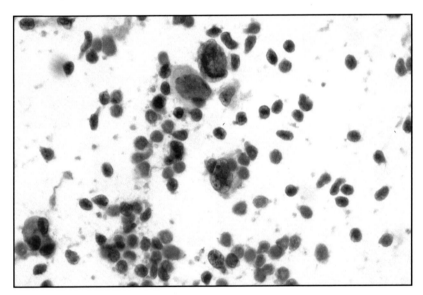

Image 9.11
Hodgkin's disease. Reed-Sternberg variants are randomly scattered in a polymorphous background of lymphocytes. (Papanicolaou).

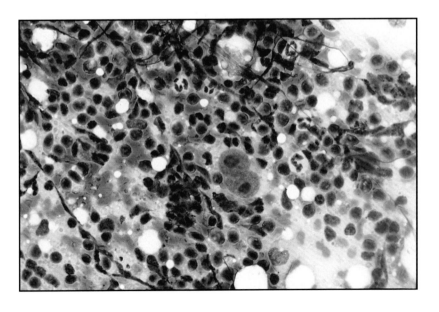

Image 9.12
Hodgkin's disease. Classic binucleated Reed-Sternberg cells. (Romanowsky).

Image 9.13
Hodgkin's disease. (Romanowsky).

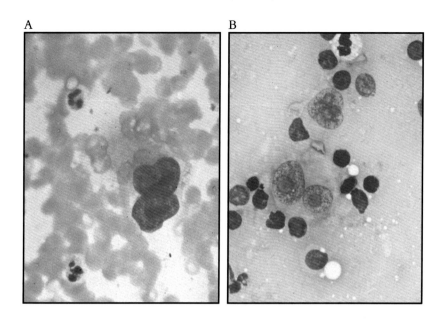

Image 9.14
Hodgkin's disease. Reed–Sternberg cell variants. (Romanowsky).

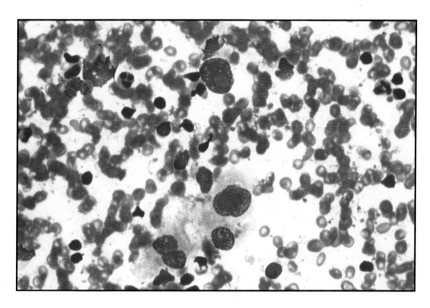

Image 9.15
Hodgkin's disease. (H&E).

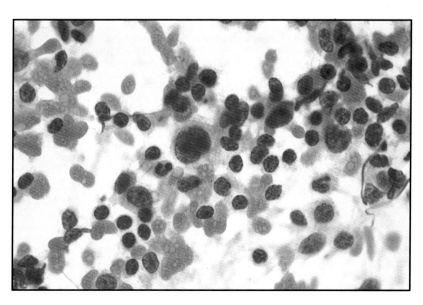

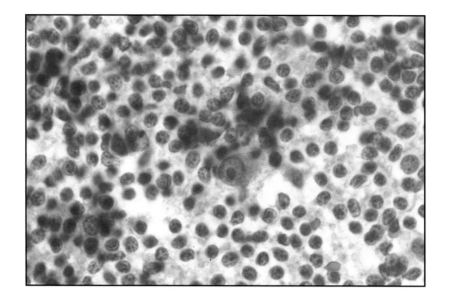

Image 9.16
Hodgkin's disease. (Papanicolaou).

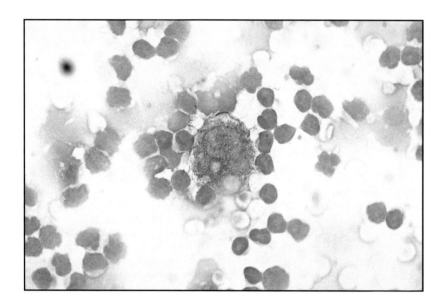

Image 9.17
Hodgkin's disease. Positive CD15 (Leu-M1) staining of Reed-Sternberg cell.

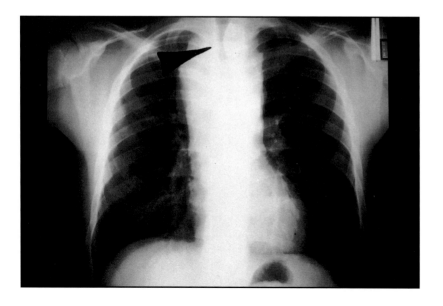

Image 9.18
Lymphoblastic lymphoma. Chest x-ray from 15-year-old male who presented with shortness of breath. Note tracheal compression (arrowhead) by a large anterior mediastinal mass.

Image 9.19
Lymphoblastic lymphoma.
A Monomorphous population of relatively uniform blasts.
B High power from another case showing bland nuclear chromatin. Note the prominent lymphoglandular bodies (Courtesy of Dr M Almeida). (Romanowsky).

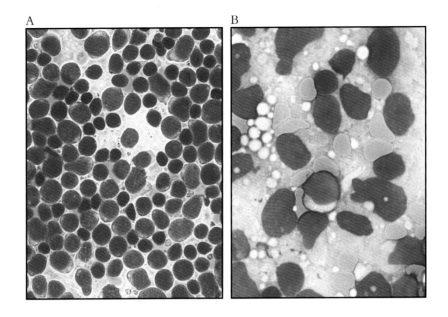

Image 9.20
Lymphoblastic lymphoma. Positive nuclear staining for TDT (terminal deoxynucleotidyl transferase).

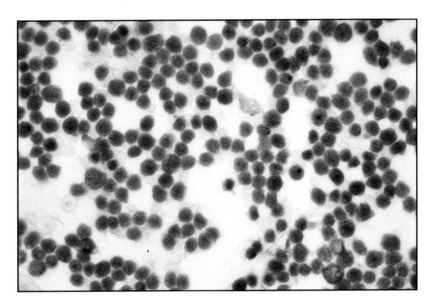

Image 9.21
Small non-cleaved cell lymphoma [Burkitt's]. A monomorphous sheet of lymphoid cells with coarse shromatin and obvious nucleoli is interrupted by a tingible-body macrophage (Courtesy of Dr M Almeida). (Papanicolaou).

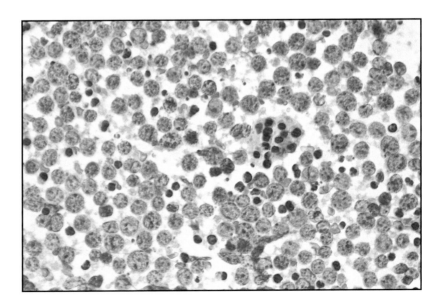

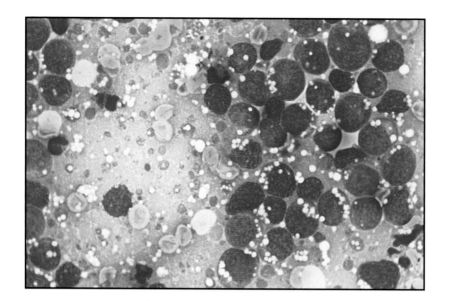

Image 9.22
Small non-cleaved cell lymphoma [Burkitt's]. Cytoplasmic vacuoles are obvious as are background lymphoglandular bodies (Courtesy of Dr M Almeida). (Romanowsky).

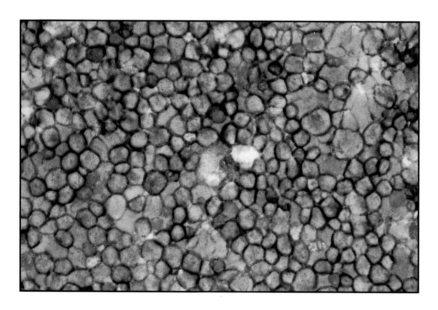

Image 9.23
Small non-cleaved cell lymphoma [Burkitt's]. Positive cell surface staining with B-cell marker CD19.

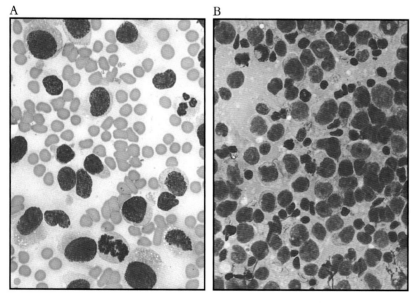

Image 9.24
Large cell lymphoma.
A Large cells – compare with neutrophil (arrowhead) – having a moderate amount of finely vacuolated cytoplasm. Note mitotic figure to the left of center.
B Obvious nucleoli in many cell nuclei. (Romanowsky).

Image 9.25
Metastatic nasopharyngeal carcinoma (lymphoepithelioma). Clustering of cells with nuclear overlapping and prominent nucleoli.
A Romanowsky.
B Papanicolaou.
C Cytokeratin immunostain.

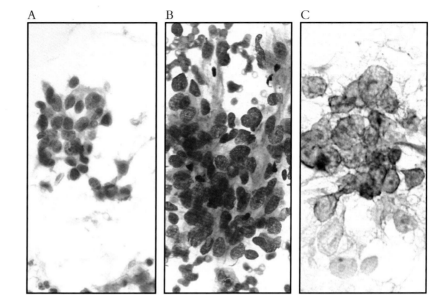

References

1. Wakely PE, Kardos TF, Frable WJ. Application of fine needle aspiration biopsy to pediatrics. *Hum Pathol* 19:1383-1386, 1988.

2. Silverman JF, Gurley AM, Holbrook CT, Joshi VV: Pediatric Fine Needle Aspiration Biopsy. *Am J Clin Pathol* 95:653-659, 1991.

3. Slap GB, Connor JL, Wigton RS, Schwartz JS: Validation of a Model to Identify Young Patients for Lymph Node Biopsy. *JAMA* 255:2768-2773, 1986.

4. Lake AM, Oski FA. Peripheral Lymphadenopathy in Childhood. *Amer J Dis Child* 132:357-359, 1978.

5. Kardos TF, Maygarden SJ, Blumberg AK, Wakely Jr. PE, Frable WJ. Fine Needle Aspiration Biopsy in the Management of Children and Young Adults With Peripheral Lymphadenopathy. *Cancer* 63:703-707, 1989.

6. Stanley MW, Knoedler JP. Skeletal structures that clinically simulate lymph nodes. Encounters during fine-needle aspiration. Diagn Cytopathol 9:86-88, 1993.

7. Tsang WYW, Chan JKC. Spectrum of Morphologic Changes in Lymph Nodes Attributable to Fine Needle Aspiration. *Hum Pathol* 23:562-565, 1992.

8. Frable WJ, Kardos TF. Fine Needle Aspiration Biopsy. Applications in the Diagnosis of Lymphoproliferative Diseases. *Amer J Surg Pathol* 12 (Suppl 1):62-72, 1988.

9. Söderstrom N. The Free Cytoplasmic Fragments of Lymphoglandular Tissue (Lymphoglandular Bodies). A Preliminary Presentation. *Scand J Haemat* 5:138-152, 1968.

10. Flanders E, Kornstein MJ, Wakely PE, Kardos TF, Frable WJ. Lymphoglandular bodies in Fine Needle Aspiration Cytology. *Amer J Clin Pathol* (In Press).

11. O'Dowd GJ, Frable WJ, Behm FG: Fine Needle Aspiration Cytology of Benign Lymph Node Hyperplasia. Diagnostic Significance of Lymphohistiocytic Aggregates. *Acta Cytol* 29:554-558, 1985.

12. Stani J. Cytologic Diagnosis of Reactive Lymphadenopathy in Fine Needle Aspiration Biopsy Specimens. *Acta Cytol* 31:8-13, 1987.

13. Silverman JF. Fine Needle Aspiration of Cat-Scratch Disease. Acta Cytol 29:542-547, 1985.

14. Christ ML, Feltes-Kennedy M. Fine Needle Aspiration Cytology of Toxoplasmic Lymphadenitis. *Acta Cytol* 26:425-428, 1982.

15. Maygarden SJ, Flanders E. Mycobacteria can be seen as "Negative Images" in Cytology Smears from Patients with Acquired Immunodeficiency Syndrome. *Mod Pathol* 2:239-243, 1989.

16. Stanley MW, Horwitz CA, Burton LG, Weisser JA. Negative images of bacilli and mycobacterial infection: A study of fine-needle aspiration smears from lymph nodes in patients with AIDS. *Diag Cytopathol* 6:118-121, 1990.

17. Silverman JF. Fine Needle Aspiration of Cat-Scratch Disease. Acta Cytol 29:542-547, 1985.

18. Schuster V, Kreth HW. Epstein-Barr Virus Infection and Associated Diseases in Children. *Eur J Pediatr* 151:794-798, 1992.

19. Kardos TF, Kornstein MJ, Frable WJ. Cytopathology and Immunopathology of Infectious Mononucleosis. *Acta Cytol* 32:722-726, 1988.

20. Stanley MW, Steeper TA, Horwitz CA, Burton LG, Strickler JG, Borken S. Fine Needle Aspiration of Lymph Nodes in Patients with Acute Infectious Mononucleosis. *Diag Cytopathol* 6:323-329, 1990.

21. Layfield LJ. Fine Needle Aspiration Cytologic Findings in a Case of Sinus Histiocytosis With Massive Lymphadenopathy (Rosai-Dorfman Syndrome). *Acta Cytol* 34:767-770, 1990.

22. Trautman BC, Stanley MW, Goding GS, Rosai J. Sinus Histiocytosis With Massive Lymphadenopathy (Rosai-Dorfman Disease): Diagnosis by Fine Needle Aspiration. *Diag Cytopathol* 7:513-516, 1991.

23. Kardos TF, Vinson JH, Behm FG, Frable WJ, O'Dowd G. Hodgkin's Disease: Diagnosis by Fine Needle Aspiration Biopsy: Analysis of Cytologic Criteria from a Selected Series. *Amer J Clin Pathol* 86:286-291, 1986.

24. Moriarty A, Banks E, Bloch T. Cytologic Criteria for Subclassification of Hodgkin's Disease Using Fine Needle Aspiration. *Diag Cytopathol* 5:122-125, 1989.

25. Das DK, Gupta SK. Fine Needle Aspiration Cytodiagnosis of Hodgkin's Disease and Its Subtypes. II. Subtyping by Differential Cell Counts. *Acta Cytol* 34:337-341, 1990.

26. Kjeldsberg CR, Wilson JF, Berard CW. Non-Hodgkin's Lymphomas in Children. Hum Pathol 14:612-627, 1983.

27. Jacobs J, Katz R, Shabb N, El-Naggar A, Ordonez N, Pugh W. Fine Needle Aspiration of Lymphoblastic Lymphoma: A Multiparameter Diagnostic Approach. *Acta Cytol* 36:887-894, 1992.

28. Nathwani BN, Diamond LW, Winberg CD, Kim H, Bearman RM, Glick JH, Jones SE, Gams RA, Nissen NI, Rappaport H. Lymphoblastic Lymphoma: A clinicopathologic study of 95 patients. *Cancer* 48:2347-2357, 1981.

29. Griffith RC, Kelly DR, Nathwani BN, Shuster JJ, Murphy SB, Hvizdala E, Sullivan MP, Berard CW. A Morphologic Study of Childhood Lymphoma of Lymphoblastic Type. *Cancer* 59:1126-1131, 1987.

30. Kardos TF, Sprague RI, Wakely Jr. PE, Frable WJ. Fine Needle Aspiration Biopsy of Lymphoblastic Lymphoma and Leukemia. A Clinical, Cytologic, and Immunologic Study. *Cancer* 60:2448-2453, 1987.

31. Brownell MD, Sheibani K, Battifora H, Winberg CD, Rappaport H. Distinction between Undifferentiated (Small Noncleaved) and Lymphoblastic Lymphoma. *Amer J Surg Pathol* 11:779-787, 1987.

32. Hutchison RE, Murphy SB, Fairclough DL, Shuster JJ, Sullivan MP, Link MP, Donaldson SS, Berard CW. Diffuse Small Noncleaved Cell Lymphoma in Children, Burkitt's versus Non-Burkitt's Types. *Cancer* 64:23-28, 1989.

33. Das DK, Gupta SK, Pathak IC, Sharma SC, Datta BN. Burkitt-Type Lymphoma. Diagnosis by fine needle aspiration cytology. Acta Cytol 31:1-7, 1987.

34. Sneige N, Dekmezian RH, Katz R, Fanning TV, Lukeman JL, Ordonez NF, Cabanillas FF. Morphologic and Immunocytochemical Evaluation of 220 Fine Needle Aspirates of Malignant Lymphoma and Lymphoid Hyperplasia. *Acta Cytol* 34:311-322, 1990.

35. Agnarsson BA, Kadin ME: Ki-1 positive large cell lymphoma. A morphologic study of 19 cases. *Amer J Surg Pathol* 12:264-274, 1988.

36. Gordon BG, Weisenberger DD, Warkentin PI, Anderson J, Sanger WG, Bast M, Gnarra D, Vose JM, Bierman PJ, Armitage JO, Coccia PJ. Peripheral T-Cell Lymphoma in Childhood and Adolescence. A Clinicopathologic Study of 22 Patients. *Cancer* 71:257-263, 1993.

37. Koo CH, Rappaport H, Sheibani K, Pangalis GA, Nathwani BN, Winberg CD. Imprint Cytology of Non-Hodgkin's Lymphomas. Based on a Study of 212 Immunologically Characterized Cases. Hum Pathol 20 (Suppl.):1-137, 1989.

38. Akhtar M, Ali MA, Haider A, Antonius J, Hainau B, Dayel FA. Fine Needle Aspiration Biopsy of Ki-1 Positive Anaplastic Large-Cell Lymphoma. *Diag Cytopathol* 8:242-246, 1992.

39. Grenko RT, Schabb NS. Metastatic Nasopharyngeal Carcinoma: Cytologic Features of 18 Cases. *Diagn Cytopathol* 7:562-566, 1991.

40. Chan MKM, McGuire LJ, Lee JCK. Fine Needle Aspiration Cytodiagnosis of Nasopharyngeal Carcinoma in Cervical Lymph Nodes. A Study of 40 Cases. *Acta Cytol* 33:344-350, 1989.

41. Feinmesser R, Miyazaki I, Cheung R, Freeman JL, Noyek AM, Dosch HM. Diagnosis of Nasopharyngeal Carcinoma by DNA Amplification of Tissue Obtained by Fine Needle Aspiration. *New Engl J Med* 326:17-21, 1992.

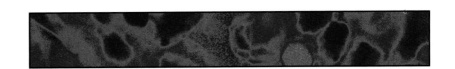

CHAPTER TEN

Head and Neck

Fine needle aspiration (FNA) biopsy of the head and neck region in children has several merits. First, it is reliable for distinguishing a benign lesion from a malignant one. In a recent review, sensitivity and specificity rates of 97% and 99%, respectively, were obtained from 165 such aspirates in patients less than 16 years old.[1] It can provide information that may negate the need for surgical biopsy in benign, as well as in metastatic conditions in which surgery is also not usually needed. We reported another series of 89 aspirates of which 67 cases (including 11 metastatic or locally recurrent tumors) did not require subsequent surgery.[2] FNA biopsy of this region also can provide material for culture of infectious lesions, initiating a prompt, informed workup in certain diseases (eg, infectious mononucleosis), and identifying the nature of the mass.

As previously stressed, an enlarged lymph node is the most common reason for a superficial head and neck mass in children and adolescents. It can easily be confused with other entities in this age group. Among these are congenital cysts, salivary gland lesions and soft tissue tumors.

Cysts

The neck is the site for several benign cystic lesions in children. They can be medial (thyroglossal [T-G] duct cyst, dermoid cyst) or lateral (branchial cleft cyst, parathyroid cyst).

Branchial Cleft Cyst

Branchial cysts are uncommon in childhood, representing mainly remnants of the second branchial cleft. They are generally painless, and because they may sometimes arise suddenly, parents and patients are frequently anxious. The typical location of cysts is at the anterior border of the sternocleidomastoid muscle. The mass may be firm, but not rock hard. It is not uncommon to drain the cyst entirely during the aspiration procedure. FNA biopsy usually retrieves semiliquid yellowish purulent material. Due to this macroscopic appearance, a portion of the aspirate is usually submitted for culture even though most cases of branchial cleft cyst are sterile. Smears show numerous nucleated and anucleated squamous cells, amorphous cellular debris, notched rectangular or rhomboid cholesterol crystals, and inflammatory cells – primarily neutrophils and histiocytes (Image 10.1) (Table 10.1).[3,4] Infrequently, ciliated respiratory cells are found. While lymphoid follicles with well-developed germinal centers frequently surround such cysts, these are not generally encountered in smears, but may be occasionally seen. If the cyst ruptures, multinucleated giant cells from the attendant foreign body response may be captured in the aspirate.

The major differential diagnosis of a branchial cleft cyst in adults – cystic degeneration of a metastatic squamous cell carcinoma – is not a consideration in children. Suppurative lymphadenitis with abscess formation may mimic an inflamed branchial cleft cyst. Squamous cells, which are a consistent component of branchial cleft cyst, are not, however, found in cystic degeneration of metastatic squamous cell carcinoma.

The major differential diagnosis of a branchial cleft cyst in adults-cystic degeneration of a metastatic squamous cell carcinoma-is not a consideration in children

T-G Duct and Dermoid Cysts

These cysts typically have a cytologic appearance similar to that described for branchial cleft cyst (Table 10.1). Distinction is usually based on anatomic location, with the T-G duct cyst almost always in the midline, dermoid cyst more often slightly to one side of center and branchial cleft cyst always a lateral structure. The T-G duct cyst represents cystic enlargement of an abnormally persistent embryologic tract that extends from the base of the tongue through the hyoid bone to the thyroid gland. Because of this embryologic connection, a T-G duct cyst ordinarily moves in a cranial direction with swallowing, or if the child is asked to stick out his tongue. Such movement does not occur

Table 10.1
Branchial Cleft and Thyroglossal Duct Cysts-Cytomorphology

Variable amount of liquid contents, frequently purulent in appearance.

Nucleated and anucleated benign squamous cells.

Amorphous proteinaceous debris.

Thyroid follicular cells usually absent.

Table 10.2
Thyroid Cyst-Cytomorphology

Variable amount of fluid which is generally dark brown.

Benign thyroid follicular cells in small clusters or as single cells.

Colloid (variable in amount).

Numerous hemosiderin-laden macrophages.

with dermoid or branchial cleft cysts. Thick mucoid (colloid-like) material may be expressed onto the slide from a T-G duct cyst aspirate. Anucleated and nucleated squamous cells are randomly scattered and occur with foamy histiocytes (Image 10.2).[5] Rupture may induce a foreign body reaction, which leads to occasional findings of benign multinucleated giant cells and mixed acute and chronic inflammatory cells in smears. Some aspirates of T-G duct cysts contain ciliated respiratory cells; one must be sure, however, that tracheal epithelium has not been aspirated. It is distinctly unusual to see thyroid follicular cells in such aspirates. T-G duct cysts may become secondarily infected; if so the cytologic picture is that of an abscess.

Parathyroid Cyst

These cysts are most common during middle age, but we have encountered an example in a 5-year-old girl. They are usually lateral to the midline, and confused with thyroid nodules. The key to their recognition is that the aspirated liquid is clear. For definitive diagnosis, a portion of the fluid should be sent for parathyroid hormone analysis.[6] Few cells are found on the slide even with cytospin preparations. Most are round bare nuclei, but some cells have a small amount of cytoplasm; others appear histiocytic (Image 10.3). No background elements are seen.

Thyroid Cyst

Cyst formation within the thyroid gland is usually a secondary degenerative phenomenon occurring within a benign nodular goiter. The fluid is typically a light brown or brownish-black liquid rather than the semi-transparent or sometimes thick yellowish mucoid material obtained from T-G duct cysts or colloid nodules. Smears contain numerous macrophages both with and without cytoplasmic debris and hemosiderin (Table 10.2). Follicular thyroid cells and colloid are limited. If, after evacuation of the cyst fluid a nodule remains, it must be re-aspirated. Rarely in this population, papillary carcinoma with cystic degeneration occurs.

Rarely in this population, papillary carcinoma with cystic degeneration occurs

Cystic Lymphangioma (Hygroma)

When cystic transformation of the lymphatics occurs in the head and neck region, it is usually localized to the carotid triangle. In the great majority of patients, it exists at birth or develops within the first 6 months of life (see Chapter 12, Soft Tissue).

Thyroid

Diffuse enlargement of the thyroid or a discrete mass lesion involving the thyroid gland is extremely uncommon in the 1st decade and somewhat less so in the 2nd. Most thyroid disease in this age group is brought to medical attention because of a hyper- or hypothyroid state. FNA biopsy has a very limited role, if any, in the diagnosis of primary hyperplasia (eg, Graves' disease).

Conversely, FNA biopsy has demonstrated great practical utility and should be considered one of the first steps in the evaluation of a solitary or large thyroid nodule.[7-10] Many of the advantages listed for lymph node FNA biopsy (see Table 9-1) also apply to thyroid, such as the ability of thyroid FNA biopsy to triage properly the child into the surgical versus nonsurgical treatment group. In the pediatric age group, one is most likely to encounter a thyroid nodule in adolescent females. The cytomorphology of thyroid lesions is similar to that of adults. Since several chapters and texts have appeared on thyroid FNA biopsy,[5,11-13] we will not attempt an all-inclusive discussion of the subject, but rather concentrate on those lesions one is more apt to encounter in the pediatric population.

In our experience, adolescents are quite cooperative when the FNA biopsy procedure is calmly and intelligently described to them. FNA biopsy is usually performed with the adolescent patient in the supine position rather than sitting up. Normally, a pillow is placed under the lower neck and upper shoulders to allow the head to fall back slightly and thus accentuate the thyroid gland. Patients less than 10 years of age normally have to be held, again in a supine position, but the procedure can usually be performed with a minimum of difficulty.

Criteria to determine whether an aspirate is sufficiently cellular to constitute a satisfactory specimen have been presented in the literature of benign thyroid lesions. Hamburger et al feel that 6 clusters of benign follicular cells on 2 separate slides are required to reduce significantly false-negative diagnoses.[14] One should be cautious of minimal numerical figures, because in some colloid nodules this number may not be achieved even though the nodule is thoroughly sampled. We are unaware of any similar study restricted to the pediatric group.

FNA biopsy has demonstrated great practical utility and should be considered one of the first steps in the evaluation of a solitary or large thyroid nodule

Goiter

Benign nodular goiter, usually of the colloid type, appears as a slowly growing increase in thyroid gland size seen primarily in adolescent females. Thyroid enlargement is usually asymmetrical and diffuse, but a single nodule may also develop. Patients are euthyroid, and the enlargement is painless.

Histologically, the classic colloid goiter shows follicle hyperplasia with a range in follicle size. Many follicles are markedly distended by amorphous eosinophilic colloid. Degenerative changes include parenchymal fibrosis, fresh and old hemorrhage with hemosiderin deposits and numerous macrophages.

Aspiration smears are typically rich in background colloid, which can appear either as an amorphous background film of material, or, if thicker, as rounded and well-defined masses.[5,13] Colloid is better seen in air dried MGG-stained smears where it has a lilac or deep blue coloration (depending on its thickness). With the Papanicolaou stain, it appears pale green. Linear "cracks" simulating the appearance of broken panes of glass, are a common artifact within colloid (Image 10.3).

Follicular epithelial cells are smeared both as isolated single cells and as aggregates. The former often appear as uniform bare round nuclei with a homogeneous fine chromatin. Cellular aggregates may be distributed in sheets that have regular cell spacing producing a "honeycomb" structure (Image 10.4). They may also be distributed as irregular, loosely cohesive aggregates, and occasionally as single intact follicles. Atypical follicular cells characterized by nucleomegaly and irregular nuclear membrane contours may be found, but they are an isolated phenomenon. Small numbers of Hürthle (Askanazy) cells exist separately and within clusters of follicular epithelial cells. They are recognized by their larger nuclei, distinct single nucleoli, and abundant finely granular cytoplasm. Hemosiderin-laden macrophages indicate a degenerative process usually from prior hemorrhage into the gland and are commonly associated with cyst formation.

Chronic Lymphocytic Thyroiditis (Hashimoto's)

Most often, chronic lymphocytic thyroiditis is considered an autoimmune disease with a wide clinical spectrum of severity. The thyroid is usually diffusely enlarged, but on occasion, chronic thyroiditis presents as a firm solitary mass. In the pediatric population, the disease principally affects teenage girls who are usually euthyroid.

Macroscopically, the gland is firm and the cut surface is a smooth, dull white. A lymphocytic inflammatory infiltrate is histologically pre-

Table 10.3
Chronic Thyroiditis-Cytomorphology

Heterogeneous mixture of single lymphoid cells analogous to the picture of a reactive lymph node.

Benign thyroid follicular cells.

Colloid (variable in amount).

Variable amount of Hürthle (Askenazy) cell change: large polygonal cell with abundant fine granular cytoplasm.

---

sent throughout the gland (Image 10.5). Secondary lymphoid follicle formation with germinal centers is common. Thyroid follicles show a range in size and colloid content. Some follicles show hyperplastic epithelial changes. Random Hürthle (Askanazy) cell metaplasia of follicular cells often develops. A recent study showed no difference in the histopathologic changes of chronic thyroiditis between children and adults.[15] Prolonged destruction of thyroid parenchyma leads to fibrosis within the gland.

Typically, a mixture of heterogeneous lymphoid cells and thyroid follicle cells are seen in aspiration smears (Table 10.3).[16] The number and variety of lymphoid cells is dependent on the severity of the inflammatory process. In minimally inflamed glands it may be difficult to distinguish mature lymphocytes from bare follicular cell nuclei. In contrast, inflammation may be so florid that residual epithelial cells are obscured, and the aspirate mimics a reactive lymphadenopathy with a wide range of lymphoid cells and numerous tingible-body macrophages. Plasma cells and histiocytes may be present in smears, but in much smaller numbers than lymphocytes. The amount of colloid on the smear is inversely related to the intensity of the inflammation.

Readily identifiable Hürthle cells are used as a benchmark for the diagnosis of Hashimoto's thyroiditis. It is not unusual for some follicular cell nuclei, especially Hürthle cell nuclei, to be markedly enlarged and show some degree of pleomorphism. This is not a reason to suspect malignancy. The Hürthle cells tend to be arranged in groups, in contrast to Hürthle cell neoplasms, which have a dissociated pattern. It must be mentioned nonetheless that papillary carcinoma can sometimes be associated with a lymphocytic thyroiditis, and follicular cells need to be closely examined. Rarely, potential confusion with non-Hodgkin's lymphoma may occur in florid cases of chronic thyroiditis, but this occurs almost exclusively in adults.

Papillary Carcinoma

Of the thyroid cancers, papillary carcinoma is the most common type in both children and adults. Adolescent females constitute the susceptible population in the pediatric age group. It is not infrequent that the neoplasm is clinically discovered as a lymphadenopathy containing metastatic deposits. Historically, papillary thyroid carcinoma in children is strongly associated with prior radiation therapy to the neck and mediastinum.

The gross appearance of most papillary thyroid carcinomas is a firm, ill-defined grey-white area that contrasts with the surrounding reddish-brown nonneoplastic parenchyma. Histopathologically, papillary fronds of epithelium lining thin fibrovascular cores project into gland lumens or dilated cystic spaces. Fibrosis and hemorrhage are consistent features. Key to the diagnosis are the nuclear features of dispersed chromatin, thickened nuclear membranes, cytoplasmic pseudoinclusions and longitudinal grooves. The chromatin clearing produces what have become widely known as "orphan Annie" or "ground glass" nuclei, a diagnostic feature in tissue sections that is only rarely appreciated in cytologic preparations.[17]

Historically, papillary thyroid carcinoma in children is strongly associated with prior radiation therapy to the neck and mediastinum

Table 10.4
Papillary Thyroid Carcinoma-Cytomorphology

Generally, numerous follicular epithelial cells on smears.

Branching, papillary shaped aggregates and sheets of epithelial cells.

Follicular cells show nucleomegaly, linear nuclear grooves, intranuclear cytoplasmic inclusions, dense "metaplastic" cytoplasm.

When present, background colloid is very opaque, with a smeared quality ("pulled taffy or chewing gum").

Psammoma bodies (infrequent).

Numerous clusters of thyroid epithelial cells are dispersed in the aspiration smear (Table 10.4). Some of these have a monolayered branching papillary configuration, while others are arranged in loose, irregular sheets (Image 10.6). Occasionally the flat sheets will be folded or twisted. Cell cluster size is extremely variable. Nuclei are irregular and slightly larger than normal. Very characteristic of this carcinoma are the nuclear features of linear "grooves" and cytoplasmic pseudoinclusions.[11-13,18,19] The latter are not universally present, but common if diligently searched for. They appear as round, sharply demarcated pale areas within nuclei that are identical in color and texture to the cell cytoplasm (Image 10.7). Nuclear grooves are best seen in alcohol-fixed smears, but can also be appreciated in the Romanowsky-stained smears (Image 10.8). Cell cytoplasm is moderate and denser (so-called metaplastic change) than that seen in nonneoplastic follicular cells.

Of note is the relative lack or complete absence of background colloid. When colloid is present, it has a dense, viscous appearance which has led some to label this "chewing gum" or "taffy-like" colloid (Image 10.9). On air-dried, Romanowsky-stained smears, this colloid is usually metachromatic rather than blue. Finding psammoma bodies (round concentrically laminated calcific structures) in the smear greatly assists in the diagnosis, but these are seen at most in only about $1/3$ of cases.

Salivary Gland

Acute Sialadenitis

Acute purulent sialadenitis is much less common than the chronic form, and is usually bacterial in origin. This entity occurs more often in adults than in children. The aspiration biopsy sample is highly cellular and contains primarily neutrophils.[19] Lesser numbers of macrophages, lymphocytes and fibroblasts are present. Individual cell necrosis and background amorphous proteinaceous debris is common. Fragments of salivary gland acinar cells and duct epithelium are infrequent.

Chronic Sialadenitis

Nonspecific chronic sialadenitis exceeds all other reasons for salivary gland enlargement in children. It most often manifests as chronic parotiditis characterized by a unilateral swelling of the parotid gland. Histopathology shows a chronic inflammatory infiltrate dispersed throughout the ducts and exocrine tissue of the gland with a variable degree of atrophy and replacement fibrosis of acinar units which is dependent on the duration and severity of the inflammatory process. Aspiration cytology reflects the histologic landscape, and reveals mature lymphocytes, some plasma cells and histiocytes admixed with fragments or normal acinar cells and duct epithelium of the parotid gland.[5,19]

Granulomatous inflammation secondary to sarcoidosis, tuberculosis and cat-scratch disease may also involve the salivary glands, although less commonly than lymph nodes.[5,20] Again, the parotid gland is most commonly involved. The cytopathology of these granulomatous processes is identical to that described for granulomatous lymphadenitis, except that one will not find ductal or acinar cells in the latter.

Juvenile Hemangioma

Juvenile hemangioma (hemangioendothelioma) is the most frequent pediatric salivary gland tumor. Many consider this a hamartoma rather than a true neoplasm. It occurs largely as a soft mass in the parotid gland of female infants. Because this tumor may rapidly enlarge, it can be a source of parental concern. The overlying skin may exhibit bluish or reddish-blue discoloration that can be accentuated when the child cries. Crying or straining by the child also increases the size and firmness of the mass. On occasion, a cutaneous hemangioma overlying the mass may be present. The diagnosis is usually clinically evident to the experienced pediatrician, and FNA biopsy is not generally requested or necessary.

Juvenile hemangioma is the most frequent pediatric salivary gland tumor

Our experience (in those cases in which the clinical diagnosis is not obvious) is that aspiration smears are generally bloody with only a few isolated polygonal and spindle cells, which may be loose or tightly clustered. Cell nuclei are bland, and a moderate amount of cytoplasm is present. Others have described similar findings.[21] Although the FNA biopsy features are nondiagnostic, aspiration smears are helpful in ruling out other conditions when the clinical diagnosis is in doubt. It can confirm the benign nature of the mass when conservative (nonoperative) management is desired.

Neoplasms

Other than the commonplace hemangioma, salivary gland neoplasms are rare in children. In most large series, fewer than 5% of salivary gland tumors involve patients less than 18 years old.[22] They typically arise within the parotid gland as opposed to the minor salivary glands. There is no sex predilection. Pleomorphic adenoma (mixed tumor) and mucoepidermoid carcinoma are, respectively, the most common benign and malignant salivary gland tumors of this age group.[23] The cytopathology is identical in children to that seen in adults. Both benign and malignant lesions present as gradually enlarging masses.

Pleomorphic Adenoma (Benign Mixed Tumor)

Within the pediatric population, children in their early teens are more commonly affected. As in adults, the mass is not tender and frequently firm to palpation.

A blend of mesenchymal and epithelial elements is seen histologically. Epithelial cells are arranged in solid sheets, cords and ducts which are randomly scattered in a myxoid stroma which frequently transforms into foci of epithelial squamous metaplasia and/or mesenchymal (chondroid or osseous) metaplasia.

Myoepithelial cells are common throughout mixed tumors and may assume a spindle or plasmacytoid configuration.

Aspirate smears are moderate to highly cellular (Table 10.5). Cells from the myoepithelial component are relatively monotonous, oval and arranged either as single cells or loose sheets.[24,25] Cells have round to oval bland nuclei, and a moderate amount of cytoplasm with discrete cell boundaries (Image 10.10). Spindle shaped cells are more common within the mesenchymal component of these smears (Image 10.11). This chondromyxoid stroma is more evident in Romanowsky-stained smears in which it is displayed as hypocellular opaque fragments with a deep magenta color (Image 10.12). With alcohol-fixed smears, a fine fibrillary structure is noted at the edges of these fragments. Infrequently, isolated pleomorphic cells can be seen. The diagnosis is usually straightforward when the mesenchymal portion is abundant.

Mucoepidermoid Carcinoma

While mucoepidermoid carcinoma most commonly involves the parotid gland, the minor salivary glands are not exempt as primary sites. Boys and girls are almost equally affected.

The histopathology varies depending on the degree of differentiation. Well-differentiated neoplasms are usually cystic with easily identifiable mucinous cells. The inverse occurs in poorly differentiated forms that are solid and dominated by undifferentiated cells with epidermoid features.

Table 10.5
Benign Mixed Tumor, Salivary Gland-Cytomorphology

Myoepithelial cells arranged singly or in sheets and cords.

Ductal cell nuclei round to oval, finely granular chromatin, moderate amount of cytoplasm.

Chondromyxoid stroma, typically abundant, containing variable numbers of spindle cells.

Aspirates are often very cellular. Cells are disseminated in loose nondescript aggregates and singly. In the low-grade form, both glandular and squamous cells coexist on the same slide ordinarily in close proximity to one another.[24] The former are relatively uniform in size, polygonal or columnar (Image 10.13). The cytoplasm is coarsely vacuolated, or contains a large single cytoplasmic mucin vacuole. The squamous component has more opaque cytoplasm with discrete cell borders. The smear background is "dirty" containing granular pyknotic cellular debris and mucin. In cystic lesions, it is possible to aspirate large amounts of mucin which may overshadow a meager cell population. This can lead to an incorrect diagnosis of mucocele. Stains for mucin can be performed directly on aspirate smears.

The cells in poorly differentiated carcinoma show a high N/C ratio with coarse nuclear chromatin and visible nucleoli, and they generally lack mucin (Image 10.14). Such cells are difficult to separate from other undifferentiated primary or metastatic carcinomas. Because of inherent problems with adequate sampling, one should be cautious in assigning definitive grades to aspirates of mucoepidermoid carcinoma.

Eye

While we have no personal experience with intraocular FNA biopsy in children, in those centers that perform this procedure, the diagnostic accuracy is high.[26] Most physicians in this country do not routinely perform ocular FNA biopsy on suspected retinoblastomas due to potential seeding of malignant cells along the needle tract.

Retinoblastoma is the most common intraocular neoplasm encountered in children. In the orbital and periorbital region, rhabdomyosarcoma is a common primary malignant neoplasm, particularly in infants and young children. The orbital and periorbital region is also a not uncommon location for metastatic neuroblastoma.

Dermoid cysts are among the benign entities occurring in this anatomic site. They occur along the eyebrow and on the eyelid, but may extend into the orbit. Their cytologic morphology is as described above.

In the orbital and periorbital region, rhabdomyosarcoma is a common primary malignant neoplasm, particularly in infants and young children

Retinoblastoma

Retinoblastoma occurs in both sporadic and hereditary forms. It is primarily a sporadically occurring unilateral neoplasm. Bilateral cases are almost always hereditary, that is, associated with a family history of the tumor. The typical age at presentation is between 1 and 3 years: hereditary retinoblastoma ordinarily develops in the 1st year.

Leukocoria (white pupillary reflex) is the typical presenting clinical sign. Extensive cytogenetic studies have localized the retinoblastoma gene in the q14 region of chromosome 13. The gene is thought to be recessive, and deletion of both alleles is required for tumor formation. Because it may invade the optic nerve and spread into the subarachnoid space, the cytopathologist may occasionally encounter this neoplasm in CSF fluid (see Chapter 3, Cerebrospinal Fluid and the Central Nervous System, p 55).

Table 10.6
Retinoblastoma-Cytomorphology

Very cellular smears.

Monotonous small rounded cells with high N/C ratios.

Hyperchromatic nuclei, coarse nuclear chromatin, indistinct nucleoli, nuclear molding.

Mitoses numerous and individual cell necrosis common.

Rossette formation.

Histologically, retinoblastoma is composed of solid sheets of uniform small "blue" cells punctuated by islands of necrosis and dystrophic calcification. Cells have hyperchromatic round nuclei, indistinct nucleoli, and scant cytoplasm. Evidence of neural differentiation can be recognized by the variable presence of Flexner-Wintersteiner rosettes, fleurettes, and Homer Wright rosettes.[27,28] Mitoses are numerous.

Relatively uniform round small cells dominate the densely cellular aspiration smears (Table 10.6). Cells are dispersed in both clusters and as single cells.[29,30] Not uncommonly, in the better differentiated forms, discrete rosette formation is found.[31,32] Molding of cell nuclei to one another is common. Nuclei are hyperchromatic with coarsely granular chromatin and inconspicuous nucleoli (Image 10.14). There is scant cell cytoplasm and bare nuclei are ubiquitous. Mitotic figures are numerous as is individual cell necrosis.

Potential Problems in Diagnosis: The cytomorphology is nearly identical to that described for the other malignant small round cell tumors. In particular, medulloepithelioma is extremely difficult to distinguish from retinoblastoma by light microscopy alone.

If needed, immunostaining will reveal expression of neural differentiation in this neoplasm with positive staining for neuron-specific enolase, retinal S-protein, and synaptophysin, and negative staining for glial fibrillary acid protein and S-100. Ultrastructure of these cells demonstrates features of retinal photoreceptors.[32] Cytogenetic mapping shows the characteristic chromosomal deletion.

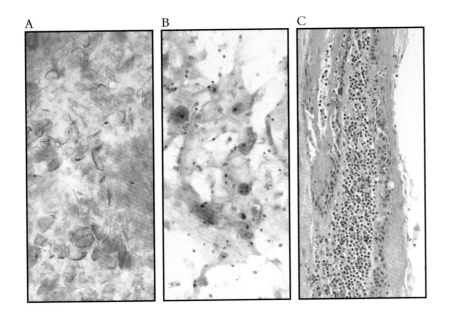

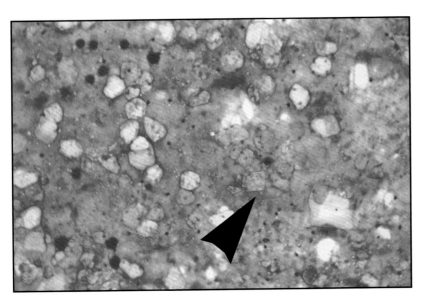

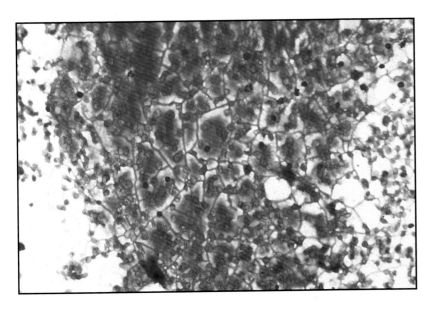

Image 10.1
Branchial cleft cyst.
A Numerous anucleate squamous cells. (Romanowsky).
B Pigmented histiocytes and cellular debris. (Papanicolaou).
C Histologic section of wall of cyst showing surface keratinization and underlying lymphoid tissue. (H & E).

Image 10.2
Thyroglossal duct cysts. Pigmented macrophages, anucleated squamous cells, notched cholesterol crystals (arrowhead) and cellular debris are present. (Romanowsky).

Image 10.3
Normal thyroid. "Cracking artifact" within colloid. (Romanowsky).

Image 10.4
Benign nodular goiter.
A Uniformly arranged sheet of monotonous follicular epithelial cells. (Romanowsky).
B The 3-dimensional nature of benign thyroid follicles is better appreciated in this alcohol-fixed smear. (Papanicolaou).

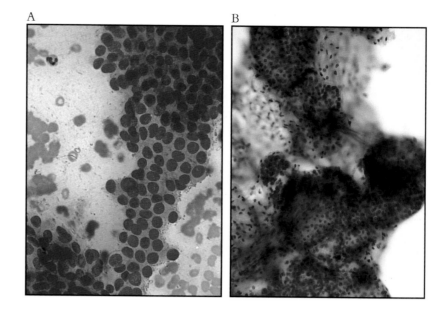

Image 10.5
Hashimoto's thyroiditis. There is an admixture of mature lymphocytes with follicular cells that have oncocytic change. (Romanowsky).

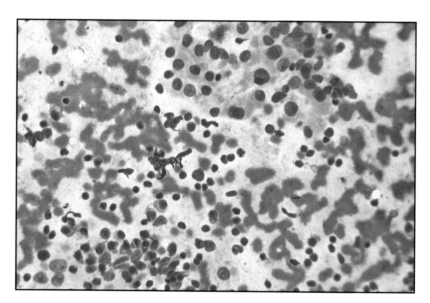

Image 10.6
Papillary carcinoma, thyroid. Low-power magnification shows papillary cords and sheets of epithelial cells. (Papanicolaou).

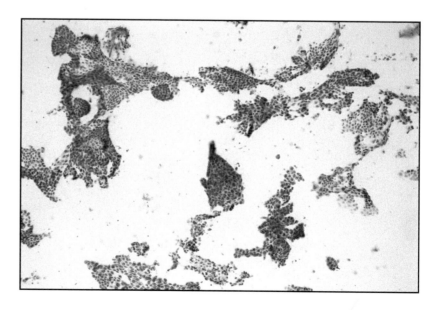

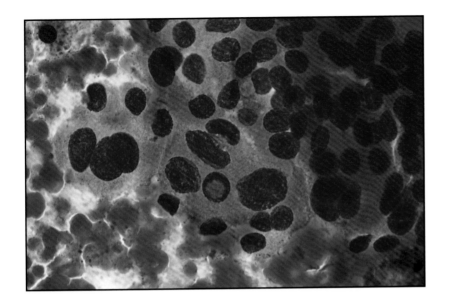

Image 10.7
Papillary carcinoma, thyroid. Prominent nuclear pseudoinclusion. (Romanowsky).

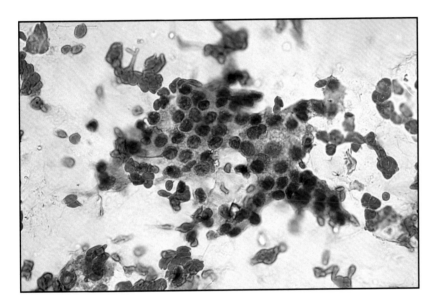

Image 10.8
Papillary carcinoma, thyroid. Linear nuclear grooves are seen in a few cells. (Papanicolaou).

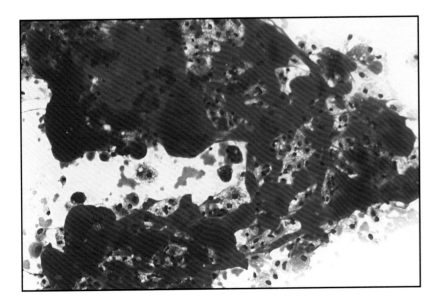

Image 10.9
Papillary carcinoma, thyroid. Thick, viscous appearing colloid has obscured most of the cells in this field. (Romanowsky).

Image 10.10
Benign mixed tumor, salivary gland. Monotonous cells with eccentric nuclei and bland chromatin are surrounded by metachromatic material. (Romanowsky).

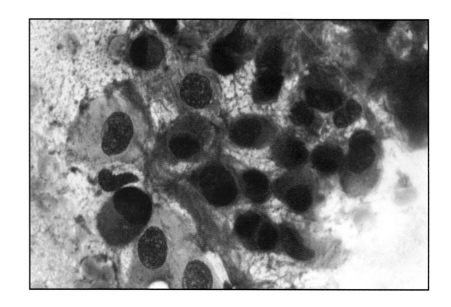

Image 10.11
Benign mixed tumor, salivary gland. Stromal cells display elongated nuclei embedded within fibromyxoid fragment. (Papanicolaou).

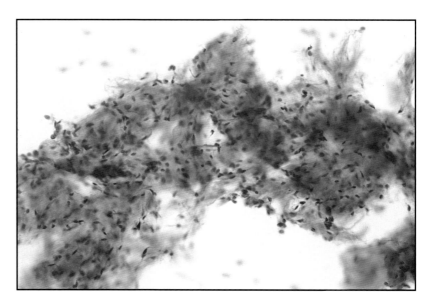

Image 10.12
Benign mixed tumor, salivary gland. Low-power view of small cell clusters embedded within metachromatic stroma. (Romanowsky).

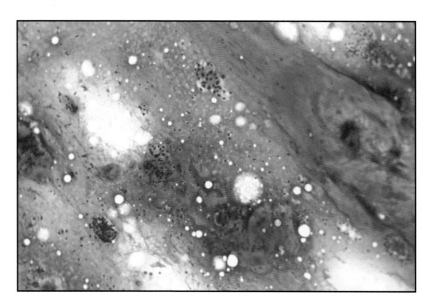

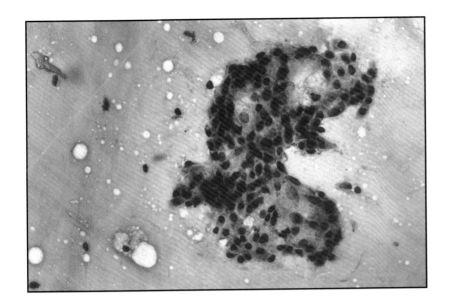

Image 10.13
Mucoepidermoid carcinoma, salivary gland. Low-grade carcinoma shows bland cells within a myxoid background. (Romanowsky).

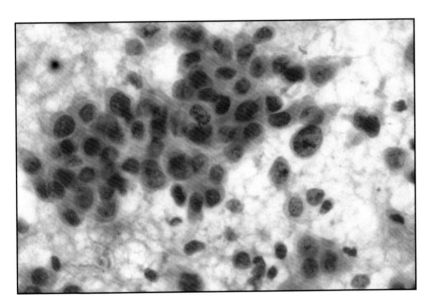

Image 10.14
Mucoepidermoid carcinoma, salivary gland. Cells of high-grade carcinoma are more pleomorphic with larger nuclei and discrete nucleoli. (Papanicolaou).

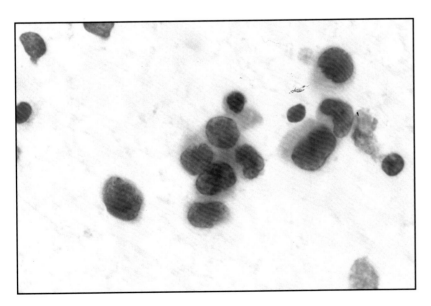

Image 10.15
Retinoblastoma, eye. Small cells with high N/C ratios and coarse nuclear chromatin are loosely aggregated together. (Papanicolaou). (Courtesy of Dr H Ehya).

References

1. Wakely Jr PE. Merits of fine needle aspiration biopsy in children. Head and neck. *Diag Cytopathol* 8:299-301, 1992.
2. Mobley DL, Wakely Jr. PE, Frable MAS. Fine needle aspiration biopsy. Application to pediatric head and neck masses. *Laryngoscope* 101:469-472, 1991.
3. Clark OH, Okerlund MD, Cavalieri RR, Greenspan FS. Diagnosis and treatment of thyroid, parathyroid, and thyroglossal cysts. *J Clin Endocrinol Metab* 48:983-988, 1979.
4. Engzell U, Zajicek J. Aspiration biopsy and cytologic findings in 100 cases of congenital cysts. *Acta Cytol* 14:51-57, 1970.
5. Feldman PS, Covell JL, Kardos TF. Fine Needle Aspiration Cytology. Lymph Node, Thyroid, and Salivary Gland. ASCP Press, Chicago, 1989.
6. Silverman JF, Prabhaker KG, Morris MT. Parathyroid Hormone (PTH) assay of parathyroid cysts examined by fine needle aspiration biopsy. *Amer J Clin Pathol* 86:776-780, 1986.
7. Van Vliet G, Glinoer D, Verelst J, Spehl M, Gompel C, Delange F. Cold thyroid nodules in childhood. Is surgery always necessary? *Eur J Pediatr* 146:378-382, 1987.
8. Mazzaferri EL, de los Santos ET, Rofagha-Keyhani S. Solitary thyroid nodule. Diagnosis and management. *Med Clini North Am* 72:1177-1211, 1988.
9. Sheppard MC, Franklyn JA. Management of the single thyroid nodule. *Clin Endocrinol* 37:398-401, 1992.
10. Layfield LJ, Reichman A, Bottles K, Giuliano A. Clinical determinants for the management of thyroid nodules by fine needle aspiration cytology. *Arch Otolaryngol Head Neck Surg* 118:717-721, 1992.
11. Frable WJ. The thyroid. In:Thin Needle Aspiration Biopsy. Major Problems in Pathology, vol. 14. Bennington JL, ed. WB Saunders Co, Philadelphia, 1983.
12. Kini SR. The thyroid. In: Guides to Clinical Aspiration Biopsy. TS Kline, ed. Igaku-Shoin, Tokyo, 1987.
13. Orell SR, Sterrett GF, Walters MN, Whitaker D. The thyroid glands. In: Manual and Atlas of Fine Needle Aspiration Cytology 2nd ed. Churchill Livingstone, New York, 1992:chap 6.
14. Hamburger JI, Husain M. Semiquantitative criteria for fine needle biopsy diagnosis. Reduced false negative diagnoses. *Diag Cytopathol* 4:14-17, 1988.
15. Mizukami Y, Michigishi T, Kawato M, Sato T, Nonomura A, Hashimoto T, Matsubara F. Chronic thyroiditis. Thyroid function and histologic correlations in 601 cases. *Hum Pathol* 23:980-988, 1992.
16. Guarda LA, Baskin HJ. Inflammatory and lymphoid lesions of the thyroid gland. cytopathology by fine needle aspiration. *Amer J Clin Pathol* 87:14-22, 1987.
17. Hapke MR, Dehner LP. The optically clear nucleus. A reliable sign of papillary carcinoma of the thyroid? *Amer J Surg Pathol* 3:31-38, 1979.
18. Deligeorgi-Politi H. Nuclear crease as a cytodiagnostic feature of papillary thyroid carcinoma in fine needle aspiration biopsies. *Diag Cytopathol* 3:307-310, 1987.
19. Droese M. Cytological diagnosis of sialadenosis, sialadenitis, and parotid cysts by fine needle aspiration. *Adv Otorhinolaryngol* 26:49-96, 1981.

20. Wakely Jr PE, Silverman JF, Holbrook CT, Fairman RP, Daeschner CW, Joshi VV. Fine needle aspiration biopsy as an adjunct in the diagnosis of childhood sarcoidosis. *Pediatr Pulmonol* 13:117–120, 1992.

21. Hilborne LH, Glasgow BJ, Layfield LJ. Fine needle aspiration cytology of juvenile hemangioma of the parotid gland. A case report. *Diag Cytopathol* 3:152-155, 1987.

22. Callender DL, Frankenthaler RA, Luna MA, Lee SS, Goepfert H. Salivary gland neoplasms in children. *Arch Otolaryng Head Neck Surg* 118:472-476, 1992.

23. Schuller DE, McCabe BF. Salivary gland neoplasms in children. Otolaryngol Clinics North Amer 10:399-412, 1977.

24. Orell SR, Sterrett GF, Walters MN, Whitaker D. Head and neck: salivary glands. In: Manual and Atlas of Fine Needle Aspiration Cytology. 2nd ed. Churchill Livingstone, New York, 1992:chap 4.

25. Webb AJ. Cytologic diagnosis of salivary gland lesions in adult and pediatric surgical patients. *Acta Cytol* 17:51-58, 1973.

26. Arora R, Rewari R, Betharia SM. Fine needle aspiration cytology of orbital and adnexal masses. *Acta Cytol* 36:483-491, 1992.

27. Sang D, Albert DM. Retinoblastoma. Clinical and histopathologic features. *Hum Pathol* 13:133-147, 1982.

28. He W, Hashimoto H, Tsuneyoshi M, Enjoji M, Inomata H. A reassessment of histologic classification and an immunohistochemical study of 88 retinoblastomas. A special reference to the advent of bipolar-like cells. *Cancer* 70:2901-2908, 1992.

29. O'Hara BJ, Ehya H, Shields JA, Augsberger JJ, Shields CL, Eagle RC. Fine needle aspiration biopsy in pediatric ophthalmic tumors and pseudotumors. *Acta Cytol* 37:125-130, 1993.

30. Char DH, Miller TR. Fine needle biopsy in retinoblastoma. *Amer J Ophthalmol* 97:686-690, 1984.

31. Das DK, Das J, Chachra KL, Natarajan R. Diagnosis of retinoblastoma by fine-needle aspiration and aqueous cytology. *Diag Cytopathol* 5:203-206, 1989.

32. Akhtar M, Ali MA, Sabbah R, Sackey K, Bakry M. Aspiration cytology of retinoblastoma. Light and electron microscopic correlations. *Diag Cytopathol* 4:306-311, 1988.

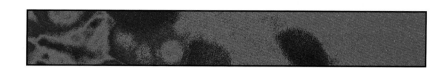

CHAPTER ELEVEN

Bone

In this country, fine needle aspiration (FNA) biopsy has been limited principally to an adjunct procedure for the diagnosis of presumed bone tumors, not as a replacement for tissue histopathology. It expands the pathologist's morphologic horizon by giving the cellular detail not possible in paraffin sections. In certain circumstances, however, eg, differentiation of acute osteomyelitis from a neoplasm, FNA biopsy may obviate the need for surgical biopsy.

Direct FNA biopsy may be performed on lytic bone lesions that have destroyed the cortex. In cases where the bony cortex is intact, a fine needle may be passed secondarily through a larger cutting needle that has penetrated the cortical bone. FNA biopsy of bone in children ordinarily requires local or general anesthesia, and is performed under radiographic guidance. Interpretation of the aspiration cytology (or tissue histopathology, for that matter) should not be attempted without full knowledge of the radiologic appearance, radiologic differential diagnosis and clinical considerations.

It should be remembered that as in adults, metastatic tumors to bone are more common than primary malignant bone tumors.[1] Only the more common primary bone tumors, or those that are somewhat specific to children will be discussed in this section (Table 11.1). Metastatic nonlymphoreticular neoplasms to bone, except for neuroblastoma, are rare in children. As with many other organ s

Table 11.1

Cytologic Features of Selected Childhood Bone Neoplasms

Features	Osteosarcoma	Eosinophilic Granuloma	Ewing's Sarcoma	Chondroblastoma
Typical age group	10-30 years	5-15 years	8-18 years	10-20 years
Anatomic site	long bones (diaphysis)	skull, pelvis, long bones	pelvis, long bones	long bones (epiphysis)
FNA biopsy-cytology				
Cell size	intermediate to large	intermediate	small	intermediate
Pleomorphism	frequent	minimal	absent	minimal
Cell shape	variable	round, oval	rounded	round, oval
Nuclei	pleomorphic linear groove	reniform, oval,	rounded	rounded, reniform
Nucleoli	prominent	small	inconspicuous	indistinct
Cytoplasm	moderate to abundant	moderate to abundant	meager	moderate
Background	metachromatic material	eosinophils, osteoclasts,	metachromatic	
Immunochemistry		none CD1-, S-100-positive	Vimentin-, HBA 71-, PAS-positive	S-100-positive

ystems, malignant tumors of bone in children, both primary and metastatic, are quite different from those in adults. For eg, multiple myeloma is almost unheard of in children. Metastatic neoplasms in adults are usually epithelial neoplasms, eg, carcinomas of the breast, prostate and kidney.

Osteosarcoma

Osteosarcoma is the most common malignancy of bone in children (about 2/3 of all malignant bone neoplasms), which peaks in the 2nd decade of life with a slight predominance in males. The long bones and pelvis are most frequently involved in the following descending order: distal femur, proximal tibia, humerus, pelvic bones.

Several histologic variants exist; all are required to have sarcomatous stroma admixed with tumor osteoid production, even if only focally. Conventional osteosarcoma contains malignant cells intimately associated either individually or in groups with osteoid. About 1/2 of conventional osteosarcomas contain chondroblastic or fibrosarcomatous stroma.

The cell yield is variable and dependent on the amount of sclerotic osteoid obtained and the degree of dilution by blood (Table 11.2). However, smears are usually moderately to highly cellular, and consist of cells that are dispersed in both clusters and as isolated cells.[2-4] The most common cell is a pleomorphic intermediate to large cell (Image 11.1). Nuclei are generally oval, but may be pleo-

Table 11.2
Osteosarcoma-Cytomorphology

Cells dispersed in both clusters and as isolated cells.

Pleomorphic intermediate to large cells with variable shapes.

Multinucleated cells common.

Nuclei generally oval, but may be pleomorphic; dense nuclear chromatin. Nucleoli may be prominent.

Mitotic figures common.

Moderate to large amount of finely granular cytoplasm.

Metachromatic staining osteoid present in cell clusters or isolated (best seen in Romanowsky stained smears).

Table 11.3
Ewing's Sarcoma-Cytomorphology

Highly cellular smear.

Cells dispersed as single, isolated cells with a minority arrayed in loose clusters.

Monotonous small cells (2 to 3 times a mature lymphocyte) which are fragile; bare nuclei common.

Uniform round to oval nuclei with finely granular chromatin. Nucleoli small or absent.

Cytoplasmic vacuoles or blebs variable.

Mitoses usually frequent.

Absent background material.

---

morphic and eccentrically located within the cell. Occasionally, 2 or more nuclei are present. Nuclear chromatin is dense and coarse with prominent nucleoli. Normal and abnormal mitotic figures are common. There is a moderate to large amount of finely granular cell cytoplasm. Dense metachromatic staining amorphous material, presumably osteoid or chondroid stroma, is admixed with these pleomorphic cells or may be smeared as isolated fragments. This material is best seen in air-dried, Romanowsky-stained smears. Multinucleated osteoclasts vary in number. In our limited experience, cytopathology alone is not reliable in splitting osteosarcoma into histologic subtypes.

Knowledge of the x-ray features and review of roentgenograms with a qualified radiologist is the most important ancillary study for the pathologist to perform prior to issuing a diagnosis of a malignant bone tumor. Immunochemistry is not particularly helpful or needed. Electron microscopy may be required to demonstrate tumor osteoid, which appears as hydroxyapatite crystals superimposed on mature collagen.

Ewing's Sarcoma

Second in incidence only to osteosarcoma among the primary malignant childhood tumors of bone, Ewing's sarcoma has a predilection for children in their early to mid-adolescent years. It is rare in the non-white population. The long bones of the leg (femur greater than tibia or fibula), and the pelvic bones are most commonly involved.

Histologically, sheets of monotonous small rounded cells (2 to 3 times the diameter of a mature lymphocyte) with a meager amount of cytoplasm are found within the bone. Ordinarily, a dimorphic population of pale cells are mixed with smaller darkly stained pyknotic nuclei. In some cases, cells having a moderate amount of cytoplasm are present. Cells of Ewing's sarcoma typically (but not always) contain abundant glycogen as demonstrated by the periodic acid-Schiff (PAS) stain. Individual cell and group necrosis is common. There is a perceptible lack of stromal matrix.

This neoplasm is the paradigm of the so-called "malignant small round cell tumor" group. As such, aspirate smears are very cellular (Table 11.3).[5] Monotonous small cells about 2 to 3 times the size of a mature lymphocyte are dispersed primarily as single cells with a minority arrayed in loose clusters (Image 11.2). Sporadically, rosette-like structures may be seen. Cells are fragile, and aspirates typically contain many bare nuclei. Cell nuclei are uniform, round to oval, with finely granular chromatin that has a coarse appearance in Papanicolaou-stained smears. Nucleoli are inconspicuous. A meager amount of cytoplasm is present, and cytoplasmic vacuoles and blebs may be seen (Image 11.3). Mitoses are frequent. Background material is absent.

Potential Problems in Diagnosis: Metastatic tumors of the malignant small round cell syndicate (particularly neuroblastoma and lymphoma), and primitive neuroectodermal tumor of bone may be confused with Ewing's sarcoma. Some argue that primitive neuroectodermal tumor of bone and Ewing's sarcoma are very closely related, and represent different points along the spectrum of the same tumor.[6] In some cases their differentiation may be unsolvable. Both small cell osteosarcoma and mesenchymal chondrosarcoma can be differentiated from Ewing's sarcoma if their background matrix material is present.

Cytoplasmic glycogen content of Ewing's sarcoma is variable. It is usually present and, in some cases, may be abundant. Because of this, a positive PAS stain which can be performed directly on smears is helpful. Other small round cell tumors, however, may also contain glycogen, notably rhabdomyosarcoma, neuroblastoma and primitive neuroectodermal tumor of bone, thus precluding use of this stain as the sole marker for differentiating among this group of neoplasms.

Immunophenotyping and electron microscopy are important and necessary to exclude the primitive neural, myogenic and lymphoid tumors that are part of the malignant small round cell tumor category. Positive immunoreactivity in Ewing's sarcoma occurs almost exclusively with vimentin. An occasional case may demonstrate cytokeratin staining in isolated cells. Enthusiasm has recently been expressed for monoclonal antibodies to the glycoprotein product of the MIC 2 gene as a sensitive immunologic marker for Ewing's sarcoma.[7] Most studies have

Immunophenotyping and electron microscopy are important and necessary to exclude the primitive neural, myogenic and lymphoid tumors that are part of the malignant small round cell tumor category

been performed on paraffin-embedded tissue. Strong immunoreactivity to the MIC 2 gene, however, has also been reported in primitive neuroectodermal tumor of bone, rhabdomyosarcoma and lymphoblastic lymphoma, thus emphasizing that an antibody panel rather than a single antibody be used in immunodiagnosis.[8-10]

Ultrastructurally, Ewing's sarcoma tumors contain few organelles and no evidence of specific differentiation. Typically a small dark and larger light cell population is seen by electron microscopy with primitive cell junctions and no intervening collagenous stroma. Cytoplasmic pools of glycogen, and evenly distributed nuclear euchromatin are present. Chromosomal analysis consistently displays a t(11;22) translocation in the great majority of cases - the same chromosomal defect typical of primitive neuroectodermal tumor of bone.[11] It has been argued that because no specific immunohistochemical for Ewing's sarcoma exists, the single most reliable tissue marker for Ewing's sarcoma and its congeners (ie, primitive neuroectodermal tumor of bone) is cytogenetic instead of morphologic.[6]

Eosinophilic Granuloma

This lesion currently is classified as one of the Langerhans cell histiocytosis (LCH). It is characterized by an idiopathic proliferation of Langerhans histiocytes which is broadly divided into three overlapping clinical variants: eosinophilic granuloma, Hand-Schuller-Christian disease, and Letterer-Siwe disease. Eosinophilic granuloma is considered the localized and least aggressive form of LCH. Although eosinophilic granuloma may be monostotic or polyostotic, a solitary osteolytic defect of the skull, femur or ribs occurring between 5 years and 16 years of age is the most common mode of presentation. Radiographically, these bony defects are sharply circumscribed. The skin and lymph nodes are other anatomic sites that may be affected by Langerhans cell histiocytes.

Table 11.4
Eosinophilic Granuloma-Cytomorphology

Moderately to highly cellular smears.

Large, sometimes vacuolated histiocytes.

Histiocyte nuclei rounded or folded/reniform, finely granular chromatin, linear nuclear grooves.

Histiocyte cytoplasm abundant, granular and sometimes vacuolated.

Multinucleated osteoclast-type giant cells variable in number.

Variable number of eosinophils. Other inflammatory cells may exist in smaller amounts.

Light microscopy reveals a patternless mixture of mature histiocytes and eosinophils with a smaller population of plasma cells, lymphocytes and/or neutrophils. Histiocyte nuclei are rounded as well as slightly indented producing a reniform appearance. A longitudinal nuclear groove can be found in many of the histiocytes. Although usually numerous, the eosinophil population is variable and may occasionally be sparse.

Moderately to highly cellular smears are obtained from aspiration (Table 11.4). Cells are dispersed singly and as loose aggregates (Image 11.4). The predominant cell is the Langerhans histiocyte which has an oval, rounded or reniform nucleus.[12-15] A prominent nuclear groove is seen in some Langerhans histiocytes (Image 11.5). Infrequently, such cells are binucleated. Nuclear chromatin is finely granular with an indistinct nucleolus. Histiocyte cytoplasm is typically abundant, finely granular and sometimes vacuolated. Multinucleated osteoclasts are generally found, but not usually in large numbers. There is a wide range in the number of eosinophils. Eosinophils typically have bilobed nuclei, but they may also be multilobed or unlobed. Other inflammatory cells, principally neutrophils and foamy histiocytes, may also exist in smaller amounts.

Potential Problems in Diagnosis: Because both the Langerhans histiocyte and the chondroblast may display a prominent nuclear groove, chondroblastoma may be mistaken for eosinophilic granuloma. The latter, however, has a polymorphous population of eosinophils, neutrophils and foamy histiocytes while the former does not. Osteoclasts are also generally more numerous in chondroblastoma. Radiographic location for these two entities is, of course, vastly different. Osteomyelitis may also enter into the differential diagnosis of the disease. In the acute form, neutrophils predominate while plasma cells are markedly increased in chronic osteomyelitis. When present, the histiocytes in osteomyelitis are almost always rounded rather than reniform, and consistently fail to demonstrate a nuclear groove. In unusual instances, immunophenotyping or electron microscopy are necessary to be certain of the diagnosis.

Langerhans histiocytes routinely express S-100 (as do chondroblasts), and CD1 (OKT-6) (Image 11.6). Ultrastructurally, the Birbeck granule is diagnostic of the Langerhans histiocyte. It is a cytoplasmic organelle frequently seen invaginating from the plasmalemma membrane, as a pentalaminar rod-shaped structure which not uncommonly has a bulbous expansion at one end of the rod producing a "tennis racket" configuration (Image 11.7).

Chondroblastoma

This uncommon benign neoplasm of bone has a peak incidence during adolescence. It occurs in the epiphysis, and involves most frequently the proximal humerus, proximal tibia, and both proximal and distal ends of the femur. Radiographic features demonstrate a lytic, frequently expansile lesion with a thin intact rim of bony sclerosis.

Radiographic features of chondroblastoma demonstrate a lytic, frequently expansile lesion with a thin intact rim of bony sclerosis

In tissue sections, a diffuse, patternless sheet of round to polygonal cells is interrupted in areas by osteoclast-type giant cells, calcification, and sometimes by small deposits of chondroid stroma. Calcium deposition is typically arrayed in a pericellular, honeycomb pattern invoking the image of "chicken wire." Cells have a moderate amount of cytoplasm, and distinct cell borders. Nuclei may be rounded, reniform and occasionally lobulated. Mitoses are noticeably absent.

Aspiration smears may be very cellular. Intermediate-size mononuclear polygonal chondroblasts with polygonal contours are arranged in loose clusters and as isolated cells.[16] Some cells are binucleated. There is only a slight variation in nuclear size, with round, oval or reniform shapes present (Image 11.8). Nuclei are characterized by a prominent nuclear groove, fine chromatin and indistinct nucleoli. Cells have a moderate amount of cytoplasm. Multinucleated osteoclasts are numerous. Occasionally, background chondroid matrix and calcified material may be found.

Potential Problems in Diagnosis: Although not considered a neoplasm of children, giant cell tumor of bone can occasionally occur in this age group and needs to be considered in the differential diagnosis if large numbers of osteoclast-type giant cells exist in the smears. Fanning et al stress that the key to differentiating these two entities lies in recognizing that the mononuclear cells of chondroblastoma are rounded, while those of giant cell tumor are spindle shaped with tapered cytoplasm.[13] Also, the obvious nuclear groove of chondroblasts is absent in giant cell tumor. The distinction between chondroblastoma and eosinophilic granuloma has been previously discussed.

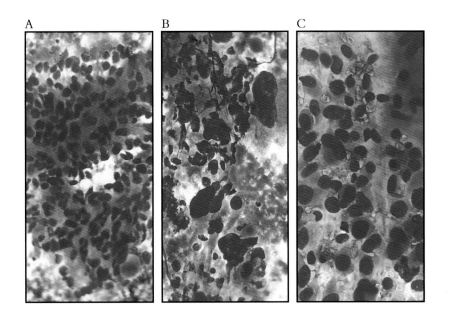

Image 11.1
Osteosarcoma.
A Malignant cells embedded within an osteoid matrix.
B and **C** Marked cellular pleomorphism. (Romanowsky).

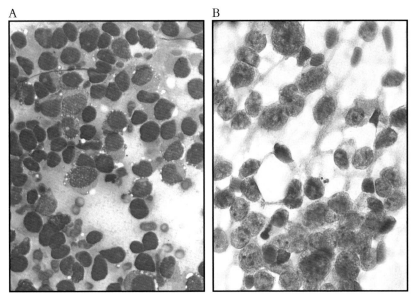

Image 11.2
Ewing's sarcoma. Patternless sheet of monomorphous small cells with some nuclear molding.
A Romanowsky.
B Papanicolaou.

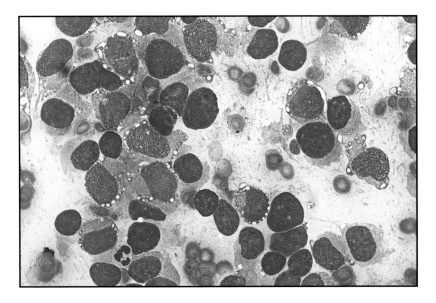

Image 11.3
Ewing's sarcoma. Small cells (compare with neutrophil in the photograph) have finely granular nuclear chromatin and a modest amount of cytoplasm. Some cells are vacuolated. Note absence of lymphoglandular bodies. (Romanowsky).

Image 11.4
Eosinophilic granuloma. Histiocytes are admixed with eosinophils.
A H & E.
B Romanowsky.

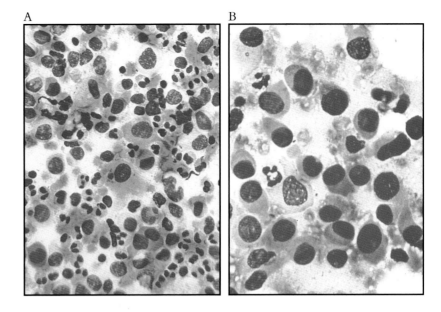

Image 11.5
Eosinophilic granuloma. Linear nuclear groove (arrowhead) and reniform shape of some histiocytes. (Papanicolaou).

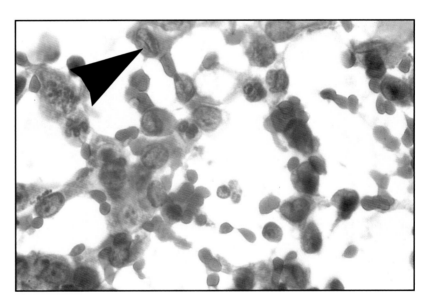

Image 11.6
Eosinophilic granuloma. Positive cytoplasmic staining of Langerhans' histiocytes with S-100 antigen.

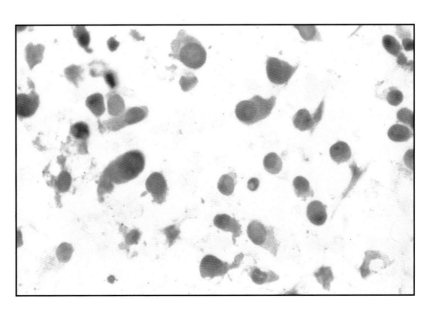

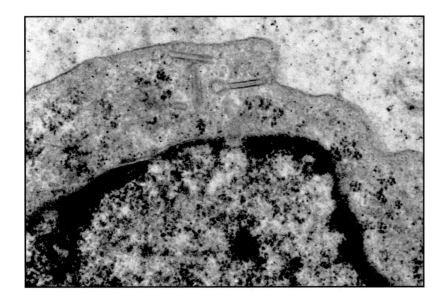

Image 11.7
Eosinophilic granuloma. Birbeck granule with bulbous enlargement at one end in a Langerhans histiocyte.

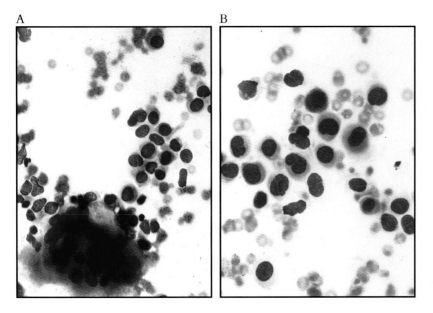

Image 11.8
A Chondroblastoma. A multinucleated osteoclast is seen.
B Some cells have a reniform nuclear shape. (Romanowsky).

References

1. Sanerkin NG, Jeffree GM. Cytology of Bone Tumors. A Colour Atlas With Text. JB Lippincott, Philadelphia, 1980.

2. Walaas L, Kindblom LG. Light and electron microscopic examination of fine-needle aspirates in the preoperative diagnosis of osteogenic tumors. A study of 21 osteosarcomas and two osteoblastomas. *Diag Cytopathol* 6:27-38, 1990.

3. White VA, Fanning CV, Ayala AG, Raymond AK, Carrasco CH, Murray JA. Osteosarcoma and the role of fine-needle aspiration. A study of 51 cases. *Cancer* 62:1238-1246, 1988.

4. Layfield LJ, Glasgow BJ, Anders KH, Mirra JM. Fine needle aspiration cytology of primary bone lesions. *Acta Cytol* 31:177-184, 1987.

5. Akhtar M, Ali MA, Sabbah R. Aspiration cytology of Ewing's sarcoma. Light and electron microscopic correlations. *Cancer* 56:2051-2060, 1985.

6. Ewing's sarcoma and its congeners. An interim appraisal [editorial]. *Lancet* 339:99-100, 1992.

7. Fellinger EJ, Garin-Chesa P, Glasser DB, Huvos AG, Rettig WJ. Comparison of cell surface antigen HBA71 (p30/32mic2), neuron-specific enolase, and vimentin in the immunohistochemical analysis of Ewing's sarcoma of bone. *Amer J Surg Pathol* 16:746-755, 1992.

8. Riopel MA, Dickman PS, Link M, Perlman EJ. MIC 2 analysis in pediatric lymphomas. *Lab Invest* 68:128A, 1993. (Abst.)

9. Perlman EJ, Dickman PS, Askin FB, Grier HE, Miser JS, Link MP. Ewing's sarcoma-routine diagnostic utilization of MIC2 analysis. A Pediatric Oncology Group/Children's Cancer Group Intergroup Study. *Hum Pathol* 25:304-307, 1994.

10. Weidner J, Tjoe J. Immunohistochemical profile of monoclonal antibody 013. Antibody that recognized glycoprotein p30/32 MIC2 and is useful in diagnosing Ewing's sarcoma and peripheral neuroepithelioma. *Am J Surg Pathol* 18:486-494, 1994.

11. Turc-Carel C, Aurias A, Mugneret F, Lizard S, Sidana I, Volk C, Thiery JP, Olschwang S, Philip I, Berger MP, Philip T, Lenoir GM, Mazabrand A. Chromosomes in Ewing's sarcoma. I. An evaluation of cases and remarkable consistency of t(11;22) (q24;q12). *Cancer Genet Cytogenet* 32:229-238, 1988.

12. Elsheikh T, Silverman JF, Wakely Jr. PE, Holbrook T, Joshi VV. Fine-needle aspiration cytology of Langerhans cell histiocytosis (eosinophilic granuloma) of bone in children. *Diag Cytopathol* 7:261-266, 1991.

13. Katz RL, Silva EG, DeSantos LA, Lukeman JM. Diagnosis of eosinophilic granuloma of bone by cytology, histology, and electron microscopy of transcutaneous bone-aspiration biopsy. *J Bone Joint Surg [Amer]* 62:1284-1290, 1980.

14. Shabb N, Fanning CV, Carrasco CH, Guo SQ, Katz RL, Ayala AG, Raymond AK, Cangir A. Diagnosis of eosinophilic granuloma of bone by fine-needle aspiration with concurrent institution of therapy. A cytologic, histologic, clinical, and radiologic study of 27 cases. *Diag Cytopathol* 9:3-12, 1993.

15. Akhtar M, Ali MA, Bakry M, Sackey K, Sabbah R. Fine needle biopsy of Langerhans histiocytosis (histiocytosis X). *Diagn Cytopathol* 9:527-533, 1993

16. Fanning CV, Sneige NS, Carrasco CH, Ayala AG, Murray JA, Raymond AK. Fine needle aspiration cytology of chondroblastoma of bone. *Cancer* 65:1847-1863, 1990.

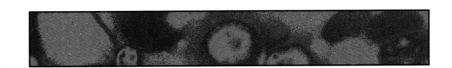

CHAPTER TWELVE

Soft Tissue

Soft tissue neoplasms are an important aspect of childhood disease. It has been stated that nearly 15% of all pediatric neoplasms in the US are derived from mesenchymal tissue.[1] Fine needle aspiration (FNA) biopsy, however, remains an underutilized procedure in the evaluation of soft tissue masses from infants and children. Possible explanations are that the vast majority of childhood soft tissue masses are benign, and will be entirely removed regardless of the cytology. In addition, because of the heterogeneous nature of soft tissue tumors, aspiration cytology from this site is among the most difficult to interpret.

Many surgeons contend that open biopsy is the only appropriate procedure for the initial diagnosis of a sarcoma.[2] Nonetheless, the principal goal of separating benign lesions (cysts, benign tumors and localized infectious processes) from malignant tumors, can be accomplished with a high degree of accuracy by FNA biopsy.[3-6] Classifying lesions into definitive histopathologic subtypes is more difficult, and, admittedly, not possible in the initial setting for some neoplasms, but still achievable in several instances. In this anatomic region particularly, cytopathologists need to be cautious, but not timid in the diagnostic interpretation of aspiration smears of a soft tissue mass.

The evaluation of histologic architecture necessitating it, open biopsy remains the "gold standard" for pathologic subclassification of primary childhood soft tissue tumors, therefore follow-up surgical biopsy is usually necessary for most *initial* primary malignant tumors. However, FNA biopsy has other roles in the evaluation of soft tissue masses. First,

Table 12.1
Aspiration Cytology of Selected Malignant Childhood Soft Tissue Tumors

	RMS	FS	SS	MPNST	EOE	ASPS	CCS	EpS
Typical age group	< 15 yrs	infantile & early teens	late teens & young adults	teens	teens	older	older teens	late teens teens & young adults
Anatomic site	H & N, extremity, trunk	extremity	knee	extremity	chest wall	H & N, extremity	foot, knee	fingers, hands
FNAB Cytology								
Cell size	small to intermed	small	small	small	small	large	intermed	large
Pleomorphism	0 to +++	±	0 to +	+ to +++	±	±	± to +	+ to +++
Cell shape	mainly round to polygonal	spindle	spindle	spindle	rounded	rounded to oblong	rounded	rounded to polygonal
Nuclei	round to elongated	elongated	elongated	elongated	round	round to oval	round to oval	oval
Nucleoli	± to +++	±	±	+ to ++	±	++ to +++	± to +	++ to +++
Cytoplasm	± to ++	± to +	± to +	± to +	± to +	+++	+ to ++	++ to +++
Mitoses	+ to ++	± to +	± to +	+ to ++	+ to ++	±	± to +	± to +
Immunophen-otype (positive staining)	Vimentin, desmin, actin, MyoD1	Vimentin only	Vimentin CK (epithelial cells)	Vimentin, S-100 (sporadic)	Vimentin only	Vimentin rarely S-100	Vimentin S-100	Vimentin CK, EMA HMB 45

RMS = rhabdomyosarcoma; FS = fibrosarcoma; SS = synovial sarcoma; MPNST = malignant peripheral nerve sheath tumor; EOE = extraosseous Ewing's;
ASPS = alveolar soft part sarcoma; CCS = clear cell sarcoma; EpS = epithelioid sarcoma; CK = cytokeratin; EMA = epithelial membrane antigen.

not all soft tissue masses need to be excised - eg, hematoma formation without an antecedent clinical history, the sternomastoid tumor (fibromatosis colli) of infancy, and some benign vascular tumors.

FNA biopsy can also help direct the surgical approach to a particular lesion, especially if a clinically innocuous mass turns out to be cytologically malignant. FNA biopsy can document recurrent or metastatic tumor in soft tissue[7]; in many instances this will completely obviate the need for surgical exploration or excision. As in other body sites, FNA biopsy has the advantages of low cost, speed, minimal trauma to the child, relief of parental anxiety in many cases and performance ability in an outpatient setting.

A different menu of diagnostic entities, as contrasted with adults, must be entertained by the cytopathologist when confronted with a potentially malignant soft tissue mass in the first 2 decades of life (Table 12.1). For example, one is not ordinarily required to consider carcinoma or malignant fibrous histiocytoma (the most common adult sarcoma) in the differential diagnosis of soft tissue tumors in this age group. The category of malignant small round cell tumors is one of the most intriguing in pediatric neoplasia. Although their recognition as a group is not particularly difficult cytologically, the challenge lies in separating them into clinically meaningful pathologic types because of their primitive cellular nature. Techniques ancillary to light microscopy are almost always necessary to accomplish this whether one is dealing with

Table 12.2
Fibromatosis-Cytomorphology

Cellularity low to moderate.

Acellular or hypocellular fragments of collagen or mucoid ground substance.

Spindle cells lie free or in loose clusters.

Spindled or oval nuclei with smooth nuclear contours; bare nuclei common. Homogeneous nuclear chromatin. Nucleoli small or absent.

Thin, delicate unipolar and bipolar tapered strands of pale cytoplasm.

Atrophic myofibers with clustered nuclei may be present.

Isolated macrophages, lymphocytes and plasma cells.

Knowledge of the age, anatomic location, clinical examination and any radiographic information is mandatory to acheive a consistently accurate interpretation of smears

the paraffin tissue section or the cytologic smear. One of the more difficult aspects of soft tissue aspiration cytology remains (as it does in adults) the separation of a benign, but cytologically exuberant and atypical reactive process from a malignant neoplasm. It cannot be overemphasized that knowledge of the age, anatomic location, clinical examination and any radiographic information is mandatory to achieve a consistently accurate interpretation of smears.

Benign Soft Tissue Tumors

Fibromatosis

Fibromatosis may occur at any age, and involve almost any body site including intrathoracic and intra-abdominal locations as well as the somatic soft tissue. Several classifications have been offered for the various fibromatoses of childhood. Because of unique histologic characteristics, anatomic location or age at onset, specific diagnostic terms are awarded to certain fibrous proliferations (Table 12.2). For example, fibromatosis colli or digital fibroma are defined by their anatomic site. Nonetheless, the largest number of these occur as fibromatoses, not otherwise specified. Clinical signs and symptoms are nonspecific since most fibromatoses appear as a nondescript mass. All are characterized by their lack of metastatic potential, despite their infiltrative pattern. Yet, repeated local recurrence can be a major problem with incompletely excised neoplasms.

Although fibromatoses consist of a proliferation of spindled fibroblasts and myofibroblasts, many have certain histologic characteristics that set them apart, eg, calcification and chondroid matrix in juvenile aponeurotic fibroma and cytoplasmic inclusions in recurrent digital fibroma (Image 12.1). Those fibromatoses that have no special designation consist of uniform fibroblasts embedded in a collagenous stroma showing infiltration of muscle at their periphery.

Smear cellularity varies from low to moderate (Table 12.2). The collagenous matrix produced by these lesions frequently precludes aspirating large numbers of cells. Fibroblasts are spindled cells lying free or in loose clusters with uniform oval or elongated nuclei with smooth nuclear contours.[8-12] Bare nuclei are common. Some aspirates contain plump stellate or polygonal cells. Polygonal cells typically have a rounded nucleus with loose, finely granular chromatin and small nucleoli. Nucleoli are normally indistinct in spindle cell nuclei that have generally smudged nuclear chromatin. Thin, tapering unipolar and bipolar strands of pale cytoplasm with ill-defined cell borders are characteristic of fibroblasts (Image 12.2). Acellular or hypocellular fragments of collagenous stroma or mucoid ground substance (metachromatic in Romanowsky smears) may be found. Atrophic and degenerating skeletal myofibers with closely clustered sarcolemmal nuclei are frequently present, and may simulate multinucleated giant cells. Mitotic figures are very infrequent.

Potential Problems in Diagnosis: As in tissue histopathology, the greatest dilemma lies in differentiating highly cellular fibromatoses from low-grade fibrosarcoma. The latter are more richly cellular, but the distinction from a very well-differentiated fibrosarcoma may be formidable. Other diagnostic considerations include nodular fasciitis, leiomyoma, exuberant granulation tissue reaction and benign neural tumors. Nuclei in the latter have a more wavy and serpentine border than those of fibroblasts. Reactive fibroblasts with "open" nuclei, and discrete nucleoli may evoke suspicions of a malignant process, but significant nuclear pleomorphism is rare, if it exists at all. The fibroblasts in nodular fasciitis are more likely to demonstrate multi- or binucleation; mature lymphocytes and plasma cells are almost always found.[13]

Ancillary studies are not particularly helpful. Fibroblasts express the intermediate filament vimentin by immunochemistry, but little else. Electron microscopy will confirm the fibroblastic or myofibroblastic nature of cells, but not necessarily provide a definitive diagnosis.

The fibroblasts in nodular fasciitis are more likely to demonstrate multi- or binucleation; mature lymphocytes and plasma cells are almost always found

Schwannoma (Neurilemoma)

In the pediatric population, schwannoma is more likely to occur in older children and adolescents. It is primarily a solitary mass affecting the head and neck region and upper extremities. Unfortunately, FNA biopsy will ordinarily cause sharp pain in the patient.

This tumor is truly encapsulated, and composed of crowded spindle cells with elongated frequently wavy nuclei that are often arranged in parallel rows (Antoni A pattern). Cells may also be widely separated by a loose fibrous matrix containing coarse collagen bands (Antoni B pattern). Hyalinized blood vessels and mast cells are frequent.

Cellularity of smears ranges from sparse to moderately cellular. Schwann cells are distributed both singly and as aggregates with the former being more common.[14,15] Aggregates may contain nuclei crowded together and arrayed in parallel palisading groups simulating the Antoni A pattern seen in tissue sections (Image 12.3). Rarely, Verocay body formations (two groups of cells in "picket fence" arrangement separated by acellular fibrillar material) may be found.[16]

Schwann cell nuclei are uniform, oval and spindled. Only sporadically are they wavy with tapered ends. Nuclei have a bland, homogeneous chromatin and indistinct nucleoli. Cytoplasm consists of elongated thin strands with tapered processes. Cell boundaries are indistinct and the cytoplasm becomes confluent with that of other cells in a cluster. Bare, tapered nuclei are also present. Rarely, isolated pleomorphic nuclei are seen. Metachromatic, amorphous background material can be prominent in Romanowsky-stained smears.

Positive immunoreactivity of cell smears with S-100 will help confirm the neural nature of this neoplasm. Electron microscopy demonstrates spindle cells with elongated, frequently interdigitating cell processes enveloped by a thin basal lamina. Extracellular long spacing collagen (Luse bodies) may be seen.

Neurofibroma

Neurofibroma may exist as a single lesion or as part of the stigmata of von Recklinghausen's disease. Solitary neurofibroma presents as a nontender mass in the skin or subcutis. Sharp stinging pain may occur during the FNA biopsy procedure. We have witnessed the multinodularity of a plexiform neurofibroma confused clinically and radiologically with lymphadenopathy.

Spindle and stellate cells are admixed with cords of collagen in a myxoid or loose fibrous stroma in histologic sections. Hyalinization is common. Segments of normal nerve may be found in the plexiform type.

To the naked eye, the aspirate often has a water-clear slightly gelatinous appearance because of the abundant myxoid stroma in this neoplasm (Table 12.3). Cell yield is variable, but usually there is a paucity of cells. Most cells are isolated, but small aggregates are not uncommon. Spindle and stellate cells possess markedly elongated, sometimes wavy, twisted and curved nuclei (Image 12.4).[10,12] Nuclear chromatin is bland, and nucleoli are absent or indistinct. Stripped nuclei with tapered ends are common. Individual cell cytoplasm is meager, and frequently confluent with that of other cells in a cluster. Metachromatically stained background material (myxoid matrix) is usually conspicuous (Romanowsky stain). Mitotic figures and mast cells are seldom seen.

Table 12.3
Neurofibroma-Cytomorphology

Cell yield variable, generally a hypocellular smear.

Cells isolated and in small aggregates.

Slim and elongated spindle and stellate shaped cells.

Wavy, twisted, or curved spindled nuclei with bland chromatin, and absent nucleoli.

Scant cell cytoplasm; frequently confluent with that of other cells in a cluster.

Myxoid stroma generally abundant.

Potential Problems in Diagnosis: At times, the cytologic distinction between these two benign neural neoplasms (schwannoma and neurofibroma) can be difficult, if not impossible. A key difference is in the nuclei wherein twisted, curved nuclei are more characteristic of neurofibroma, while the uniform schwann cell nuclei can be confused with those of fibroblasts or leiomyocytes; this distinction, however, is not absolute. The lack of extreme cellularity, cellular pleomorphism, background necrosis, and mitoses is usually sufficient to safeguard one from calling these entities malignant.

S-100 expression by spindle cells will help confirm the neural nature of the neoplasm. Ultrastructural study shows spindled cells with long cell processes that are separated by bundles of collagen fibrils and invested by a discontinuous, fragmented external basal lamina. Subplasmalemmal pinocytotic vesicles are common.

Table 12.4
Lymphangioma-Cytomorphology

Straw-colored or clear fluid; amount is variable.

Uniform, small mature lymphocytes; occasional macrophage.

Amorphous proteinaceous background.

Hemangioma

This is the most common soft tissue neoplasm of childhood. FNA biopsy is not recommended for the clinically obvious cutaneous or subcutaneous hemangioma, which frequently regresses in infants and young children. Deeper hemangiomas usually relinquish blood as soon as the aspiration procedure is begun; hence the mass may decrease in size after the FNA biopsy procedure.

Capillary, cavernous and intramuscular types occur. Common to all types is a proliferation of vascular spaces lined by flattened endothelial cells. Subtyping is based on vessel caliber and location.

Smears consist almost entirely of blood. Occasional isolated or small groups of polygonal cells are seen.[10,12] In the intramuscular variant, smears are moderately cellular with clusters of oval and spindle cells (Image 12.5). Degenerating skeletal myofibers may also be present in the intramuscular form. Hemosiderin-laden macrophages may be seen. Immunostaining for CD31, CD34, Factor VIII and/or Ulex europeus antigens may be helpful in recognizing cells as endothelial in origin.

Lymphangioma

The majority of lymphangiomas occur before 2 years of age, occur in the head, neck and axillary region and are usually readily identified clinically because of their fluctuant nature. Clear, colorless or straw-colored fluid is typically obtained with FNA biopsy although these aspirates are frequently contaminated with fresh or brown hemolyzed blood. Although the mass may disappear after drainage by FNA biopsy, fluid typically reaccumulates in the area.

Cystically dilated vascular spaces are lined by a flattened endothelium in histologic preparations. Vascular lumens contain proteinaceous fluid in which variable numbers of mature lymphocytes are present. Lymphoid aggregates including some with germinal centers may exist in the interstitial connective tissue.

Because of the extremely low cell yield, we recommend cytocentrifugation preparations of the fluid rather than conventional smears. Small collections of mature lymphocytes, erythrocytes and occasional monocytes and histiocytes are seen with a background of amorphous proteinaceous material (Image 12.6) (Table 12.4). Ancillary studies are not particularly helpful.

Lipoma

Lipomas are uncommon in pediatrics, customarily being a neoplasm of adults beyond the 3rd decade of life. When they do occur, one is more apt to encounter them on the extremities of adolescents. They are soft to palpation, movable and localized to the subcutaneous tissue. Paraffin-embedded tissue demonstrates a thin fibrous capsule surrounding mature adipose tissue that envelopes a subtle vascular pattern.

In cytologic smears mature adipose tissue readily recapitulates its histologic counterpart.[17] Lipocytes are gathered into tight clusters separated from one another by thin, delicate cell boundaries. The obvious cytologic feature is the large, clear cytoplasmic vacuole, which dwarfs the small, round and peripherally (sometimes centrally) located nucleus.

Because an intact fibrous capsule cannot be appreciated cytologically, one can only state that smears contain mature adipose tissue, and the diagnosis of lipoma is inferred by the presence of a soft, freely movable mass.

Potential Problems in Diagnosis: The differential diagnosis of lipoma in children includes lipoblastoma. Lipoblastoma is a rare benign tumor of adipose tissue that is unique to children during the first 3 years of life, and is located primarily in the extremities. Tissue pathology demonstrates lobules of fat with mature lipocytes toward the center of lobules and multivacuolated lipoblasts and spindle cells at the periphery. FNA biopsy cytology displays fragments of fibrofatty tissue with spindle cells, stellate cells and monovacuolated and multivacuolated lipoblasts in a myxoid background.[18]

Because an intact fibrous capsule cannot be appreciated cytologically, one can only state that smears contain mature adipose tissue, and the diagnosis of lipoma is inferred by the presence of a soft, freely movable mass

Malignant Soft Tissue Tumors

Rhabdomyosarcoma

Rhabdomyosarcoma is the most common primary soft tissue malignancy in children. Estimated annual incidence is about 5 per mil-

Table 12.5
Rhabdomyosarcoma-Cytomorphology

Very cellular smears in either crowded aggregates with piling up of cells on one another or as single cells.

Small to intermediate sized cells with binucleated and multinucleated forms.

Cells are rounded, polygonal or spindle shaped with high N/C ratios.

Nuclei are oval, moderately pleomorphic, hyperchromatic, frequently eccentric. Nucleoli are variable in size.

Cytoplasm is meager to moderate in amount; extends from the nucleus in a tapered, unipolar ("tadpole-shape") fashion. Cytoplasmic cross-striations very rare.

Mitoses variable.

Background necrosis may be present.

lion children. Peak incidence occurs between 2 and 6 years and late adolescence. The conventional pathologic classification is divided into embryonal, alveolar and pleomorphic subtypes. Botryoid rhabdomyosarcoma is considered a special subepithelial form of embryonal rhabdomyosarcoma and arises in mucosa lined hollow viscera. Tsokos et al have introduce the term "solid alveolar" type in their description of the National Cancer Institute classification of this tumor.[19] Their study reiterated that the alveolar subtype is an independently unfavorable and statistically significant prognostic factor, even if only focally present within the tumor.

The embryonal subtype is more likely to occur in the head and neck, genitourinary and retroperitoneal regions of young children, while the alveolar subtype favors the extremities and perineal regions of older children, adolescents and young adults.

Rhabdomyosarcoma has a varied histologic picture dependent upon the type and degree of differentiation. The histologic appearance ranges from primitive small cells with rounded contours, no visible nucleoli, and meager cytoplasm to well-differentiated forms with spindled or oval forms with vesicular nuclei, prominent nucleoli and abundant eosinophilic cytoplasm — uncommonly with visible cross-striations. The alveolar subtype is characterized by thick fibrous septa segregating cells into loose nests in which better differentiated rhabdomyoblasts are found at center.

FNA biopsies of rhabdomyosarcoma produce highly cellular smears that show cells disseminated as crowded aggregates, with piling of cells one upon another or, more commonly, as single cells (Table 12.5).[12,20,21] Rhabdomyoblasts are small to intermediate. Most are round or polygonal: few cells are spindled. Binucleation and multinucleation are characteristic (Image 12.7). Nuclei are oval, moderately pleomorphic and frequently eccentric (Image 12.8). Stripped nuclei are common due to the fragility of cells. Nuclear chromatin is usually very dense; nucleoli may be prominent. Cytoplasm is meager to abundant, depending on the degree of differentiation, and frequently extends from the nucleus in a unipolar tapered fashion (Image 12.9). Cytoplasmic vacuoles are common. In well-differentiated forms, markedly

Rhabdomyosarcoma has a varied histologic picture dependent upon the type and degree of differentiation

Table 12.6
Fibrosarcoma-Cytomorphology

Variable cell yield.

Cells arranged in both clusters and as single forms.

Oval or spindle cells with variable, usually minimal nuclear pleomorphism.

Cytoplasm is frequently tapered, bipolar or unipolar and meager.

Nucleoli small or indistinct; mitotic figures inconsistently present.

Metachromatic staining collagenous stroma may be found.

---

elongated ribbon-like cytoplasmic tails may be present; rarely, we have encountered a "tigroid" background similar to that described for seminoma in the Romanowsky-stained smears (Image 12.10). Cytoplasmic cross-striations are extremely unusual (Image 12.11). Background necrosis and mitoses are variable but generally are common.

Potential Problems in Diagnosis: Of all the malignant small round cell tumors, rhabdomyosarcoma displays the widest range of cytologic morphology. The most primitive are nearly indistinguishable from Ewing's sarcoma or primitive neuroblastoma, while the more differentiated forms show obvious "strap" cells. We have found binucleated and multinucleated cells to be a helpful clue in segregating rhabdomyosarcoma from other forms.[22] Akhtar et al[23] have cytologically grouped rhabdomyoblasts into early, intermediate and late forms based primarily on the amount of cytoplasm. As a general rule, immunochemistry or electron microscopy are required for definitive diagnosis of rhabdomyosarcoma, particularly the primitive small cell variety. We have not been able to subtype consistently alveolar from embryonal rhabdomyosarcoma in most instances by FNA biopsy. Recurrent or or metastatic neoplasms can usually be diagnosed with confidence without ancillary studies.[7]

Most rhabdomyosarcomas express the immunocytochemical markers actin and desmin (Image 12.12).[24,25] Although it is a very specific antigenic marker of skeletal muscle differentiation, we have found myoglobin to be too insensitive in most instances. Recently, MyoD1 has been reported to be a reliable antigen for rhabdomyosarcoma.[26] Ultrastructural diagnostic features include the presence of alternating thin and thick cytoplasmic filaments and/or rudimentary Z-band formation. Cytogenetic studies have revealed chromosome 11q deletion and chromosome 2;13 translocation.

Fibrosarcomas

Fibrosarcomas appears to have 2 incidence peaks in children: in the first few years of life, and again in early adolescence. It affects the extremities more commonly than the torso. It is a histologically monotonous tumor with more or less uniform, densely packed spindle cells arranged in interweaving parallel bundles — the classic herringbone pattern. The well-differentiated variant may have an abundant collagen matrix.

There is a variable cell yield depending on cellular differentiation and stromal collagenization in FNA biopsy, but cells are plentiful from moderate and poorly differentiated forms of this tumor (Table 12.6). Cells are arranged in both clusters and as single forms.[10-12] They are nearly all oval or spindled with variable nuclear pleomorphism dependent on the degree of differentiation (Image 12.13). Cytoplasm is frequently tapered, bipolar or unipolar and meager. Nucleoli are small or indistinct and mitotic figures are inconsistent. Metachromatic-staining collagenous stroma may be found.

Relatively consistent positive immunoreactivity to vimentin, and negative immunostaining for neural (S-100, neurofilament), myogenic (desmin and muscle-specific actin) and epithelial (cytokeratin, epithelial membrane antigen) markers helps confirm the diagnosis. A recent review of congenital and infantile fibrosarcomas substantiates the hypothesis that they are characterized by a nonrandom gain of chromosomes.[27]

Synovial Sarcomas

About ⅓ of synovial sarcomas occur in patients less than 20 years of age, typically in adolescence. The knee and thigh are the most common sites, followed by the upper extremity.

Synovial sarcomas occur as both biphasic and monophasic types. The latter closely simulates fibrosarcoma with spindle cells arranged in sheets and fascicles. Biphasic synovial sarcomas have both a distinctive epithelial component, and a spindle cell component that mimics fibrosarcoma. The epithelial component may be laid out in solid cords or glandular nests. Calcification is not uncommon, but collagen production is sparse. Pleomorphic giant cells are rare.

A rich cell yield is dispersed as single cells or thick closely packed clusters of cells (Table 12.7).[10-12,28] Relatively uniform spindled and oval cells possess rounded or oblong monotonous nuclei (Image 12.14). Nuclear chromatin is bland, and typically the smooth nuclear rim is blunted rather than tapered at each pole. Nucleoli are small or indistinct, and mitoses are common. Cells contain only a small amount of pale cytoplasm. Parallel arrangement of cuboidal or columnar nuclei representing the glandular (epithelial) component of a biphasic tumor may be seen, but this is distinctly unusual, and subtle. A moderate amount of background metachromatic staining material may be seen.

Potential Problems in Diagnosis: If a biphasic pattern exists, one can be more confident in the diagnosis. Fibrosarcoma and malignant peripheral nerve sheath tumor are major diagnostic considerations when only the spindle cell component is present, as in tissue histopathology. In one study, synovial sarcomas could not be reliably distinguished from fibrosarcoma and malignant peripheral nerve sheath tumor using smears alone.[11] Most authors agree that metastatic or locally recurrent synovial sarcomas can be readily recognized, but subtyping of an initial lesion is difficult. Ancillary studies can be extremely helpful since epithelial cells and some spindle cells consistently exhibit positive immunoreactivity to cytokeratin. Spindle cells also stain with vimentin. Ultra-

Fibrosarcoma and malignant peripheral nerve sheath tumor are major diagnostic considerations when only the spindle cell component is present, as in tissue histopathology

Table 12.7
Synovial Sarcoma-Cytomorphology

Rich cell yield dispersed as single cells or closely packed clusters.

Relatively uniform spindle and oval cells possess rounded or oblong monotonous nuclei.

Bland nuclear chromatin; smooth nuclear rim blunted rather than tapered at each pole.

Nucleoli small or indistinct; mitoses common.

Only a small amount of pale staining cytoplasm.

Parallel arrangement of cuboidal or columnar nuclei representing the glandular (epithelial) component of a biphasic tumor (unusual).

Moderate amount of background metachromatic staining material.

---

structurally, the epithelial cells have junctional complexes and microvilli.[11]   An X;18 chromosomal translocation is characteristic of this neoplasm.[29,30]

Extraosseous Ewing's Sarcoma

Extraosseous Ewing's sarcoma affects the same patient group as its counterpart in bone.   The chest wall, lower extremity, and paravertebral region are involved (see Chapter 11, Bone, p 249).[31,32]

Alveolar Soft Part Sarcoma

Alveolar soft part sarcoma is typically a tumor of older teenagers and young adults, but as many as $1/5$ of cases occur in younger patients.[33]   The head and neck is a usual site in children, while the thigh is affected in adults.   The histogenesis of ASPS remains a mystery, although a muscle origin has been suggested due to positive staining of cells with the myogenic marker MyoD1.[34]

Histologically, the large monotonous cells of alveolar soft part sarcoma are arrayed into well-defined nests surrounded by thin fibrous septa.   Cells are ordinarily loosely cohesive within these nests.

Loosely aggregated and single very large rounded cells are found in moderately to highly cellular smears (Table 12.8).[7,12,35]   Nuclei are round and eccentrically placed with dense nuclear chromatin and single very large prominent nucleoli (Image 12.15).   Occasional cells are binucleated.   Due to the fragility of tumor cells, bare nuclei are common. Cells contain voluminous finely granular cytoplasm with some showing faint linear cytoplasmic striations. Mitotic figures are rare.

Characteristic membrane bound crystals with rectangular or rhomboid shapes are found by electron microscopy.   Immunochemistry is largely nonreactive for markers of epithelial and neuroendocrine differentiation.   Rare cells within a few cases have demonstrated positive staining for S-100[33] and MyoD1,[34] but it remains premature to rely on these antibodies to establish a diagnosis of ASPS at this time.

Table 12.8

Alveolar Soft Part Sarcoma-Cytomorphology

Single and loosely aggregated large, rounded cells.

Round and eccentric nuclei with dense nuclear chromatin and single prominent nucleoli.

Occasional binucleated cells. Bare nuclei common.

Voluminous finely granular cytoplasm, some with faint linear cytoplasmic striations.

Mitotic figures rare.

Malignant Peripheral Nerve Sheath Tumor

In the pediatric age group, this uncommon neoplasm is more frequent in the 2nd decade. In a large series from the Mayo Clinic, almost 13% of malignant peripheral nerve sheath tumor occurred in children.[36] The soft tissues of the lower extremity and trunk are the principal sites affected. A strong association exists with von Recklinghausen's disease, and it is common for malignant peripheral nerve sheath tumor to arise in a nerve trunk or pre-existing neurofibroma. An enlarging mass is the most common mode of presentation. The prognosis is poor. Spindle cells with uniform, smooth and sometimes serpentine nuclei arranged in fascicles is the typical pattern found in tissue sections. However, as recently demonstrated by Meis et al, a wide spectrum of morphologic patterns can be seen.[37]

Moderately to highly cellular smears have cells arranged singly and in clusters (Image 12.16). Cellular pleomorphism is variable. Spindle shaped cells display elongated nuclei many with tapered ends, and delicate bipolar or unipolar cytoplasmic processes.[10-12] The nuclear border is slightly wavy and twisted in some nuclei. Nuclear chromatin is finely granular, and some cells possess prominent nucleoli. Anisonucleosis and bare nuclei are common. Polygonal cells are common in the epithelioid variant. Individual cell necrosis and mitoses are variable.

Problems in Diagnosis: Malignant spindle cell tumor is usually as diagnostically specific as possible from the aspirate using light microscopy alone. Knowledge of a clinical history of von Recklinghausen's disease or evidence of the mass arising from a nerve or neurofibroma allows one to suggest the diagnosis of malignant peripheral nerve sheath tumor. Vendraminelli et al emphasized the twisted, comma or pear-shaped configuration of cell nuclei as being highly characteristic of malignant peripheral nerve sheath tumor.[38]

Fibrosarcoma and synovial sarcoma (monophasic type) are the principal differential diagnostic considerations. The degree of cellular and nuclear pleomorphism is usually greater in malignant peripheral nerve sheath tumor than in these other two neoplasms. Although the twisted configuration of nuclei in malignant peripheral nerve sheath tumor contrasts with the smoother and more regular nuclear outline of synovial sarcoma and fibrosarcoma, this can be an extremely subtle distinction. S-100 staining of cells is common, but not universal. Electron microscopy is sometimes helpful, and may be definitive.

A strong association exists with von Recklinghausen's disease, and it is common for malignant peripheral nerve sheath tumor to arise in a nerve trunk or pre-existing neurofibroma

Table 12.9
Clear Cell Sarcoma-Cytomorphology

Highly cellular smears with cells dispersed singly and in loose aggregates.

Relatively monotonous oval and rounded intermediate-sized cells.

Nuclei often eccentric with a single nucleolus.

Moderate amount of finely granular and clear cytoplasm with well-defined cell boundaries.

Occasional mitoses and multinucleated giant cells.

Clear Cell Sarcoma of Soft Tissue

Although mainly a neoplasm of young adults, about 1/5 of patients are less than 19 years of age.[39] Soft tissues of the extremities, notably the foot and knee are the commonly affected sites. The prevailing evidence suggests that this tumor is of neural crest derivation, and shares many of the histochemical, ultrastructural and cytogenetic features of malignant melanoma. It is highly aggressive with a poor prognosis. In a recent series, tumor size (> 5 cm), and necrosis stood out as poor prognostic findings.[40]

Histologic patterns include cells arranged in cords, fascicles and rounded nests. Cells are polygonal or slightly spindled with vesicular nuclei and one or two prominent nucleoli. Mitoses are sporadic. There is a moderate amount of clear to finely granular cytoplasm. Multinucleated giant cells may exist.

Relatively monotonous oval and rounded cells (about twice the size of a neutrophil) are dispersed singly and in loose aggregates in highly cellular smears (Table 12.9).[7,12,41,42] Nuclei are often eccentric with a single nucleolus (more obvious in Papanicolaou-stained smears). There is a moderate amount of finely granular and clear cytoplasm with well-defined cell boundaries (Image 12.17). Occasional mitoses and multinucleated giant cells are present, while markedly pleomorphic cells are absent.

The cells in a large percentage of cases express S-100 and HMB-45 antibodies. Histochemical staining for melanin is also positive in a large percentage of cases. Premelanosomes can be found in the majority of cases using electron microscopy.

Epithelioid Sarcoma

Epithelioid sarcoma is a well-delineated clinicopathologic entity that occurs chiefly in the 2nd and 3rd decades of life. The extremities, particularly the hands and forearm, are the principal sites of involvement. Single or multiple firm, discrete masses develop in the subcutis, dermis, or deeper soft tissue; a small number are ulcerated at the time of presentation.

The neoplasm is histologically arranged in nodules, some of which are well defined and contain central areas of necrosis.[43] Due to this deceptively benign arrangement, diagnostic confusion with granulomatous inflammation is frequently mentioned in the literature. Epithelioid sarcoma is composed of polygonal epithelial-like cells intermingled with areas of spindle cells. Cytoplasm is plentiful with discrete cell boundaries. Nuclei are often vesicular, containing single, easily visible nucleoli. Smears are very cellular with cells in both aggregates and distributed as single cells.[10,12] Large polygonal cells have moderate to abundant cytoplasm, which is frequently tapered, and sharp cell boundaries. Nuclei are eccentric in most cells. Nuclei are pleomorphic with prominent nucleoli (Image 12.18). Background necrosis may be evident. Immunophenotyping of epithelioid sarcoma shows a high percentage of cells that express epithelial membrane antigen, vimentin and cytokeratin.[44] The latter two antibodies are almost invariably present. Integration of the clinical features, cytomorphology and this immunoprofile virtually guarantees diagnosis of epithelioid sarcoma.

Image 12.1
Spindle shaped fibroblasts display delicate tapering strands of cytoplasm. Note the completely spherical sky-blue, glassy cytoplasmic inclusions characteristic of this subtype of childhood fibromatosis. (Romanowsky).

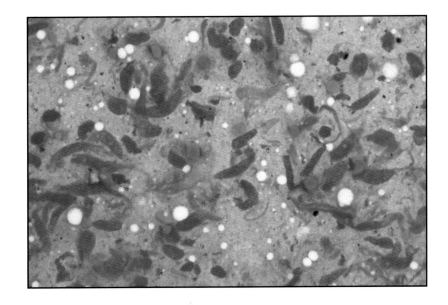

Image 12.2
Fibromatosis. Fibroblasts with unipolar and bipolar elongated cytoplasm.
A Romanowsky.
B Papanicolaou.

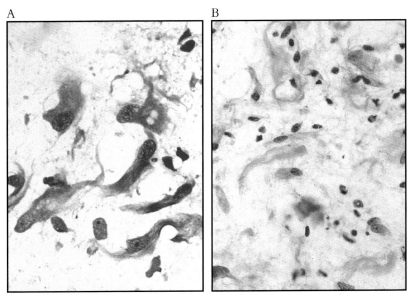

Image 12.3
Schwannoma. Spindle cells with stripped nuclei are loosely scattered and embedded within metachromatic stroma. (Romanowsky).

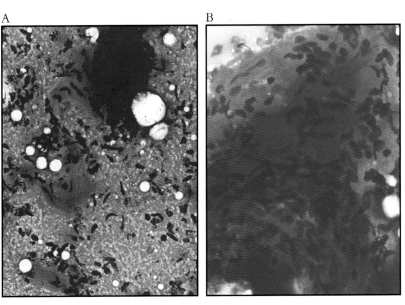

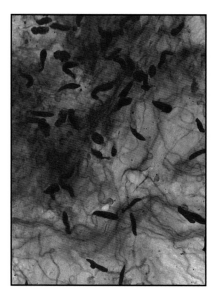 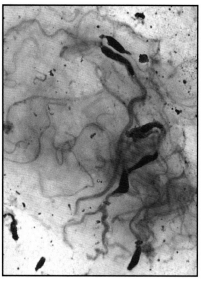

Image 12.4
Neurofibroma. Slender, twisted and curved cell nuclei are entrapped within a translucent metachromatic stroma. (Romanowsky).

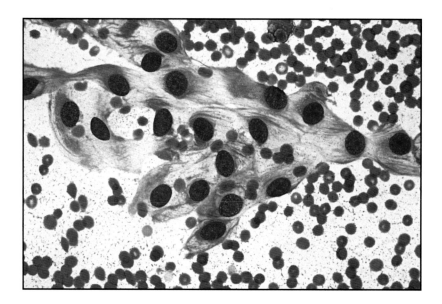

Image 12.5
Hemangioma. A loose group of oval cells has rounded, bland nuclei and delicate wisps of cytoplasm. (Romanowsky).

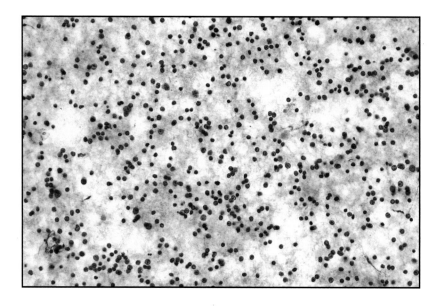

Image 12.6
Lymphangioma. Cytospin preparation from FNA biopsy showing mature lymphocytes only. (Papanicolaou).

Image 12.7

Rhabdomyosarcoma. Small rounded cells, some with eccentric multiple nuclei.

A Romanowsky.
B Papanicolaou.

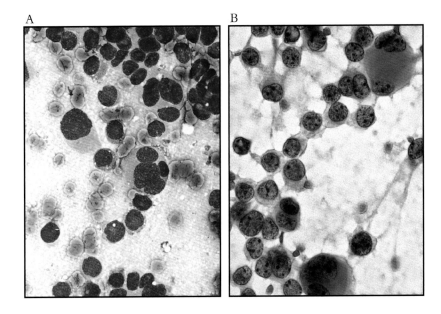

Image 12.8

Rhabdomyosarcoma. Nuclear pleomorphism and nucleoli are obvious in this field. (Romanowsky).

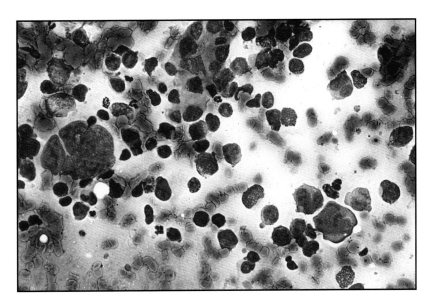

Image 12.9

Rhabdomyosarcoma. An occasional cell has a tapered cytoplasm. (Papanicolaou).

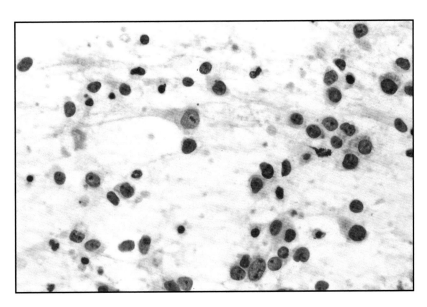

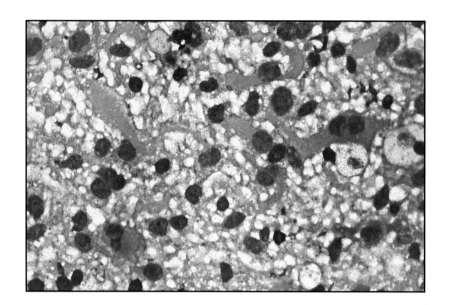

Image 12.10
Rhabdomyosarcoma. Well-differentiated, with elongated segments of cytoplasm and peripherally placed nuclei mimicking primitive myotubes. (Romanowsky). (Courtesy Dr M Almeida).

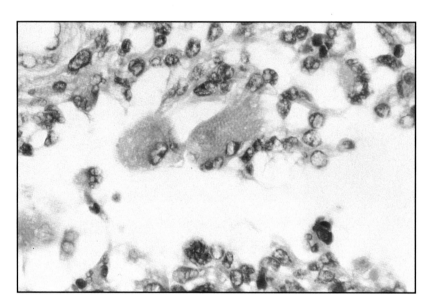

Image 12.11
Rhabdomyosarcoma. Rare strap cell with cytoplasmic cross-striations. (H&E).

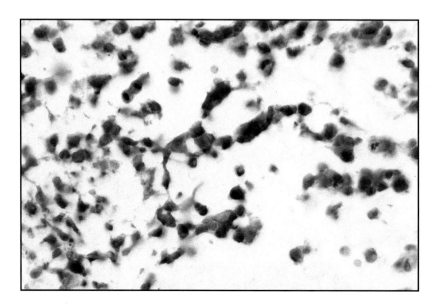

Image 12.12
Rhabdomyosarcoma. Positive staining of rhabdomyoblasts with antibody to smooth muscle actin.

Image 12.13
Fibrosarcoma. Dense clusters of stellate and spindle shaped cells.
A Papanicolaou.
B Romanowsky.

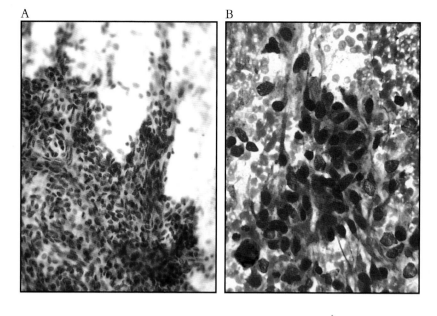

Image 12.14
Synovial sarcoma. Densely cellular clusters slightly elongated nuclei. Small nucleoli are better seen in **B**.
A Romanowsky.
B Papanicolaou.

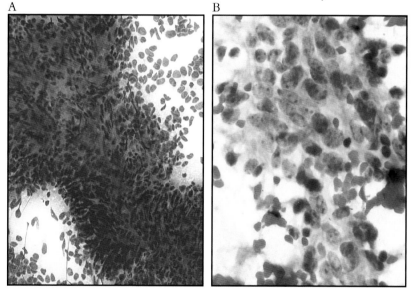

Image 12.15
Alveolar soft part sarcoma. Large cells have abundant cytoplasm and obvious single nucleoli.
A Romanowsky.
B Papanicolaou.

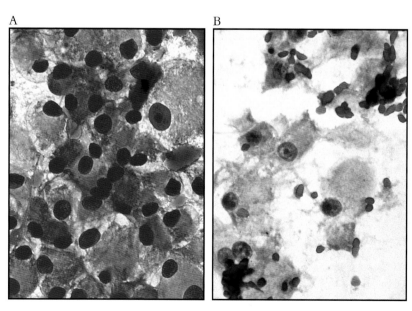

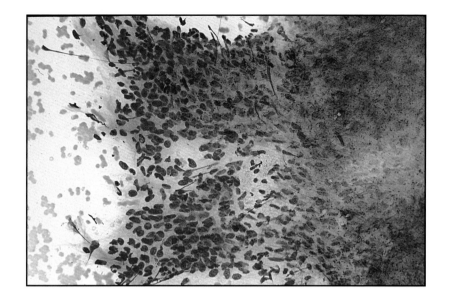

Image 12.16
Malignant peripheral nerve sheath tumor. Dense highly cellular aggregate of spindle cells. (Romanowsky).

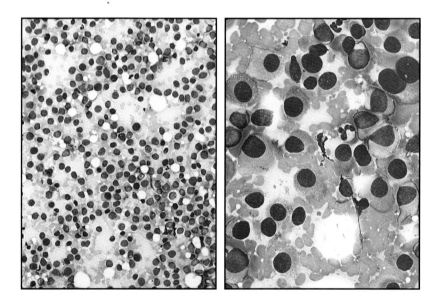

Image 12.17
Clear cell sarcoma. Uniform single cells have a moderate amount of pale staining cytoplasm. An occasional cell is binucleated. (Romanowsky).

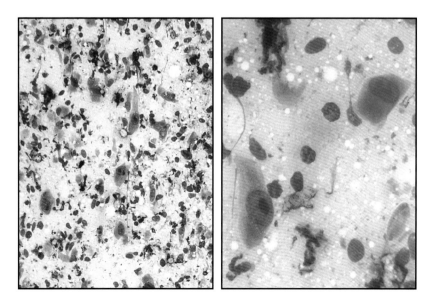

Image 12.18
Epitheliod sarcoma. Pleomorphic cells with prominent nucleoli and abundant cytoplasm. (Romanowsky).

References

1. Pui CH, Crist WM. Pediatric solid tumors. In: American Cancer Society Textbook of Clinical Oncology. Holleb AI, Fink DJ, Murphy GP, eds. The American Cancer Society, Atlanta, 32:453-480, 1991.

2. Posner MC, Brennan MF. Soft tissue sarcomas. In: American Cancer Society Textbook of Clinical Oncology. Holleb AI, Fink DJ, Murphy GP, eds. The American Cancer Society, Atlanta, 27:359-376, 1991.

3. Akerman M, Rydholm A, Persson BM. Aspiration cytology of soft tissue tumors. The 10-year experience at an Orthopedic Oncology Center. *Acta Orthop Scand* 56:407-412, 1985.

4. Wakely Jr PE, Kardos TF, Frable WJ. Application of fine needle aspiration biopsy to pediatrics. *Hum Pathol* 19:1383-1386, 1988.

5. Fraser-Hill MA, Renfrew DL. Percutaneous needle biopsy of musculoskeletal lesions. I. Effective accuracy and diagnostic utility. *Amer J Roentgenol* 158:809-812, 1992.

6. Layfield LJ, Anders KH, Glasgow BJ, Mirra JM. Fine needle aspiration of primary soft tissue lesions. *Arch Pathol Lab Med* 110:420-424, 1986.

7. Wakely Jr PE, Powers CN, Frable WJ. Metachronous soft tissue masses in children and young adults with cancer: Correlation of histology and aspiration cytology. *Hum Pathol* 21:669-677, 1990.

8. Wakely Jr PE, Price WG, Frable WJ. Sternomastoid tumor of infancy (fibromatosis colli). Diagnosis by aspiration cytology. *Mod Pathol* 2:378-381, 1989.

9. Raab SS, Silverman JF, McLeod DL, Benning TL, Geisinger KR. Fine needle aspiration biopsy of fibromatosis. *Acta Cytol* 37:323-328, 1993.

10. Willems JS. Aspiration biopsy cytology of soft-tissue tumors. In: Clinical Aspiration Cytology. 2nd ed. Linsk JA, Franzen S, eds. JB Lippincott Co, Philadelphia, p. 365-397, 1989.

11. Kindblom LG, Walaas L, Widehn S. Ultrastructural studies in the preoperative cytologic diagnosis of soft tissue tumors. *Sem Diag Pathol* 3:317-344, 1986.

12. Hajdu SI, Hajdu EO. Cytopathology of soft tissue and bone tumors. Monographs in Clinical Cytology. Vol. 12. Weid GL, ed. S. Karger, Basel, 1989.

13. Dahl I, Akerman M. Nodular fasciitis. A correlative cytologic and histologic study of 13 cases. *Acta Cytol* 25:215-222, 1981.

14. Dahl I, Hagmar B, Idvall I. Benign solitary neurilemmoma (schwannoma). A correlative aspiration cytology and histologic study of 28 cases. *Acta Pathol Microbiol Scand* [A] 92:91-101, 1984.

15. Zbieranowski I, Bedard YC. Fine needle aspiration of schwannomas. *Acta Cytol* 33:381-384, 1989.

16. Ramzy I. Benign schwannoma. Demonstration of Verocay bodies using fine needle aspiration. *Acta Cytol* 21:316-319, 1977.

17. Akerman M, Rydholm A. Aspiration cytology of lipomatous tumors. A 10-year experience at an Orthopedic Oncology Center. *Diag Cytopathol* 3:295-302, 1987.

18. Talwar MB, Misra K, Marya SKS, Dev G. Fine needle aspiration cytology of a lipoblastoma. *Acta Cytol* 34:855-857, 1990.

19. Tsokos M, Webber BL, Parham DM, Wesley RA, Miser A, Miser JS, Etcubanas E, Kinsella T, Grayson J, Glatstein E, Pizzo PA, Triche TJ. Rhabdomyosarcoma. A new classification scheme related to prognosis. *Arch Pathol Lab Med* 116:847-855, 1992.

20. Seidal T, Walaas L, Kindblom L, Angervall L. Cytology of embryonal rhabdomyosarcoma. A cytologic, light microscopic, electron microscopic, and immunohistochemical study of seven cases. *Diag Cytopathol* 4:292-299, 1988.

21. Seidal T, Mark J, Hagmar B, Angervall L. Alveolar rhabdomyosarcoma. A cytogenetic and correlated cytological and histological study. *Acta Path Microbiol Scand [A]* 90:345-354, 1982.

22. Almeida M, Stastny JF, Wakely PE, Frable WJ. Fine needle aspiration biopsy of childhood rhabdomyosarcoma. Reevaluation of the cytologic criteria for diagnosis. *Acta Cytol* 36:600, 1992.

23. Akhtar M, Ali MA, Bakry M, Hug M, Sackey K. Fine needle aspiration biopsy diagnosis of rhabdomyosarcoma. Cytologic, histologic, and ultrastructural correlations. *Diag Cytopathol* 8:465-474, 1992.

24. deJong ASH, Vark M, Heerde P. Fine needle aspiration biopsy diagnosis of rhabdomyosarcoma. An immunocytochemical study. *Acta Cytol* 31:574-577, 1987.

25. Pettinato G, Swanson PE, Insabato L, De Chiara A, Wick M. Undifferentiated small round-cell tumors of childhood. The immunocytochemical demonstration of myogenic differentiation in fine needle aspirates. *Diag Cytopathol* 5:194-199, 1989.

26. Dias P, Parham DM, Shapiro DN, Webber BL, Houghton PJ. Myogenic regulatory protein (MyoD1) expression in childhood solid tumors. Diagnostic utility in rhabdomyosarcoma. *Amer J Pathol* 137:1283-1291, 1990.

27. Argyle JC, Tomlinson GE, Steward D, Schneider NR. Ultrastructural, immunocytochemical, and cytogenetic characterization of a large congenital fibrosarcoma. *Arch Pathol Lab Med* 116:972-975, 1992.

28. Sapi Z, Bodo M, Megyesi J, Rahoty P. Fine needle aspiration cytology of biphasic synovial sarcoma of soft tissue. Report of a case with ultrastructural, immunohistologic and cytophotometric studies. *Acta Cytol* 34:69-73, 1990.

29. Sonobe H, Manabe Y, Furihata M, Iwata J, Oka T, Ohtsuki Y, Mizobbuchi H, Yamamoto H, Kumano O, Abe S. Establishment and characterization of a new human synovial sarcoma cell line, HS-SY-II. *Lab Invest* 67:498-506, 1992.

30. Dal Cin P, Rao U, Jani-Sait S, Karakousis C, Sandberg AA. Chromosomes in the diagnoses of soft tissue tumors. I. Synovial sarcoma. *Mod Pathol* 5:357-362, 1992.

31. Akhtar M, Ali M, Sabbah R. Aspiration cytology of Ewing's sarcoma. Light and electron microscopic correlations. *Cancer* 56:2051-2060, 1985.

32. Akhtar M, Ali M, Sabbah R, Bakry M, Nash JE. Fine needle aspiration biopsy of round cell malignant tumors of childhood. A combined light and electron microscopic approach. *Cancer* 55:1805-1817, 1985.

33. Lieberman PH, Brennan MF, Kimmel M, Erlandson RA, Garin-Chesa P, Flehinger BY. Alveolar soft-part sarcoma. A clinico-pathologic study of half a century. *Cancer* 63:1-13, 1989.

34. Rosai J, Dias P, Parham DM, Shapiro DN, Houghton P. MyoD1 protein expression in alveolar soft part sarcoma as confirmatory evidence of its skeletal muscle nature. *Amer J Surg Pathol* 15:974-981, 1991.

35. Uehara H. Cytology of alveolar soft part sarcoma. *Acta Cytol* 22:191-192, 1978.

36. Ducatman BS, Scheithauer BW, Piepgras DG, Reiman HM. Malignant peripheral nerve sheath tumors in childhood. *J Neuro-Oncol* 2:241-248, 1984.

37. Meis JM, Enzinger FM, Martz KL, Neal JA. Malignant peripheral nerve sheath tumors (malignant schwannomas) in children. *Amer J Surg Pathol* 16:694-707, 1992.

38. Vendraminelli R, Cavazzana AO, Poletti A, Galligioni A, Pennelli N. Fine needle aspiration cytology of malignant nerve sheath tumors. *Diag Cytopathol* 8:559-562, 1992.

39. Chung EB, Enzinger FM. Malignant melanoma of soft parts. A reassessment of clear cell sarcoma. *Amer J Surg Pathol* 7:405-413, 1983.

40. Lucas DR, Nascimento AG, Sim FH. Clear cell sarcoma of soft tissues. Mayo Clinic experience with 35 cases. *Amer J Surg Pathol* 16:1197-1204, 1992.

41. Maruyama R, Nakano M, Yamashita S, Morooka K, Daimon Y, Tsuchimochi T, Ochiai T, Koono M. Fine needle aspiration cytology of clear cell sarcoma. Report of a case with immunocyto-chemical, immunohistochemical and ultrastructural studies. *Acta Cytol* 36:937-942, 1992.

42. Caraway NP, Fanning CV, Wojcik EM, Staerkel GA, Benjamin RS, Ordoñez NG. Cytology of malignant melanoma of soft parts: fine needle aspirates and exfoliative specimens. *Diagn Cytopathol* 9:632-638, 1993.

43. Chase DR, Enzinger FM. Epithelioid sarcoma. Diagnosis, prognostic indicators, and treatment. *Amer J Surg Pathol* 9:241-263, 1985.

43. Manivel JC, Wick MR, Dehner LP, Sibley RK. Epithelioid sarcoma. An immunohistochemical study. *Amer J Clin Pathol* 87:319-326, 1987.

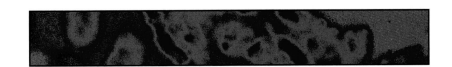

CHAPTER THIRTEEN

Breast and Skin

Breast

The breast is an uncommon site for fine needle aspiration (FNA) in the pediatric age group. Most breast masses in children are benign and occur in adolescent females. The most common entity is fibroadenoma.[1] A recent review of pediatric breast aspirates from both males and females in our own institution found that 9 of 11 were benign with fibroadenoma and gynecomastia as the most common entities. The two malignant aspirates in the group were metastatic rhabdomyosarcoma and granulocytic sarcoma. A larger review of breast FNA biopsy in patients extending to 30 years of age also identified fibroadenoma as the most common lesion in this age group.[2,3]

Inflammatory and Cystic Lesions

Inflammatory and cystic lesions are very uncommon in the pediatric breast. Fat necrosis may be clinically detected as a discrete mass. Aspirates of fat necrosis are characterized by many foamy histiocytes mixed with or without fragments of adipose tissue, inflammatory cells (neutrophils, lymphocytes) and sometimes multinucleated cells (Image 13.1). Amorphous cellular debris is a common background feature.

Simple cysts are uncommon in this age group. They can be completely evacuated by FNA biopsy. The fluid may be clear, straw-colored or brown, and turbid. It is best if a portion of the aspirate fluid is centrifuged to concentrate the cellular contents. Slides principally contain foamy and hemosiderin-laden macrophages, some benign duct cells and occasional metaplastic apocrine cells[4] (Image 13.2).

Fibroadenoma

Fibroadenoma presents as a discete, mobile, usually nontender breast mass that is commonly unilateral and firm to palpation. As it can be painful and associated with a history of rapid growth, a patient may be quite anxious about this lesion. Within the pediatric age group, the incidence of fibroadenoma peaks in adolescent females. Those individuals with bilateral and multiple lesions are more susceptible to develop recurrent tumors. Multiple fibroadenomas are also more likely in young black women.

Macroscopically, fibroadenoma is a firm to rubbery, spherical, frequently bosselated mass with a white or light pink cut face, which typically bulges from the surface upon sectioning. The common intercanalicular histologic pattern displays markedly elongated branching slits of epithelium in a rich myxoid stroma. Although this ordinary fibroadenoma is the most common type in adolescent girls, a so-called "juvenile" (hypercellular) subtype is nearly unique to this age group. The principal difference of this subtype from ordinary fibroadenoma is its more richly cellular stroma and exuberant epithelial hyperplasia.[5] Even with the increased cellularity, mitotic activity is typically absent or minimal when found. Because they can attain a very large size (>10 cm), some have also been designated as "giant" fibroadenomas.

Aspirate smears may be worrisome to the novice because of their marked cellularity.[6,7] The cell pattern shows randomly dispersed, tightly cohesive epithelial cell clusters with branching "finger" or staghorn-like projections of cells extending from the main body of the cluster (Image 13.3) (Table 13.1). Duct cell nuclei within these clusters, nonetheless, are uniform and oval with finely granular chromatin and small nucleoli (Image 13.4). In some cases nucleoli may be more prominent. Bare, bipolar nuclei, presumably of myoepithelial cell origin, may be numerous, and scattered randomly throughout the smear. Fragments of collagenous stroma containing spindled fibroblastic nuclei are also present. Using step-wise regression analysis, Bottles et al showed that the presence of stroma, so-called "antler horn" clusters, and marked cellularity were the key features in separating fibroadenoma from fibrocystic change of the breast.[7] Adding the finding of regular honeycomb sheets of epithelial cells to the features of stroma, and antler-horn clusters distinguished fibroadenoma from duct carcinoma in all instances in the statistical model.

The "juvenile" (giant fibroadenoma) subtype has a nearly identical appearance as the conventional type except that the stromal fragments are more prominent and exist in greater numbers; epithelial clusters may also be more numerous. Recognizing this juvenile type is not readily appreciated on aspiration smears, nor is it clinically necessary to do so.

Potential Problems in Diagnosis: As these smears are highly cellular, fibroadenomas have the potential to be confused with duct carcinoma

Within the pediatric age group, the incidence of fibroadenoma peaks in adolescent females

Table 13.1
Fibroadenoma-Cytomorphology

Randomly dispersed, tightly cohesive epithelial cell clusters with branching "finger" or staghorn-like projections.

Uniform cell nuclei; oval with finely granular chromatin and small nucleoli.

Bare, bipolar nuclei, generally numerous.

Fragments of collagenous stroma containing spindle shaped fibroblasts.

and phyllodes tumor in adults. Since carcinoma is such a rare entity in children, however, it should only rarely be considered seriously in the diagnosis. The innumerable bare nuclei, and uniform tightly cohesive cell sheets, many with staghorn or fingerlike projections, are key to recognizing the benign nature of the process.

Proliferative fibrocystic change and juvenile papillomatosis are 2 benign entities that can occur in adolescents. Both may contain numerous sheets of benign duct cells, and some may have this aforementioned branching shape. Apocrine cells are often numerous in these entities. Clinically, fibrocystic change is more a poorly defined induration of the breast than a discrete moveable mass.

Gynecomastia

In this age group, gynecomastia is most common in adolescent males. It may present as a unilateral or bilateral subareolar nodule. The clinical diagnosis is usually straightforward and FNA biopsy is unnecessary. In those males with a history of cancer, however, a breast nodule can be disconcerting, and FNA biopsy can frequently answer whether a nodule represents gynecomastia or metastatic disease. Light microscopy of tissue sections demonstrates epithelial hyperplasia of nonproliferating ducts with some perilobular stromal edema.

The smear pattern is not specific. Aspirates may have a pattern identical to that described for fibroadenoma, ie, monotonous duct cells in tight clusters and numerous, single bare nuclei.[8] The number and size of ductal cell aggregates is usually smaller than those seen in fibroadenoma (Image 13.5).

Gynecomastia is usually an easily made clinical diagnosis by the pediatrician. The cytologic morphology must be combined with the clinical history and physical examination to be definitive. FNA biopsy is particularly useful when unilateral enlargement of the breast occurs in a child known to have cancer, and the clinical question of metastatic disease is raised.

FNA biopsy is particularly useful when unilateral enlargement of the breast occurs in a child known to have cancer, and the clinical question of metastatic disease is raised

Carcinoma

Carcinoma of the breast is extremely unusual in children. As an adult neoplasm it is extensively discussed in general texts of

Table 13.2
Pilomatrixoma-Cytomorphology

Numerous small cells, uniform in size with high N/C ratios dispersed as isolated cells and as cohesive sheets.

Finely granular nuclear chromatin and small nucleoli.

Intact and degenerating squamous cells, anucleated squames, calcific debris.

Background population of lymphocytes, histiocytes, plasma cells and occasionally mult-inucleated giant cells.

"Ghost" cells grouped in pale clusters with colorless nuclei.

---

cytopathology to which the reader is referred. Lymphoma, leukemia and granulocytic sarcoma may infrequently present initially as breast masses in children.

Metastatic neoplasms in the pediatric breast are uncommon, but when they occur they are an important indication for FNA biopsy in a child with a known malignancy. Rhabdomyosarcoma, neuroblastoma and Ewing's sarcoma may all metastasize to the breast. Of these, rhabdomyosarcoma seems to be the most common.

Skin

Very few mass lesions develop in the skin of pediatric patients. Most discrete "skin" nodules are actually proliferative processes in the deeper soft tissue rather than the dermis and epidermis. We have placed the common hemangioma and less frequent lipoma in the soft tissue section.

Pilomatrixoma (Calcifying Epithelioma of Malherbe)

Pilomatrixoma presents as a localized swelling in the subcutaneous tissue. Most occur as firm nodules on the head and neck, including the face, and emerge somewhat more frequently in the 1st as opposed to the 2nd decade of life.

Histologically, sheets and islands of small round basaloid cells with high N/C ratios exist within the dermis and subcutaneous tissue. An abrupt transition to eosinophilic cells that retain the "ghost" cellular outlines of their basaloid neighbors and undergo frequent calcification occurs. Squamous metaplasia occurs within areas of basal cell proliferation. A foreign body giant cell response is common.

Numerous intact basaloid cells, uniform in size with high N/C ratios, fine nuclear chromatin, and nucleoli, are dispersed both as isolated cells and as cohesive sheets throughout the smear (Image 13.6) (Table 13.2). The great danger in FNA biopsy of this lesion is to mistake these basaloid cells for a malignant small round cell tumor of childhood.[9-12] Additional features on the smear that will help prevent that error include nucleated intact and degenerating squamous cells, anucleated squames, calcific debris and a background population of lymphocytes, histiocytes, plasma cells and occasionally multinucleated giant cells. "Ghost" cells are grouped in pale staining clusters with colorless nuclei where only nucleoli and nuclear membranes are visible. In one study these were only visible on the Romanowsky- and not the Papanicolaou-stained smears.[11]

Malignant Melanoma

Malignant melanoma (MM) is a rare malignancy of childhood. Although most reported cases occur de novo, risk factors include congenital nevus, xeroderma pigmentosum and dysplastic nevus syndrome.[13] We have recently accumulated 3 cases of pediatric MM that show its cytomorphologic heterogeneity—2 are aspiration smears of MM metastatic to lymph node and 1 is a primary MM recovered from the eye.[14] The cytopathology is similar to that described in the aspiration smears and ocular aspiration specimens of adults (Image 13.7). MM is distributed as both loose clusters and as isolated cells. Cells are large with variable shapes that range from spindled to round and polygonal. Mirror image nuclei and multinucleation are generally readily found. Nuclei are typically large and irregular, and nucleoli, although usually large and prominent, may be indistinct. The amount of melanin deposition is variable.

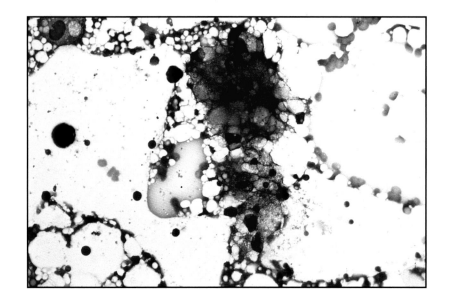

Image 13.1
Fat necrosis. Foamy histiocytes and adipose tissue. (Romanowsky).

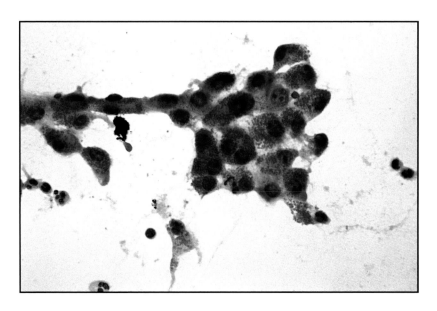

Image 13.2
Apocrine metaplasia. Uniform cells with small nuclei and granular cytoplasm. (Papanicolaou).

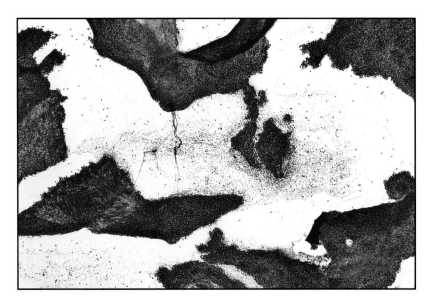

Image 13.3
Fibroadenoma. Hypercellular smear on low power showing sheets of uniform cells some of which have finger-like projections. (Romanowsky).

Image 13.4
Fibroadenoma. Tightly clustered uniform cells. Note bare nuclei in the background. (Romanowsky).

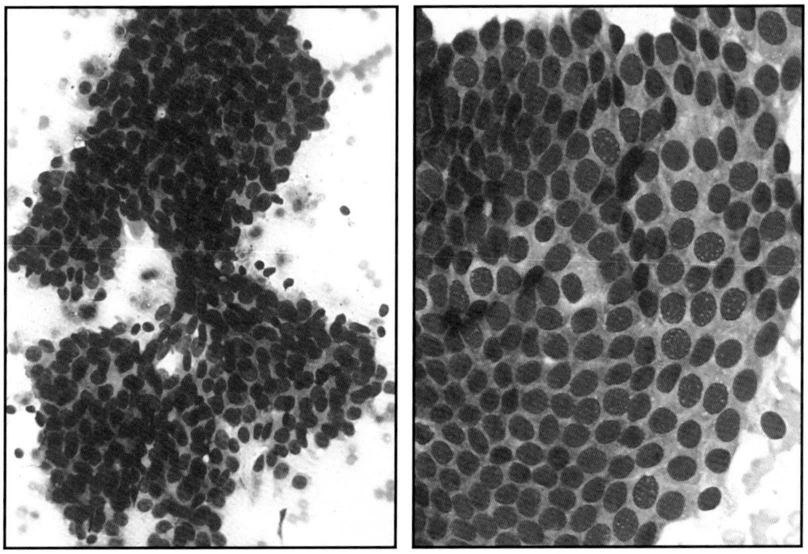

Image 13.5
Gynecomastia. Benign duct cells similar to those seen in fibroadenoma. Note bare (myoepithelial cell) nuclei. (Papanicolaou).

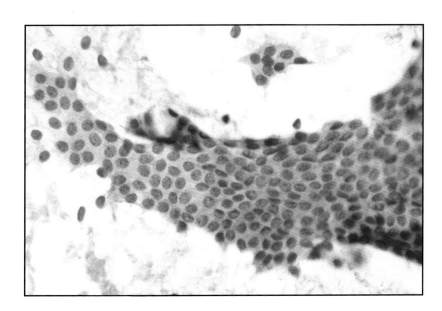

Image 13.6
A Pilomatrixoma. Uniform small cells distributed as single cells and cohesive clusters mimic a malignant small cell tumor. Note the portion of a multinucleated giant cell at lower left (Papanicolaou). (Courtesy Dr C Powers).
B "Ghost" cells grouped together in pale clusters with colorless nuclei. (Romanowsky).

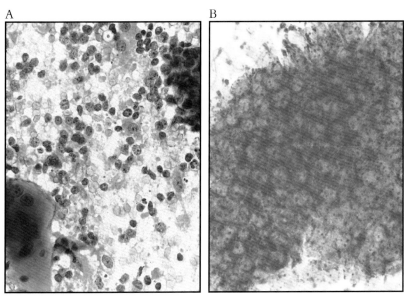

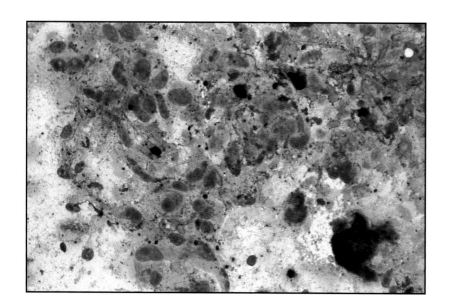

Image 13.7
Malignant melanoma. Polygonal and spindle shaped cells are loosely clustered together in this aspirate from the lymph node of a 9-year-old child. Nucleoli are large and easily seen. Melanin is disseminated as both coarse and fine granules. A heavily pigmented melanophage is seen at one corner of the photograph. (Romanowsky).

References

1. Dehner LP. Breast. In: Pediatric Surgical Pathology. 2nd ed. Williams and Wilkins, Baltimore, 1987:chap 2.

2. Gupta RK, Dowle CS, Simpson JS. The value of needle aspiration cytology of the breast, with an emphasis on the diagnosis of breast disease in young women below the age of 30. *Acta Cytol* 34:165-168, 1990.

3. Maygarden SJ, McCall JB, Frable WJ. Fine needle aspiration of breast lesions in women aged 30 and under. *Acta Cytol* 35:687-694, 1991.

4. McSwain GR, Valicenti JF, O'Brien PH. Cytologic evaluation of breast cysts. *Surg Gynec Obstet* 146:921-925, 1978.

5. Pike AM, Oberman HA. Juvenile (cellular) adenofibromas. *Amer J Surg Pathol* 9:730-736, 1985.

6. Linsk J, Kreuzer G, Zajicek J. Cytologic diagnosis of mammary tumours from aspiration biopsy smears. II. Studies on 210 fibroadenomas and 210 cases of benign dysplasia. *Acta Cytol* 16:130-138, 1972.

7. Bottles K, Chan JS, Holly EA, Chiu SH, Miller TR. Cytologic criteria for fibroadenoma. A step-wise logistic regression analysis. *Amer J Clin Pathol* 89:707-713, 1988.

8. Russin VL, Lachowicz C, Kline TS. Male breast lesions. Gynecomastia and its distinction from carcinoma by aspiration biopsy cytology. *Diag Cytopathol* 5:243-247, 1989.

9. Woyke S, Olszewski W, Eichelkraut A. Pilomatrixoma. A pitfall in the aspiration cytology of skin tumors. *Acta Cytol* 26:189-194, 1982.

10. Solanki P, Ramzy I, Durr N, Henkes D. Pilomatrixoma. Cytologic features with differential diagnostic considerations. *Arch Path Lab Med* 111:294-297, 1987.

11. Gomez-Aracil V, Azua J, San Pedro C, Romero J. Fine needle aspiration cytologic findings in four cases of pilomatrixoma (calcifying epithelioma of Malherbe). *Acta Cytol* 34:842-846, 1990.

12. Unger P, Watson C, Phelps RG, Danque P, Bernard P. Fine needle aspiration cytology of pilomatrixoma (calcifying epithelioma of Malherbe). Report of a case. *Acta Cytol* 34:847-850, 1990.

13. Roth ME, Grant-Kels JM, Kuhn MK, Greenberg RD, Hurwitz S. Melanoma in children. *J Am Acad Dermatol* 22:265-274, 1990.

14. Wakely PE, Frable WJ, Geisinger KR. Aspiration cytopathology of malignant melanoma in children. A morphologic spectrum. Submitted.

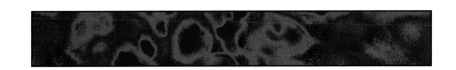

CHAPTER FOURTEEN

Abdomen and Thorax

Fine needle aspiration (FNA) cytology can be extremely useful in the workup and diagnosis of benign and malignant deep abdominal and thoracic lesions in childhood.[1-14] Many of the malignant lesions fall under the rubric of small round cell tumors of childhood which includes neuroblastoma, leukemia, lymphoma, embryonal rhabdomyosarcoma, Ewing's sarcoma and Wilms' tumor. Ancillary studies including immunocytochemistry and electron microscopy performed on the aspirated material can be quite helpful in arriving at a specific and correct diagnosis.[3,4] The following is a discussion of common and uncommon deep abdominal and thoracic lesions encountered in pediatric FNA biopsies.

Liver

Hepatoblastoma and Other Liver Malignancies

Hepatoblastoma is a tumor of young children, most often occurring in patients less than 5 years of age.[15] Hepatoblastoma is quite rare, although the most common primary hepatic malignancy in this age group, with an incidence of approximately 10% that of Wilms' tumor

Table 14.1

Hepatoblastoma - Cytomorphology

Hypercellular smears consisting of a uniform population of small to intermediate sized round to oval cells.

Cells arranged in trabeculae and rows resembling liver cords with sinusoidal lining cells as well as individually scattered cells. Occasional pseudoacinar formation. More mature fetal type and/or less mature embryonal type cells seen.

Spherical nuclei with inconspicuous nucleoli and moderate finely granular cytoplasm. Occasional stripped nuclei.

Rarely extramedullary hematopoiesis.

Mesenchymal component possible.

---

and 5% that of leukemia. Even though the frequency is estimated to be 0.85 cases/million children, it accounts for 45% of all primary liver neoplasms of childhood. The male:female ratio is approximately 1:2.5. Hepatoblastoma usually forms a solitary mass, which most often involves the right lobe of the liver (Image 14.1).[15] The tumor is often large ranging from 3 to 20 cm, and is usually unassociated with cirrhosis. Most children present with abdominal enlargement, with occasional cases associated with hemihypertrophy, precocious puberty, hypoglycemia, Wilms' tumor or the Beckwith-Wiedemann syndrome.[15]

Microscopically, hepatoblastoma is classified as either pure epithelial or mixed epithelial-mesenchymal. Epithelial hepatoblastoma is composed of either fetal or embryonal-type liver cells.[15] Tumors with predominantly fetal cells histologically resemble fetal liver with a distinctive light and dark cell pattern and foci of hematopoiesis. Embryonal cells are smaller with a more basophilic cytoplasm and higher nuclear to cytoplasmic (N/C) ratios. Embryonal cells also tend to form acini, tubules or papillary structures. In mixed epithelial-mesenchymal hepatoblastoma, the epithelial component consists either of fetal or embryonal cells and the mesenchymal elements may include primitive mesenchyme, osteoid, cartilage and/or rhabdomyoblasts. Previously, pure epithelial hepatoblastoma with only fetal-type tumor cells was believed to have a better prognosis and a higher cure rate by surgery than embryonal or mixed tumors.[16] However, a recent study for the Armed Forces Institute of Pathology (AFIP) showed that the stage at presentation was the most significant factor, while the histologic type of hepatoblastoma and DNA content did not have a significant effect.[16]

There are only a few reports of FNA cytomorphologic features of hepatoblastoma.[17-22] There have been approximately 11 prior examples of aspiration cytology of hepatoblastoma presented in the English medical literature, 4 of which were superficially described as part of larger pediatric FNA series and 2 were listed in another series.[2,21] We recently published our experience with 4 cases of histologically confirmed hepatoblastoma diagnosed by FNA biopsy.[19] The patients ranged in age from 5 months to 19 months, and consisted of 2 males and 2 females. Initial cytologic diagnosis were hepatoblastoma in 2 cases, malignant neoplasm consistent with liver cell tumor in 1 case, and probable Wilms' tumor in the 4th case. Cytologic features were similar in all cases and included hypercellular smears composed of a uniform population of small to intermediate sized round to oval cells (Image 14.2) (Table 14.1). Some cells were individually scattered, while others were arranged in trabeculae and rows resembling liver cords (Image 14.3). In occasional areas small groups of cells displayed pseudoacinar formation (Image 14.4). Stripped tumor nuclei were not uncommon (Image 14.4). Intact cells contained nuclei which were usually spherical and slightly eccentrically placed. Many nuclei had a single, frequently inconspicuous nucleolus, while uncommonly, several nucleoli were present. Intranuclear cytoplasmic inclusions were not appreciated. The cytoplasm was moderate to abundant in most cells and finely granular. A few cells contained small cytoplasmic vacuoles. Mitotic figures were not appreciated. In one of our cases, extramedullary hematopoiesis composed of eosinophils, other mature myeloid cells, and erythroid precursors was present (Image 14.4). None of our cases contained a mesenchymal component, such as acellular, metachromatically staining clumps of osteoid or cartilaginous stroma. Both embryonal and fetal differentiation were appreciated in some of our epithelial hepatoblastomas (Image 14.5). Bile pigment and/or collections of spindle cells were also not identified in the smears.

Immunocytochemical studies performed on the aspirated material revealed positive staining of the hepatocytes with low molecular weight cytokeratin markers (CAM 5.2 and 35BH11) (Image 14.6). Staining with antisera for vimentin, cytokeratin (AE-1), EMA and CEA were negative. Ultrastructural examination (EM) from the aspirate of 3 cases demonstrated features of immature hepatocytes including prominent rough endoplasmic reticulum, numerous mitochondria, conspicuous microvilli with focal canaliculus formation and well developed intercellular junctions (Image 14.6).

The cytologic differential diagnosis of hepatoblastoma includes aspirates from well differentiated hepatocellular carcinoma (hepatoma), which is the 2nd most common malignant hepatic tumor in children.[15] Most hepatomas are diagnosed after 5 years of age with a mean age between 12-14 years old.[15] Usually, aspirates from hepatocellular carcinoma consist of cells larger than normal hepatocytes and therefore differ from the slightly smaller cells seen in hepatoblastoma. Hepatocellular carcinomas also have cells with a greater degree of anisokaryosis, macronucleoli, occasional tumor giant cells and nuclear intracytoplasmic inclusions (Image 14.7). None of these features are usually present in aspirates from hepatoblastoma.[19] Immunophenotyping can be helpful in that most hepatoblastomas are AE-1–positive, whereas hepatocellular carcinomas are AE-1–negative. The fibrolamellar variant of hepatocellular carcinoma may occur in childhood and should also be considered in the differential diagnosis. However, the fibrolamellar variant contains larger cells with more abundant eosinophilic granular cytoplasm, cytoplasmic inclusions with pale bodies and enlarged nuclei with macronucleoli (Image 14.8).[23] Features similar to hepatoblastoma include the presence of mesenchymal stroma corresponding to the lamellar bands of fibrosis. However, the stromal fragments tend to be of low cellularity and show no atypical features in fibrolamellar carcinoma.

The cytologic differential diagnosis of hepatoblastoma includes aspirates from well differentiated hepatocellular carcinoma which is the 2nd most common malignant hepatic tumor in children

Aspirates from hepatic adenoma are not usually as cellular as hepatoblastoma or hepatocellular carcinoma and rarely contain extramedullary hematopoiesis. Some investigators feel that the liver cell dysplasia that occurs within hepatic adenomas or regenerative hepatic nodules makes them indistinguishable from hepatoma, but would help in differentiating them from hepatoblastoma.[24] Generally, aspirates from adenoma and focal nodular hyperplasia contain unremarkable-appearing hepatocytes.

Mesenchymal sarcoma (malignant mesenchymoma, primary sarcoma of the liver, fibromyxosarcoma) is another tumor that should be considered in the differential diagnosis since it typically occurs during the first 2 decades of life. Although quite uncommon, it is probably the 3rd most common primary malignant tumor of children, following hepatoblastoma and hepatocellular carcinoma.[25] In the Stocker and Ishak series, 16 of 31 patients with mesenchymal sarcoma were between 6 and 10 years of age.[26] Although no FNA report has been published, the anticipated cytologic findings of mesenchymal sarcoma include the presence of round, spindle and stellate-shaped cells set in a myxoid background. PAS positive intracytoplasmic pink globules may be seen. Immunoperoxidase studies performed on the aspirated material should be positive for vimentin and possibly alpha$_1$-antitrypsin and alpha$_1$-antichymotrypsin.[27] In some cases, smooth muscle or lipoblastic differentiation may be present. The histogenesis of this undifferentiated liver sarcoma is unresolved, although some believe that it may represent the malignant counterpart of the benign mesenchymal hamartoma, which is a liver neoplasm generally seen in young children. The anticipated FNA cytologic findings of mesenchymal hamartoma include the presence of benign cuboidal epithelial cells associated with bland-appearing spindle to stellate-shaped cells set in a myxoid stroma.

Other types of malignant mesenchymal tumors of the liver occurring in the pediatric age group include angiosarcoma, rhabdomyosarcoma, fibrosarcoma and leiomyosarcoma.[15] FNA cytology should reflect the characteristic cytologic features of the specific sarcoma. Often, ancillary studies including immunohistochemistry and EM will be needed to make a specific diagnosis. Parham et al believed, based on ancillary studies, that many of the hepatic sarcomas of childhood share a common histogenesis due to overlapping of immunohistochemical and ultrastructural features.[28] To the best of our knowledge, there have been no FNA cytologic reports of the other rare mesenchymal tumors of the liver in childhood.

Metastatic cancers to the liver might also enter into the differential diagnosis, since the liver is one of the most common sites for metastatic involvement in a number of childhood malignancies.[15] Metastatic neuroblastoma may cause multiple discrete tumor nodules or diffuse enlargement of the liver. Other small round cell tumors of childhood that can metastasize to the liver include Wilms' tumor, Ewing's sarcoma, embryonal and alveolar rhabdomyosarcoma and retinoblastoma.[15] The specific cytologic features of these lesions are discussed in this chapter and elsewhere in this book. However, aspirates of small cell undifferentiated (anaplastic) hepatoblastoma may show features similar to many of these lesions, since they can be composed of sheets of

Metastatic cancers to the liver might also enter into the differential diagnosis

undifferentiated small cells without any of the characteristic features of hepatoblastoma. Ancillary studies, such as positive staining of the tumor cells for low molecular weight cytokeratin and alpha fetoprotein along with EM studies can be helpful in separating the small cell undifferentiated hepatoblastoma from metastatic small round cell tumors of childhood. Malignant teratomas and endodermal sinus tumors of gynecologic or sacrococcygeal origin often spread to the liver when abdominal metastases are present.[15] Hematopoietic malignancies including acute leukemias, Hodgkin's disease and non-Hodgkin's lymphoma can also involve the liver. The cytologic features of these entities are discussed elsewhere in this book (Chapter 9).

Finally, adenoma of the adrenal cortex and paraganglioma are 2 less likely entities to be considered in the differential diagnosis of hepatoblastoma.[29,30] Aspirates of adrenal adenoma show a greater amount of cytoplasm, anisokaryosis and the presence of cellular morules characterized by several nuclei congregating in the cytoplasm of one cell without giving the appearance of a multinucleated giant cell (Image 14.9).[29,30] Ultrastructural evidence of organelles associated with steroid synthesis also favors the diagnosis of adrenal cortical adenoma. Adrenal cortical carcinomas are generally poorly differentiated malignancies that can have cells with pale lipid-laden cytoplasm (Image 14.9). Paraganglioma consists of cells showing significant anisonucleosis and nuclear atypicality with prominent intranuclear cytoplasmic inclusions (Image 14.10). EM examination demonstrates neurosecretory type granules and immunocytochemical studies are positive for neuron specific enolase (NSE) and chromogranin (Image 14.10). Of course, knowledge of the location of the lesion and clinical setting should aid in making the correct diagnosis.

Other unusual hepatic malignancies diagnosed by FNA cytology include a primary yolk sac tumor of liver.[31] Wakely et al recently reported the cytologic findings of this malignancy in a liver aspirate from a 16-month-old girl. Cytologic features consisted of single cells and loosely cohesive groups of cells having nuclei with small nucleoli and cytoplasmic vacuoles (Image 14.11). Clumps of extracellular metachromatically staining amorphous material presumably of basement membrane origin were best seen in the air-dried smears.

Benign, Non-Neoplastic Hepatic Lesions

FNA cytology has also been used to diagnose benign lesions of the liver including infiltrative processes such as storage diseases. Domanski et al recently reported the cytologic features of Gaucher's disease diagnosed by FNA biopsy of the liver and spleen,[32] which is similar to a case we encountered in which Gaucher cells were present having small, uniform, eccentrically placed nuclei and abundant cytoplasm with a fibrillary appearance (Image 14.12). We also recently diagnosed a case of familial hemophagocytic syndrome in a child by FNA biopsy.[33] Scattered histiocytic cells showing cytophagocytosis of red blood cells was found along with some admixed benign hepatocytes (Image 14.13). Other benign liver lesions that can occur in the

Table 14.2

Wilms' Tumor - Cytomorphology

Blastemal cells: small cells with high N/C ratios and scant amount of surrounding cytoplasm.

Complex, branching tubules and benign appearing stroma with bland spindle cells are often seen.

Anaplastic Wilms' has nuclear enlargement of at least 3 times the usual sized nuclei of adjacent cells, nuclear hyperchromasia and multipolar mitotic figures.

Malignant rhabdoid tumors consist of clusters and individually scattered cells with enlarged vesicular nuclei and prominent nucleoli and abundant surrounding cytoplasm. Single large intracytoplasmic eosinophilic globular structure is often present.

Clear cell sarcomas consist of singly arranged and small clusters of polygonal, stellate to spindle-shape having uniform, oval nuclei and clear cytoplasm. Mucoid material present in background of Diff-Quik-stained smears.

---

pediatric age group include liver abscesses, cysts and granulomas.[34,35] Most liver abscesses are bacterial in origin with FNA cytologic findings of sheets of neutrophils and considerable background debris. In the Diff-Quik stain, bacterial organisms are often seen, although the Gram stain will be needed for more specific classification of the bacterial population. Whenever a liver abscess is encountered, aspirated material should be submitted for microbiologic examination. Liver abscesses can also be secondary to parasites such as amoeba and fungi.[34] Liver cysts can be congenital, neoplastic or parasitic in origin.[34] Hydatid disease due to *Echinococcus granulosa* is most prevalent in sheep-raising countries and occurs quite infrequently in the US. FNA of hydatid cyst can reveal the chitinous membrane and scoleces of the tapeworm (Image 4.14).[34] Congenital cysts can be solitary or multiple.[35] Aspirates of congenital cysts generally contain unremarkable bile duct epithelium which may also show evidence of squamous metaplasia.[35]

Kidney

Wilms' Tumor and Other Primary Neoplasms

Wilms' tumor or nephroblastoma is the most frequent and important pediatric renal tumor. Wilms' tumor is defined as a mixed (triphasic) renal neoplasm composed of metanephric blastema associated with stromal and epithelial derivatives, such as tubules, glomeruli and skeletal muscle at varying stages of differentiation (Image 14.15).[15] Monophasic variants consisting exclusively or predominantly of blastemal or tubular elements are also considered to be Wilms' tumor. The incidence of Wilms' tumor is approximately 7.6 cases per million children per year. A few cases of Wilms' tumor are associated with congenital anomalies, such as hemihypertrophy, aniridia and genitourinary anomalies. Other primary renal tumors in children include cystic partially differentiated nephroblastoma, congenital (conventional) mesoblastic nephroma, atypical mesoblastic nephroma, malignant rhabdoid tumor of kidney and clear cell sarcoma of kidney.

FNA cytologic findings of Wilms' tumor include the presence of blastemal cells characterized by small cells having high N/C ratios with a scant amount of surrounding cytoplasm (Image 14.16) (Table 14.2). Nuclear molding can be seen (Image 14.16). The epithelial component consists of larger cells, some of which are arranged in tubules, which can have complex branching configurations (Image 14.17). The differential diagnosis of these epithelial tubules includes Homer-Wright rosettes seen in neuroblastoma.[36] Homer-Wright rosettes are less complex, with the cells tightly arranged around a fibrillary neuropil. In some aspirates of blastemal type Wilms' tumor, the primitive cells can be arranged around branching blood vessels simulating complex tubules (Image 14.18). This pattern can also been seen in other small round cell tumors of childhood.[36] The mesenchymal stromal component consists of fragments of fibroconnective tissue, some of which may have a myxoid appearance, with interspersed spindle-shaped cells having bland nuclear features (Image 14.19). EM examination is mainly helpful in excluding other small round cell tumors of childhood, such as neuroblastoma and rhabdomyosarcoma, by demonstrating a lack of neurosecretory granules and muscle fibrils, respectively. The ultrastructural examination of Wilms' tumor will demonstrate well formed intercellular junctions, flocculent basement membrane-like material, oligocilia, microvilli and phagolysosomes (Image 14.20). Immunocytochemical staining is mainly used to exclude other small round cell tumors such as the lack of staining for NSE (excludes neuroblastoma) and LCA (excludes lymphoma). However, Wilms' tumor will be positive for vimentin and low molecular weight cytokeratin (Image 14.21). Epithelial differentiation, by immunocytochemistry or EM, is important to recognize as it points to Wilms' tumor and not other small round cell tumors.

Anaplasia in Wilms' tumor is defined as the combination of nuclear enlargement equal to at least 3 times the usual sized nuclei of adjacent cells, nuclear hyperchromasia and multipolar mitotic figures (Image 14.22).[37] Anaplasia in Stage II-IV Wilms' tumor is associated with aggressive behavior and decreased survival. Recognition of anaplastic Wilms' tumor is important, since these neoplasms need to be treated more aggressively. FNA cytology of anaplastic Wilms' tumor will demonstrate considerable enlargement of the tumor cell nuclei that are at least 3 times the diameter of adjacent nuclei of the same cell type along with atypical mitotic figures and hyperchromasia.[37] Potential pitfalls for overdiagnosing anaplasia include confusing multinucleation with macronucleation especially when the nuclei are overlapping.[38] A number of artifacts can also contribute to overdiagnosing anaplasia such as thick sections, poor fixation or staining of histologic sections, smeared DNA strands, calcification, stain precipitate and basophilic extracellular mucinous material imitating large nuclei.[38] There is also a potential to underdiagnose anaplasia in an FNA biopsy due to sampling. However, in the study by Zuppan et

Potential pitfalls for overdiagnosing anaplasia include confusing multinucleation with macronucleation especially when the nuclei are overlapping

al of anaplastic Wilms' tumors, nearly ¹/₂ the tumors had evidence of anaplasia in at least 75% of the tumor sections; therefore, they concluded that anaplasia will often be detected in a limited biopsy. However, this study does not exclude the possibility that limited sampling by FNA biopsy may underestimate anaplasia in occasional cases. The presence of anaplasia in Wilms' tumor correlated with an extremely poor prognosis when anaplasia was present in extrarenal tumor sites and predominantly in a blastemal tumor pattern.[38]

FNA cytology can document primary and metastatic malignant rhabdoid tumor of the kidney.[39-42] Aspiration biopsy cytology of malignant rhabdoid tumor consists of cells arranged individually and in clusters having a single large nucleus with a prominent nucleolus and abundant surrounding cytoplasm (Image 14.23).[39-42] EM examination of the aspirated material will demonstrate whorled filamentous cytoplasmic inclusions (Image 14.23).[39] Malignant rhabdoid tumors account for approximately 2% of the renal tumors submitted to the National Wilms' Tumor Study (NWTS). In contrast to conventional Wilms' tumor, malignant rhabdoid tumors occur most commonly in infants or very young children with a median age of 13 months. Malignant rhabdoid tumors have a very aggressive clinical course. Malignant rhabdoid tumors can also be seen in extrarenal sites including subcutaneous tissue, thymus, heart, pelvis and liver. However, it is believed that rhabdoid tumor of the kidney represents a distinct entity, having a very high mortality rate exceeding 80%, in contrast to extrarenal rhabdoid tumors which may be a phenotype for a number of different neoplasms of various malignant potential.[43] Patients with malignant renal rhabdoid tumors also have a high probability of developing a second primary neoplasm in the central nervous system with cerebellar medulloblastoma being the most common. Immunohistochemical studies can be helpful in the workup of rhabdoid tumors.[41]

Another prognostically unfavorable renal neoplasm that has been examined by FNA biopsy is clear cell sarcoma of the kidney.[43] It also differs from conventional Wilms' tumor by its distinctive histologic appearance and an aggressive clinical course with a strong tendency to metastasize to bones.[15] FNA cytology will consist of malignant cells arranged singly and in small clusters. The tumor cells are polygonal, stellate or spindle-shaped with a pale cytoplasm and round to oval, uniform nuclei (Image 14.23). With the Diff-Quik stain, mucoid intercellular material staining light pink to deep purple will be found.[44] EM examination will show a moderate number of organelles including free ribosomes, occasional rough ER, clusters of mitochondria, and 1 or more Golgi complexes along with extracellular stroma.[44] Cells arranged in closely packed clusters with numerous desmosomal-like junctions (a feature of conventional Wilms' tumor) are not seen in clear cell sarcoma of the kidney. In addition, EM examination may exclude other types of abdominal or retroperitoneal malignancies including other malignant small round cell tumors of childhood such as rhabdomyosarcoma.

One of the current contraindications of pediatric FNA biopsy in the US is in the primary diagnosis of resectable Wilms' tumor based on the fear of tumor seeding or rupturing the capsule of the kidney and

In contrast to conventional Wilms' tumor, malignant rhabdoid tumors occur most commonly in infants or very young children with a median age of 13 months

thereby increasing the stage of Wilms' tumor as detailed by the NWTS.[45] However, in the adult FNA literature, tumor seeding along the needle tract of the fine needle has not been shown to be a complication of the procedure.[46,47] As noted by Akhtar et al, the role of FNA biopsy in the diagnosis and management of Wilms' tumor is controversial, since the majority of children with a renal mass will undergo nephrectomy regardless of the nature of the neoplasm.[48] However, FNA biopsy of Wilms' tumor may be quite beneficial in those patients with unresectable Wilms' tumor requiring chemotherapy, including some patients receiving preoperative therapy.[49-51] We believe, based on our experience with Wilms' tumor, that FNA biopsy is quite helpful in the preoperative diagnosis of Stage IV disease.[52] The International Society of Pediatric Oncology believes that preoperative chemotherapy makes subsequent surgery safer for many patients,[53,54] since chemotherapy shrinks the tumor mass and the neoplasm may become encapsulated by a dense band of fibrous connective tissue.[55,56]

Chemotherapy may also induce a more mature or atrophic appearance of the neoplasm.[56] In addition, approximately 5% of all patients present with Stage V disease, ie, bilateral nephroblastoma.[55,57,58] Preoperative chemotherapy may reduce the extent of subsequent surgery and therefore make preservation of as much functional non-neoplastic renal parenchyma possible. In another 5% of cases, extensive infiltration by neoplasm may make total resection not feasible without compromise of vital structures.[59-61] Preoperative chemotherapy may convert a patient's tumor to one that is totally resectable. Recognition of the cytologic features of Wilms' tumor and differentiation from other small round cell tumors of children will allow a correct initial FNA diagnosis of Wilms' tumor that may permit the early administration of chemotherapy. FNA biopsy may also sample Wilms' tumor in uncommon sites.[62] We believe that additional studies are needed to determine if FNA biopsy and the potential "spillage of tumor cells" should automatically increase the stage of Wilms' tumor for resectable lesions.

Recently, the FNA findings of mesoblastic nephroma has been reported.[63,64] The cytologic findings consisted of spindle cells with minimal nuclear atypia arranged individually and in clusters (Image 14.24). Correct diagnosis of this lesion is important, since the prognosis of this lesion is excellent following nephrectomy alone. The FNA findings of cystic nephroma have also been reported.[65,66] Cytologic finding of an aspirate in an adult demonstrated markedly atypical cells forming papillary clusters which potentially could be misdiagnosed as a renal cell carcinoma.[65] Cytologic features which suggested the diagnosis of cystic nephroma included low cellularity, lack of necrosis and relatively few spindle cells in an aspirate from a cystic renal mass. Drut reported an FNA cytologic finding of an aspirate of a cystic nephroma in a 3-year-old child. Benign epithelial cells were arranged in uniform sheets as well as isolated cells.[66] Another unusual lesion we have encountered in a child is an aspirate from a collecting duct carcinoma which has unique cytologic and cytogenetic characteristics.[67] FNA cytomorphologic findings of renal mass in a 10-year-old child that we recently examined revealed clusters of cells having epithelial features along with stromal cells (Image 14.25).

Correct diagnosis of this lesion is important, since the prognosis of this lesion is excellent following nephrectomy alone

Metastatic and Secondary Neoplasms

Adrenal and retroperitoneal neuroblastoma and malignant lymphoma are the most common neoplasms of childhood that can secondarily involve the kidneys.[15] Cytologic features such as neuropil and Homer-Wright rosettes may be seen in neuroblastoma.[36] Often, ancillary studies such as EM and immunocytochemistry will be needed to differentiate the blastemal type Wilms' tumor from a neuroblastoma. FNA of malignant lymphoma rarely involves the kidneys in the initial phase of the disease, although Burkitt's lymphoma can cause a nodular or diffuse infiltrate within the kidney at presentation (Image 14.26). We have encountered cases of FNA of Burkitt's lymphoma involving the kidney that demonstrated a dissociative pattern of atypical lymphoid cells showing cytoplasmic vacuolization and nuclei with 3 or 4 nucleoli. Numerous lymphoglandular bodies were present in the background (Images 14.27 through 14.31). Cytogenetic studies performed on the aspirated material demonstrated the characteristic 8:14 translocation (Image 14.26).[13]

Other Abdominal Neoplasms

Intraabdominal desmoplastic small round cell tumor of childhood is a rare malignancy consisting of nests of small cells surrounded by abundant desmoplastic stroma. Most of the patients have been between 16 and 18 years old.[68,69] The tumor predominantly involves the omentum or peritoneum with secondary invasion of the bowel wall. This intraabdominal small round cell tumor is believed to be of divergent differentiation based on coexpression of epithelial and mesenchymal markers.[68] The FNA cytologic findings have recently been reported.[69-71] Cytomorphologic findings included groups of undifferentiated tumor cells with nuclear molding as well as loose clusters and a dense desmoplastic stroma (Image 14.32). Some of the aspirated cells were larger and resembled glandular elements. Immunocytochemical studies performed on the aspirated material demonstrated positive staining of the tumor cells for cytokeratin, desmin and NSE.[69,70] EM examination demonstrated primitive junctions with paranuclear aggregates of intermediate filaments as well as rare intracellular lumina.[70,71]

Other abdominal and retroperitoneal malignancies can be sampled by FNA biopsy including soft tissue neoplasms, gynecologic malignancies and lymphomas (Image 14.33). We have had a very limited experience with FNA of pediatric retroperitoneal and intraabdominal soft tissue neoplasms. Cytologic features of these lesions will be similar to the bone and soft tissue neoplasm discussed in Chapters 11 and 12. FNA cytologic features of pediatric lymphomas are discussed in Chapter 9.

We have seen occasional cases of FNA of primary and metastatic ovarian neoplasms. The common epithelial tumors of the ovary account for only 15% to 20% of all ovarian neoplasms in children, in contrast to 60% to 70% in adults.[15] Germ cell neoplasms involve the ovary in 20% to 35% of pediatric cases with only the sacrococcygeal region exceeding the ovary in frequency in most series.[15] Benign cystic

Intraabdominal desmoplastic small round cell tumor of childhood is a rare malignancy consisting of nests of small cells surrounded by abundant desmoplastic stroma

teratomas account for 30% to 90% of germ cell tumors depending on the series, followed by teratoma, endodermal sinus tumor, embryonal carcinoma, malignant mixed germ cell tumor, choriocarcinoma and dysgerminoma. We have aspirated patients with embryonal and endodermal sinus tumors which demonstrated syncytial clusters of pleomorphic cells having vacuolated cytoplasm associated with intra- and extracellular globular material (Image 14.34). The discussion of other ovarian tumors is beyond the scope of this book due to our limited personal experience with these lesions and sparse literature on the subject. In male patients, germ cell neoplasms are the most common primary tumors of the testes in the first 2 decades of life.[15] We have had no experience with FNA of primary testicular germ cell tumors, although we have documented metastatic testicular carcinoma involving retroperitoneal lymph nodes. Yolk sac tumors are the most frequent neoplasm of the testes in childhood followed by embryonal carcinoma, teratoma, teratocarcinoma. Choriocarcinoma and seminoma are quite uncommon in the pediatric age group (Image 14.35). Other unusual lesions examined by FNA cytology include retrocystic hamartoma (tailgut cyst) in a child.[72] FNA cytology demonstrated cyst fluid contents containing numerous squamous epithelial cells, lymphocytes and neutrophils (Image 14.36). Cytologic features of other presacral cysts are discussed by Young et al.[72]

Pancreas

Pancreatoblastoma

Primary pancreatic malignancies are rare in childhood.[15,73-75] Pediatric pancreatic neoplasms show a greater tendency to originate in the islets of Langerhans', in contrast to most adult adenocarcinomas which are of ductal derivation.[15] Nonendocrine neoplasms seen in the pediatric period include the very rare conventional ductal adenocarcinoma, the cystic (papillary) solid neoplasm, acinar cell carcinoma and pancreatoblastoma. Pancreatoblastoma (pancreatic carcinoma of infantile type) is quite rare with approximately 25 cases reported in the literature.[74,76-84] In a review of 8 cases by Buchino et al, the following features of pancreatoblastoma were noted: age range of 15 months to 13 years; tumor size of 7 to 11 cm; localization in the head or tail of the pancreas and a relatively favorable clinical course (Image 14.37). However, metastatic disease and fatal outcome have been reported.[78]

Histologic examination of pancreatoblastoma reveals tall columnar or cuboidal cells having round to oval vesicular nuclei with occasional nucleoli. Tumor cells are generally uniform with only a mild to moderate degree of pleomorphism and variable mitotic activity. The tumor cells tend to be arranged in an organoid pattern characterized by nests of cells surrounded by dense fibrous stroma (Image 14.38). Focal acinar and/or tubular patterns may also be present.[74,78] Charac-

Nonendocrine neoplasms seen in the pediatric period include the very rare conventional ductal adenocarcinoma, the cystic (papillary) solid neoplasm, acinar cell carcinoma and pancreatoblastoma

Table 14.3

Pancreatoblastoma - Cytomorphology

Columnar to cuboidal cells having round to oval vesicular nuclei with occasional nucleoli and moderate amount of granular cytoplasm.

Occasional elongated spindle and triangular shaped epithelial cells as well as smaller cells with high N/C ratios and dense cytoplasm.

Abundant stromal fragments.

---

teristic squamoid nests called corpuscles lacking evidence of intracytoplasmic keratinization are usually present along with elongated spindle-shaped cells. The histogenesis of pancreatoblastoma is controversial and uncertain. Frable et al concluded that the neoplasm was of ductal cell origin with some differentiation towards acinar or central acinar cells based on EM examination.[80] Others have favored acinar derivation[81,85,86] or dual acinar and neuroendocrine derivation based on immunocytochemical and/or EM findings.[74,78] Acinar derivation has also been supported by immunocytochemical studies revealing positive staining of the cells for lipase, trypsin, chymotrypsin, alpha$_1$-antitrypsin along with negative staining for CEA, NSE, and pancreatic hormones including insulin, glucagon, somatostatin and pancreatic polypeptide.

We have examined 1 case of pancreatoblastoma by FNA biopsy.[87] The smears were hypercellular and consisted of numerous oval to cuboidal cells that had a moderate amount of granular cytoplasm (Image 14.39) (Table 14.3). Elongated spindle- and triangular-shaped epithelial cells were also seen along with smaller cells that had higher N/C ratios and denser cytoplasm (Image 14.40). In addition, abundant fragments of stroma were present including some rimmed by epithelial cells (Image 14.41). Immunocytochemical studies performed on the aspirated material revealed positive staining of the epithelial cells for cytokeratin (AE1/3, and high and low molecular weight cytokeratin markers). The tumor cells also showed intense staining for NSE (Image 14.42) and slight staining for alpha$_1$-antitrypsin. S-100, alpha-fetoprotein, and neurofilaments were nonreactive. EM examination of the aspirated specimen revealed cells with oval nuclei and moderate to abundant surrounding cytoplasm which contained well developed organelles including abundant rough ER. Numerous large electron-dense zymogen-like granules measuring 400 to 600 nanometers were seen in some of the cells. Well-defined membranes surrounding the granules were not seen. In addition, small neuroendocrine granules measuring from 100 to 200 nanometers were also present in some of the tumor cells (Image 14.43). These granules had distinct membranes and a denser quality than did the larger granules. Although most of the tumor cells contained only 1 type of granule, rare cells demonstrated amphocrine features with the presence of both the zymogen-type granules characteristic of acinar cells and the neuroendocrine granules typical of islet cells. The immunocytochemical and EM findings were supportive of a blastemal origin of the cells

Table 14.4
Acinar Cell Carcinoma - Cytomorphology

Predominantly highly cohesive groups of cells having central placed uniform hyper-chromatic nuclei with one to two prominent nucleoli and moderate amount of granular, eosinophilic cytoplasm.

Occasional 3-dimensional groups and clusters.

PAS positive cytoplasmic staining.

with bidirectional differentiation. The differential diagnosis of pancreatoblastoma should include other pancreatic neoplasms of putative acinar origin including: (1) acinar cell carcinoma, a rare highly malignant neoplasm, and (2) solid and cystic acinar cell tumor (papillary and solid neoplasm), a tumor in young women that usually has a favorable prognosis.

Acinar Cell Carcinoma

The FNA cytology of acinar cell carcinoma is characterized by numerous clusters of tumor cells showing acinar differentiation and no stromal component (Table 14.4).[88,89] The neoplastic cells are arranged in highly cohesive aggregates having uniform nuclei and a moderate amount of granular eosinophilic cytoplasm. Some groups have a 3-dimensional acinar configuration (Image 14.44). The neoplastic cells of acinar cell carcinoma have round to oval, coarsely granular, hyperchromatic nuclei that contain 1 to 2 prominent nucleoli (Image 14.44). In contrast to normal acinar cells, the malignant cells have large prominent nucleoli set within an open chromatin pattern. The nuclei range from round to irregular and are often centrally placed, in contrast to the eccentrically placed nuclei of islet cell tumors. The PAS reaction accentuates the cytoplasmic granularity which is due to abundant zymogen granules. EM examination demonstrates numerous zymogen granules but no neuroendocrine differentiation. Acinar cell carcinomas usually stain positively for alpha$_1$-antitrypsin and pancreatic enzymes and do not stain with CEA, NSE and pancreatic endocrine hormonal markers.[86,88]

In contrast to normal acinar cells, the malignant cells have large prominent nucleoli set within an open chromatin pattern

Papillary-Cystic Tumor

The papillary-cystic tumor is a very uncommon pancreatic neoplasm that occurs almost exclusively in adolescents and young adult females.[79,89-92] This pancreatic neoplasm is considered to be a low grade malignancy that can often be cured with surgical resection. However, rarely, metastatic disease has been documented, usually after a protracted clinical course.[93] Aspiration cytology of solid-cystic neoplasms reveals a cellular population of uniform cells arranged along papillary fronds having a delicate stroma (Table 14.5).[79,91-95] The papillae are lined by 1 to several layers of radially oriented uniform neoplastic cells (Image 14.45). The neoplastic nuclei are oval and pale-staining with a

Table 14.5
Papillary-Cystic Tumor - Cytomorphology

Cellular population of uniform cells arranged along delicate papillary fronds.

Papillae lined by 1 to several layers of cells.

Nuclei are oval with finely granular chromatin and inconspicuous to small nucleoli and characteristic longitudinal nuclear groove.

Cells have thin rim of amphophilic cytoplasm and can have reddish-pink hyaline globules with Romanowsky stains.

Table 14.6
Islet Cell Tumor - Cytomorphology

Cellular smears consisting of uniform population of small to medium-sized cells arranged individually and in loose clusters.

Eccentrically placed nuclei imparting a plasmacytoid appearance in Diff-Quik-stained smears.

Nuclei have characteristic "salt and pepper" chromatin with small to inconspicuous nucleoli and scant to moderate amount of granular cytoplasm.

finely granular, evenly distributed chromatin and inconspicuous to small nucleoli. Characteristically, delicate nuclear folds or grooves extend along the long axis of the nucleus. Despite these bland nuclear features, aneuploidy has been documented.[93] The neoplastic cells usually have a thin rim of surrounding amphophilic cytoplasm. With the May-Grunwald-Giemsa stain, reddish-pink staining hyaline droplets have been described.[93] Both zymogen and/or neuroendocrine granules have been appreciated with EM examination.

Islet Cell Tumor

Very infrequently, islet cell tumors occur in the pediatric population, although relatively more common vis-a-vis the adult population.[15] Aspirates of islet cell tumors are generally highly cellular, composed of a uniform population of small to medium-sized neoplastic cells (Table 14.6). The tumor cells are generally dissociative or arranged in loosely cohesive small aggregates that may show acinar or trabecular arrangements.[89,90] The neoplastic nuclei often are eccentrically placed imparting a plasmacytoid appearance to the cells with the Diff-Quik stain (Image 14.46). The nuclei have a characteristic "salt and pepper" chromatin pattern with generally small to inconspicuous nucleoli that are best appreciated in the alcohol-fixed material. A scant to moderate amount of granular cytoplasm is usually present. Occasionally, due to the fragility of the cells, naked nuclei and a granular smear pattern will be present in the background that should not be mistaken for necrosis. The cytoplasm is generally basophilic, probably reflecting the abundant rough endoplasmic reticulum frequently present in the tumor cells. EM examination may also demonstrate moderate numbers of neurosecretory type granules. Immunocytochemical studies for NSE and chromogranin are positive. Specific markers for insulin, gastrin, somatostatin, glucagon and serotonin will all be positive in selected cases.[89,90,96]

Adrenal Glands

Neuroblastoma

Neuroblastoma is the 3rd most common neoplasm of childhood and excluding central nervous system tumors, the most common solid nonlymphoreticular neoplasm of infancy and childhood. The incidence is 9/million children. The majority are diagnosed before 5 years of age with approximately $1/2$ presenting clinically before the age of 2.[97] Congenital and fetal cases exist and neuroblastoma is the most common malignant tumor in the neonate.[98] Neuroblastoma can arise from any site containing sympathetic neural tissue. The major sites include the adrenal gland and sympathetic ganglia in the retroperitoneum, accounting for 60% to 70% of the cases. Other sites are thoracopulmonary, mediastinal, cervical and pelvic regions.[97,98] Approximately 70% of the patients present with metastasis to regional lymph nodes, liver, bones and lungs. In contrast to the success in the therapy of Wilms' tumor, the survival of children over 1 year of age with metastatic neuroblastoma has remained disappointingly poor with a mortality rate of approximately 50%. The prognosis of neuroblastoma is correlated with the age of diagnosis, the primary site and the stage rather than the histologic grade.[98] However, the recent Shimada classification evaluates and grades neuroblastoma based on histologic features such as stromal development, cellular differentiation and the presence of mitotic-karyorrhectic cells as well as clinical findings.[99] Joshi et al have shown that the behavior and prognosis of neuroblastoma is related to the presence of either a stroma-rich or stroma-poor tumor, age at diagnosis, percentage of differentiating tumor cells and mitotic karyorrhectic index.[100] In general, children under 1 year of age have the best prognosis. Adrenal neuroblastomas are associated with a relatively poor prognosis, while thoracic neuroblastomas have a more favorable course.[98] Grading has some minor relationship to prognosis, with ganglioneuroblastoma having a better prognosis than well differentiated neuroblastoma. Prognosis is also related to molecular characteristics of the tumor including N-*myc* amplification, ploidy and specific chromosomal aberrations.[101] Since neuroblastoma has failed to demonstrate a dramatic clinical improvement with the use of chemotherapy, it is important that an accurate FNA diagnosis of neuroblastoma be made in order to distinguish this neoplasm from other small round cell tumors of childhood.[97]

Adrenal neuroblastoma usually presents as a discrete round mass having a smooth external surface or a large multinodular mass measuring from 5 to 10 cm in greatest dimension.[102] Some neuroblastomas demonstrate extensive necrosis with hemorrhage and cystic

It is important that an accurate FNA diagnosis of neuroblastoma be made in order to distinguish this neoplasm from other small round cell tumors of childhood

Table 14.7

Neuroblastoma - Cytomorphology

Hypercellular smears consisting of numerous individually scattered small cells with some cohesive groups.

Nuclear molding often seen.

Neuroblastic cells have oval to slightly irregular nuclei with evenly dispersed finely granular chromatin and small to inconspicuous nuclei and scant amount of cytoplasm is present. Occasional cells have delicate unipolar cytoplasmic tags.

When present, ganglion cells are binucleated to multinucleated with coarsely granular chromatin and prominent nucleoli.

Background neuropil, representing tangle of neuritic processes are an important diagnostic feature.

Homer-Wright rosettes occasionally present.

degeneration. Histologic examination reveals neuroblastic cells arranged diffusely or in nests separated by thin fibrovascular septae. By our definition, neuroblastoma is composed of greater than 50% neuroblasts and neuropil; in contrast, ganglioneuromas are composed exclusively of mature ganglion cells, neurites, Schwann cells and fibrous tissues.[103] Ganglioneuroblastoma contains more than 50% ganglioneuromatous elements with a relatively small neuroblastic component.[103]

Aspirates of neuroblastomas are hypercellular, consisting of numerous individually scattered small cells with some cohesive groups (Image 14.47) (Table 14.7). Nuclear molding is often seen (Image 14.44).[36] In some cases, larger cells having a moderate amount of surrounding cytoplasm are present corresponding to differentiating neuroblasts (Image 14.48). In addition, binucleated and multinucleated ganglion cells may be present (Image 14.49). Homer-Wright rosettes are seen in some, but not all of the cases (Image 14.50). The nuclei of neuroblastoma cells vary from oval to slightly irregular and have an evenly dispersed finely granular chromatin pattern with small to inconspicuous nucleoli (Image 14.51). In contrast, the nuclei of the ganglion cells have a more coarsely granular chromatin pattern with 1 or more prominent nucleoli (Image 14.52). Ganglion cells are usually oval to polygonal in shape with a moderate amount of amphophilic cytoplasm. In alcohol-fixed material, cellular processes extending from neuroblastic cells may be seen (Image 14.53). The most helpful diagnostic cytologic feature of neuroblastoma is recognition of the background neuropil, which represents a fibrillary tangle of neuritic processes associated with the neuroblastic cells (Image 14.54).[36] Mitotic-karyorrhectic cells (Image 14.55) as well as calcification (Image 14.56) can be appreciated in aspirated material.

Ganglioneuroblastomas consist of numerous multinucleated ganglion cells associated with scattering of neuroblastic cells (Image 14.57). In ganglionneuroblastoma and ganglioneuroma, neuronal fragments

The most helpful diagnostic cytologic feature of neuroblastoma is recognition of the background neuropil, which represents a fibrillary tangle of neuritic processes associated with the neuroblastic cells

Table 14.8
Differences Between PNET And Neuroblastoma

Feature	Neuroblastoma	PNET
Age incidence	Children, median age 2 years	Older children and adolescents, median age 14 years
Primary sites	Adrenal, retroperitoneal	Soft tissue & bone
Local recurrence	Yes	Yes
Metastatic pattern	Lymph nodes, bone marrow, liver & skin	Lung, bone, bone marrow & lymph nodes
Catecholamine secretion	Yes	No
Cytopathology	Neuropil, ganglion cells, occasional Homer-Wright rosettes	No neuropil, no ganglion cells, rare Homer-Wright rosettes, cytoplasmic vacuoles
Immunocytochemistry	NSE positive S-100 positive	NSE positive Beta$_2$ microglobulin HBA-71
EM	Neurosecretory granules, microtubules, and cell processes	Few dense core granules
Cytogenetics	No translocation	11;22 translocation
Other	N-*myc* gene with or without	C-*myc* gene amplification

Modified from Silverman JF, et al: Fine-needle aspiration cytology of primitive neuroectodermal tumor.
A report of three cases. *Acta Cytol* 36:541-550, 1992 (with permission).

consisting of bland spindle-shaped nuclei enmeshed in a pale fibrous appearing stroma will be appreciated (Image 14.58).[104]

A neoplasm related to neuroblastoma is the peripherally located, primitive neuroectodermal tumor (PNET), a small round cell malignancy arising in soft tissue and bone of predominantly older children and adolescents.[105-108] Central PNETs are those occurring in the central nervous system. Primary sites of involvement of peripheral PNET include the chest wall, trunk, retroperitoneum, pelvis and extremities.[109,110] Askin et al initially reported a unique clinicopathologic entity in 20 children characterized by a small cell malignancy arising in the soft tissue of the chest or peripheral lung.[111] The average age of the patients was 14.5 years with $3/4$ of them girls. Local recurrence was common without widespread metastasis but the median survival was still only 8 months. Additional cases of Askin's tumor have been subsequently described including 15 examples studied by light microscopy and EM examination.[112] Rosettes were not seen in all of the cases, although the tumor cells were positive for NSE and $2/3$ of the cases showed some cytoplasmic positivity with the PAS stain. EM examination usually demonstrated dense core neurosecretory granules and cell processes with intermediate filaments supportive of a neuroectodermal origin of the tumor. Most believe that the Askin tumor represents a PNET with a possible origin from an intercostal nerve.[112] Peripheral PNETs (peripheral neuroblastomas) differ from the classic neuroblastoma in that they are catecholamine negative, HLA positive, seen in adolescents, N-*myc* negative, and produce stromal collagen (Table 14.8).[97]

Table 14.9
PNET - Cytomorphology

Malignant cells with high N/C ratios, scant cytoplasm and occasional clusters showing nuclear molding.

Rare Homer-Wright rosettes (less often seen than in neuroblastoma).

No neuropil or ganglion cells, in contrast to neuroblastoma.

Fine cytoplasmic vacuolization and membranous cytoplasmic blebs in a few cases.

Occasional cells with fine, small, unipolar cytoplasmic tags.

They share some features of classic neuroblastoma, including EM findings of dense-core granules and neurites and positive staining for NSE. In addition, they share with other PNETs the same chromosomal translocation (11:22).[113-115] However, this chromosomal abnormality is not unique to PNET, since it is also found in Ewing's sarcoma, but has not been described in classic neuroblastoma.[114] In fact, there is considerable controversy concerning the relationship of Ewing's sarcoma and PNET, with some believing that Ewing's sarcoma represents an undifferentiated neuroectodermal malignancy.[116] Therefore, the separation of PNET from Ewing's sarcoma may be an academic issue, since it is now believed that both may share the same neuroectodermal histogenesis based on the presence of the same reciprocal chromosomal abnormality (11;22 translocation) and positive staining with monoclonal antibody HBA-71 to the p 30/32[MIC2] antigen, which is almost exclusively present on the cell membranes of PNET and Ewing's sarcoma, but not other small round cell tumors.[112-115,117,118]

There have been 3 case reports describing the FNA cytomorphologic appearance of peripheral PNET.[36,119,120] We recently described the cytomorphologic features and ancillary study findings of 8 FNA biopsies from 3 pediatric patients.[105] 2 of the biopsies suggested the initial diagnosis of PNET of the chest wall while the remaining 6 documented metastatic or locally recurrent disease. A primary diagnosis of PNET was made by FNA biopsy in 1 case enabling the pediatric oncologist to give specific therapy for the unresectable tumor and achieve remission. In the other cases, FNA biopsies documented local recurrences involving the chest wall (2 cases), pleura (1 case), and pericardium (1 case), and metastatic disease involving the breast and a supraclavicular lymph node. FNA cytologic findings included numerous malignant cells having high N/C ratios with a scant amount of cytoplasm (Image 14.59) (Table 14.9). Within some of the clusters, nuclear molding was identified (Image 14.60). The tumor cells had nuclei with evenly dispersed, finely granular chromatin. Although tumor cells had small nucleoli, prominent nucleoli were not appreciated. Homer-Wright rosettes were seen in 2 aspirates (Image 14.61). The Diff-Quik-stained smears showed the presence of fine cytoplasmic vacuolization of the cells associated with membranous cytoplasmic blebs in a few cases (Image 14.62).[105,120] In the Papanicolaou-stained smears, occasional cells had fine small unipolar cytoplasmic tags (Image 14.63).

Table 14.10
Cytologic Features Of Small Round Cell Tumors Of Childhood

Cytologic Features	PNET	NB	ES	BL	LL	RMS	WT
Nuclear molding	+	+	±	-	-	-	±
Nucleoli	-	-	-	+ (2-5)	-	±	-
Ganglion cells	-	±	-	-	-	-	-
Neuropil	-	+	-	-	-	-	-
Cytoplasmic vacuoles	+	-	+ (glycogen)	+ (lipid)	-	-	-
Cytoplasmic tags	±	±	-	-	-	+	-
Homer-Wright rosettes	± Rare	+	± Rare	-	-	-	-
Tubules	-	-	-	-	-	-	+
Lymphoglandular bodies	-	-	-	+	+	-	-
Macrophages	±	±	-	+	±	-	-
Myxoid matrix	-	-	-	-	-	±	-
Fibrous matrix	-	-	-	-	-	-	+
Spindle-shaped cells	-	-	-	-	-	+	±
Tadpole or ribbon-shaped cells	-	-	-	-	-	+	±
Dense cytoplasm	-	-	-	-	-	+	±
Karyorrhectic cells	-	+	-	+	±	-	-
Tigroid background	-	-	-	-	-	±	-

PNET - Primitive neuroectodermal tumor; NB - Neuroblastoma; ES - Ewing's sarcoma; BL - Burkitt's lymphoma; LL - Lymphoblastic lymphoma; RMS - Rhabdomyosarcoma; WT - Wilms' tumor; + = Frequently present or prominent; ± = May be present (rare) or inconspicuous; - = Absent. Modified from Silverman JF, et al: Fine-needle aspiration cytology of primitive neuroectodermal tumor. A report of three cases. *Acta Cytol* 36:541-550, 1992 (with permission).

Pseudorosette formation can also be present, characterized by malignant cells adhering to branching blood vessels (Image 14.64). In our experience, the major differential features separating PNET from neuroblastoma is the lack of prominent neuropil in PNET, in contrast to its presence in neuroblastoma. PNET also demonstrates prominent cytoplasmic vacuoles, while Homer-Wright rosettes are less often seen. Ganglion cells are not present in PNET.[105] When a predominantly dispersed pattern is present, the differential diagnosis of PNET also includes malignant lymphoma (Image 14.65). The cytologic features differentiating neuroblastoma from PNET and other small round cell tumors of children are summarized in Table 14.10.

A definitive diagnosis of neuroblastoma and/or peripheral neuroectodermal tumors is aided with utilization of immunocytochemistry and EM on the aspirated material.[105] The tumor cells are characteristically positive for NSE and may also stain positive for S-100 protein, neurofilaments and GFAP (Image 14.66).[97,121] In the workup of small round cell tumors of childhood, an immunoperoxidase panel that includes a panhematopoietic marker (LCA), epithelial markers (AE1/3, etc), vimentin and muscle markers (myoglobin, desmin, and muscle specific actin) can better exclude other small round cell tumors of childhood.[36,105,120,122,123] Ultrastructural features of neuroblastoma and PNET include the presence of membrane bound dense core granules measuring from 50 to 200 nanometers (catecholamine granules, neurosecretory granules) which are characteristically found in the peripherally of the cytoplasm and in cell processes (neurites) along with neurotubules and neurofilaments (Image 14.67). A variable amount of glycogen may be present in PNET,[105] while a greater number of neurosecretory granules and more prominent microtubules and cell processes are seen in neuroblastoma. Other additional ancillary studies that can be performed on aspirated specimens include cytogenetic studies to demonstrate the characteristic reciprocal translocation (11:22) seen in peripheral neuroectodermal tumors (Image 14.68).[105,113] Hyperdiploidy of tumor cells determined by flow cytometry and image analysis in neuroblastoma of infants is associated with a better response to chemotherapy than is diploidy (Image 14.69).[124,125] N-*myc* oncogene amplification studies can also be obtained from aspirated material. There is good data showing correlation between increased N-*myc* oncogene amplification and unfavorable histology subgroups.[124,126]

FNA biopsy of neuroblastoma and PNET enables a primary diagnosis before definitive staging and/or cytoreductive treatment with subsequent resection and staging.[36,105] FNA cytology is also used for documentation of tumor recurrence and metastatic disease as well as assessment of response to therapy (Image 14.70). In patients with a known history of neuroblastoma and PNET, aspiration cytology can exclude a nonneoplastic cause for a mass such as encountered in opportunistic infection or fibrosis and/or necrosis secondary to chemotherapy and/or irradiation.[36,105,127]

In patients with a known history of neuroblastoma and PNET, aspiration cytology can exclude a nonneoplastic cause for a mass such as encountered in opportunistic infection or fibrosis and/or necrosis secondary to chemotherapy and/or irradiation

Percutaneous FNA Biopsy of the Lung in Children to Evaluate Mass Lesions

In the past, some laboratories have utilized lung aspiration in the workup of acute pneumonias in infants and children.[128-130] We have not utilized FNA at our institutions for these types of cases, having reserved FNA biopsy for the evaluation of solid discrete lesions. We have encountered a few benign mass lesions, such as mycotic lung abscesses due to *Aspergillus* in the pediatric population (Images 14.71 through 14.73). A number of other non-neoplastic inflammatory and infectious lesions can potentially occur in the lungs including infectious processes secondary to other fungi, bacteria, mycobacteria and parasites. Discussion of these entities is beyond the scope of this book. The readers are referred to other sources for a more detailed elaboration of infectious and inflammatory conditions involving the lung examined by FNA biopsy.[34] Most of the lesions we have encountered represent metastatic malignancies to the lung (Image 14.74), excluding our experiences with thoracic and chest wall PNET, which are discussed above.

The more common benign lung tumors reported in the pediatric age group include plasma cell granuloma (inflammatory pseudotumor) followed by hamartoma and a number of other uncommon mesenchymal lesions.[15,131] The most common primary malignant neoplasms include bronchogenic carcinoma, bronchial neoplasms with salivary

Table 14.11
Ancillary Studies in the FNA Workup of Small Round Cell Malignancies of Childhood

Cytologic Diagnosis	EM	Immunocytochemistry	Cytogenetics
Neuroblastoma	Greater number of DCG and more prominent micro-tubules and cell processes than PNET Primitive cell junctions	NSE, S-100 Schwann cells, NF	Chromosome 1 deletion, short arm
PNET	Rare dense core granules (DCG) Glycogen in a few cases	NSE, vimentin Neurofilaments (NF Beta$_2$, microglobulin HBA-71	11;22 translocation
Ewing's sarcoma	Glycogen, cell junctions	Vimentin HBA-71	11;22 translocation
Burkitt's lymphoma	No specific EM features; lipid vacuoles	Leukocyte common antigen (LCA), B phenotype	8;14 translocation
Lymphoblastic lymphoma	No specific EM features	LCA, B or T phenotype	
Rhabdomyosarcoma	Myosin filaments Z band	Actin, myoglobin, and/or desmin	2;13 translocation in alveolar rhabdomyosarcoma

Modified from Silverman JF, et al: Fine-needle aspiration cytology of primitive neuroectodermal tumor. A report of three cases. *Acta Cytol* 36:541-550, 1992 (with permission).

gland-like features and carcinoid tumor. All of these lesions are quite unusual. In childhood, the lung can be involved with other rare malignant neoplasms, such as pulmonary blastoma (Image 14.75), sarcomas, lymphomas, teratomas and plasmacytoma.[131] We and others have had a very limited experience with FNA biopsy of primary pulmonary neoplasms in children.

Ancillary Studies in FNA of Pediatric Neoplasms

We recently evaluated the diagnostic contribution of ancillary studies performed on aspirated material in the workup of pediatric biopsies.[13] Ancillary studies were performed on 54 of 136 (39.7%) pediatric FNA biopsies during a 5-year period. Immunocytochemical studies consisting of immunoperoxidase staining of direct smears and cell blocks or immunophenotyping by flow cytometry were performed in selective cases. These studies were adequate in 14 cases (16.9%), suboptimal in 5 cases (21.7%), and inadequate in 4 cases (17.4%). Of the adequate and suboptimal cases, the immunoperoxidase studies help to narrow the differential diagnosis or classify the disease process in 8 cases (42.1%), confirm cytologic impression in 9 cases (47.4%), and gave contradictory results in 2 cases (10%). Adequate material for EM was obtained in 14 of 19 cases (73.7%). Ultrastructural studies were diagnostic or helped to classify the lesion in 5 cases (35.7%), confirmed the cytologic impression in 4 cases (28.6%), helped exclude diagnostic consideration in 3 cases (21.4%) and were judged to be noncontributory in 2 cases (14.3%). Our results were similar to other studies reporting the role of ancillary studies in the workup of pediatric FNA lesions (especially small round cell tumors of childhood).[3,4,36,44,48,87,105,122,123,132-141]

Cytogenetic studies performed on aspirated material revealed abnormal karyotypes in 6 of the 7 neoplasms studied. Especially helpful cytogenetic information is the presence of t(11:22) translocation seen in PNET and Ewing's sarcoma and t(8:14) translocation in Burkitt's lymphoma. A summary of useful EM, immunocytochemical and cytogenetic studies performed on the aspiration material is presented in Table 14.11.

In conclusion, FNA biopsy of deep pediatric lesions can be an accurate, inexpensive and rapid diagnostic procedure. We and others have demonstrated that ancillary studies have an important role in the workup of pediatric FNA biopsies, especially in the workup of abdominal and thoracic small round cell tumors. The optimal workup differs for each case and depends on the selection of cases potentially benefitting from ancillary studies based on the rapid initial morphologic examination of Diff-Quik-stained material as well as the clinical features of the particular case. Although a specific algorithm cannot be recommended, we believe that when a pathologist performs the initial morphologic assessment (analogous to a frozen section in surgical pathology) in concert with the clinical data, a critical initial differential diagnosis is generated which then prompts additional aspirated material to be obtained in order to perform these helpful ancillary studies that may contribute to making a specific final diagnosis.

Image 14.1
X-ray of hepatoblastoma revealing large mass replacing most of liver.

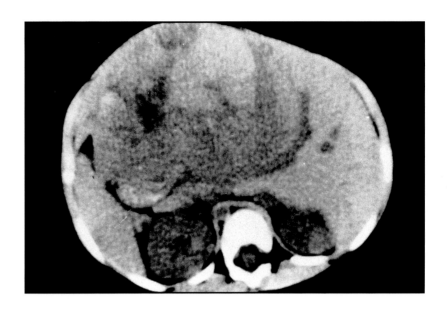

Image 14.2
Hypercellular smear of hepatoblastoma composed of uniform population of small to intermediate sized round to oval cells having a moderate amount of cytoplasm. The cells are in an anastomosing trabecular pattern. (Romanowsky).

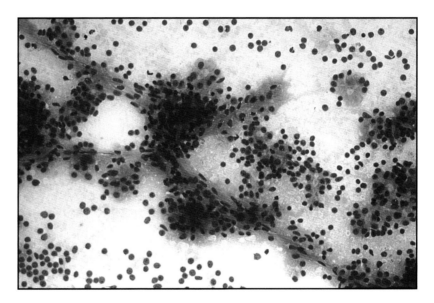

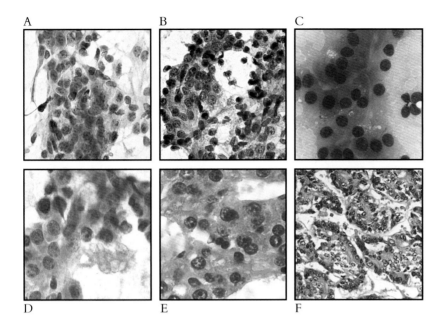

Image 14.3

A Aspirate of hepatoblastoma demonstrating cells arranged in columns resembling liver cords. (Papanicolaou).

B Cords of hepatocytes resembling immature liver tissue. (Papanicolaou).

C Cord of hepatocytes having granular cytoplasm as well as individually scattered stripped hepatocytic nuclei. (Romanowsky).

D Loosely arranged group of hepatocytes with centrally located nuclei and surrounding granular eosinophilic cytoplasm. Some spindle-shaped nuclei of sinusoidal cells are noted at the edge of the cords. (Papanicolaou).

E Cell block from aspirate of hepatoblastoma demonstrating fetal type liver cells arranged in cords. The cells have a moderate amount of granular eosinophilic cytoplasm. Along one edge of the cord there is a sinusoidal lining cell. (H&E).

F Resected hepatoblastoma showing cords of fetal-type hepatocytes corresponding to the cytologic features noted in the previous smears and cell block from the aspirate. (H&E).

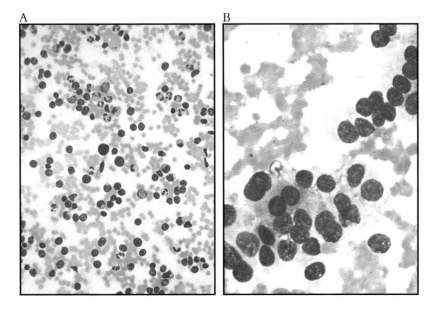

Image 14.4

A Cellular aspirate of hepatoblastoma showing groups of immature hepatocytes arranged in pseudoacinar clusters as well as single hepatocytes. Few scattered hematopoietic cells including eosinophils are present. (Romanowsky).

B Cords of hepatocytes including foci showing a pseudoacinar arrangement. (Romanowsky).

Image 14.5
Cell block revealing darker embryonal type cells in center of field, along with larger, more eosinophilic fetal cells from a FNA biopsy specimen of hepatoblastoma. (H&E).

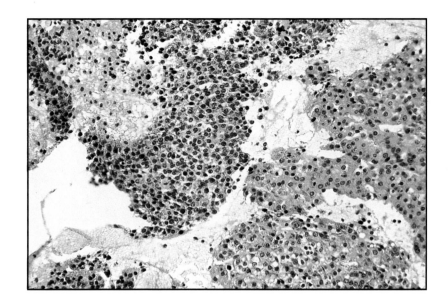

Image 14.6
A FNA of hepatoblastoma demonstrating positive cytoplasmic staining of the tumor cells for low molecular weight cytokeratin (immunoperoxidase stain).

B EM examination of aspirated cells of hepatoblastoma demonstrating canaliculus with well developed microvilli. The cells resemble immature hepatocytes and contain mitochondria, rough endoplasmic reticulin and tight intercellular junctions near the lumen. From Wakely PE et al. Fine needle aspiration biopsy of hepatoblastoma. *Mod Pathol* 3:688-693, 1990. (with permission).

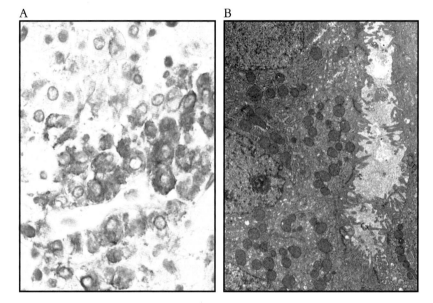

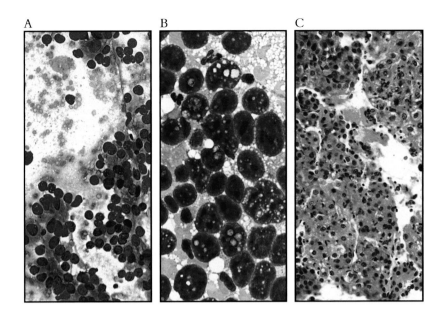

Image 14.7

A Low power of intraoperative FNA of hepatocellular carcinoma in a 10-year-old girl demonstrating numerous cords and clusters of malignant hepatocytes showing considerable variation in nuclear size. Stripped tumor nuclei are also present. (Romanowsky).

B High power of aspirate of hepatocellular carcinoma revealing pleomorphic tumor cells showing considerable variation in nuclear size and shape. Some of the tumor cells possess small intranuclear inclusions. (Romanowsky).

C Cell block from aspirate of hepatocellular carcinoma showing malignant hepatocytes demonstrating a greater degree of pleomorphism than is usually seen in a hepatoblastoma. (H&E).

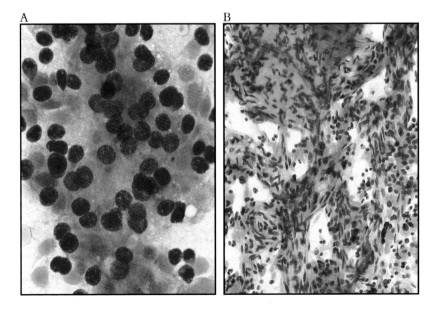

Image 14.8

A Aspirate of fibrolamellar variant of hepatocellular carcinoma revealing loosely cohesive to dissociative larger cells with abundant granular cytoplasm and cytoplasmic globules, some of which are lying free in the background. (Romanowsky).

B Low power of FNA of fibrolamellar variant of hepatocellular carcinoma showing scattered tumor cells as well as mesenchymal stroma. (Papanicolaou).

Image 14.9

A Aspirate of an adrenal adenoma showing cells stripped of cytoplasm having congregating nuclei which potentially could be confused with a small round cell tumor of childhood. The differential features include lack of nuclear molding and frothy vacuolated background consistent with an aspirate from an adrenal adenoma or adrenal cortical nodule.

B Aspirate of adrenal cortical adenoma showing stripped nuclei with some nuclear overlapping (Papanicolaou).

C Aspirate of adrenal cortical carcinoma in a 4-year-old child consisting of pleomorphic cells showing considerable variation in nuclear size. Note the pale cytoplasm and frothy vacuolated background. (Romanowsky).

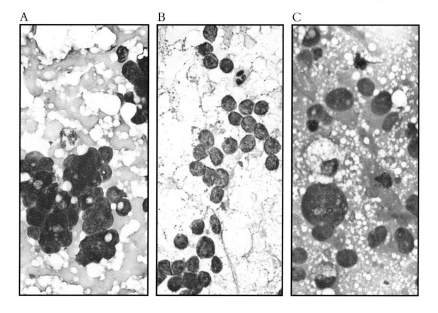

Image 14.10

A FNA of retroperitoneal paraganglioma in a 14-year-old boy presenting with a paraaortic mass. Clusters of polygonal shaped cells showing considerable anisonucleosis are noted. (Romanowsky).

B Clusters of polygonal to spindle-shaped cells having granular cytoplasm and characteristic salt and pepper type neuroendocrine nuclear chromatin. (Papanicolaou).

C Resected paraganglioma showing nests of cells with intervening fibrovascular tissue. (H&E).

D Immunoperoxidase for NSE performed on the aspirated smears

E Ultrastructure of extraadrenal pheochromocytoma (paraganglioma) demonstrating neurosecretory granules consistent with norepinephrine granules. A&B from Gurley MA, et al. The utility of ancillary studies in pediatric FNA cytology. *Diagn Cytopathol* 8:137-146, 1992 (with permission).

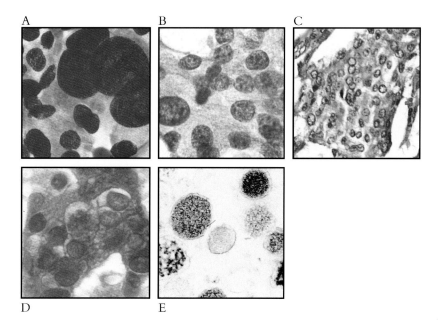

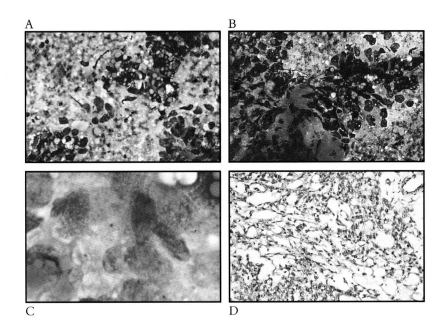

Image 14.11
A Aspirate of primary yolk sac tumor of liver consisting of loosely cohesive groups of malignant cells. (Romanowsky).
B Loose clusters of malignant cells having pale cytoplasm associated with extracellular clumps of metachromatically staining amorphous material of basement membrane origin. (Romanowsky).
C High power of malignant cells showing some air drying artifact as well as PAS-positive intracytoplasmic globules.
D Resected primary yolk sac tumor of the liver demonstrating characteristic lacy, reticulated nature of the tumor cells in a loose myxoid background. (H&E).

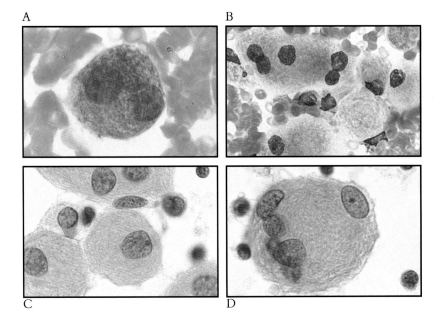

Image 14.12
A Aspirate of Gaucher's disease involving the liver, containing polygonal-shaped cells having eccentrically placed nuclei with abundant fibrillary cytoplasm. (Romanowsky).
B FNA of spleen containing numerous Gaucher's cells with uniform, small, eccentrically placed nuclei and abundant pale cytoplasm. (Romanowsky).
C Cluster of Gaucher's cells from splenic aspirate including binucleated cell. Note the abundant fibrillary pale cytoplasm as well as uniform, round nuclei. (H&E).
D Splenic aspirate in which a multinucleated Gaucher's cell is present as well as a few scattered lymphocytes. (H&E). B, C and D, courtesy of Dr A Dejmek, from Domanski H, et al. Gaucher's disease in an infant diagnosed by fine needle aspiration of the spleen. A case report. *Acta Cytol* 36:410-412, 1992 (with permission).

Image 14.13

A Aspirate of liver from patient with familial hemophagocytic syndrome demonstrating numerous histiocytes. (Romanowsky).

B Occasional histiocyte demonstrating cytophagocytosis of RBC. (Romanowsky). From Silverman JF et al. Cytomorphology of familial hemophagocytic syndrome (FHS). *Diagn Cytopathol* 9:404-410, 1993 (with permission).

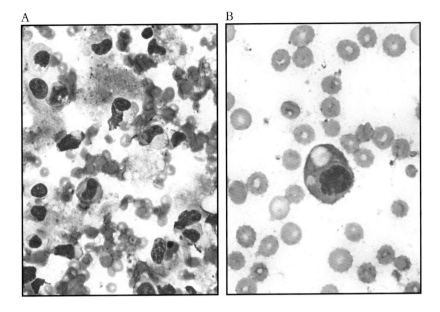

Image 14.14

This is from an aspirate of a cystic mass in the liver of a 16-year-old boy. Profiles of several embryonic tapeworms *(Echinococcus granulosus)* are present in this cell block. Inverted scolices including hooklets are seen. (H&E). (Case courtesy of Dr B Naylor).

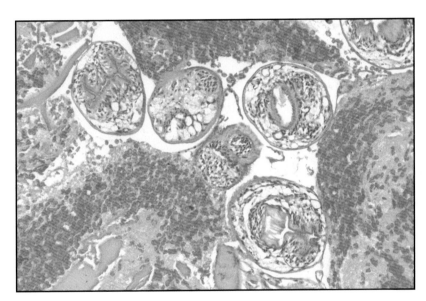

Image 14.15

Resected Wilms' tumor showing clumps of blastemal cells along with tubules and interspersed stroma. (H&E).

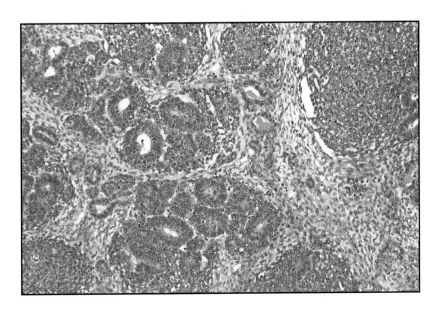

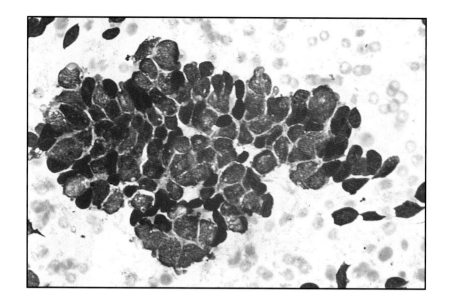

Image 14.16
Aspirate of Wilms' tumor consisting of blastemal cells characterized by small cells having high N/C ratio with a scant amount of surrounding cytoplasm. Nuclear molding is also present. (Romanowsky).

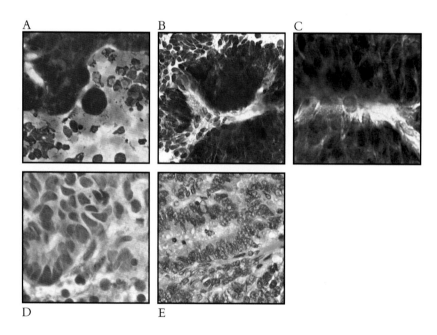

A

B

C

D

E

Image 14.17
A Aspirate of Wilms' tumor consisting of individually scattered small blastemal type cells along with complex tortuous tubules arranged in cohesive groups. (Romanowsky).
B Low power showing branching tortuous tubules with surrounding blastemal cells. (Papanicolaou).
C High power of complex tubule from aspirate of Wilms' tumor. Note also the blastemal cells arranged along luminal border. (Papanicolaou).
D Cell block from aspirate of Wilms' tumor showing scattered tubules as well as surrounding stroma. (H&E).
E Histologic correlate of branching tubules with surrounding blastemal cells. (H&E).

Image 14.18

A Blastemal cells arranged along branching blood vessels simulating complex tubules. (Papanicolaou).

B Histologic correlate of blastemal type Wilms' tumor showing blastemal cells arranged along branching blood vessels. (H&E).

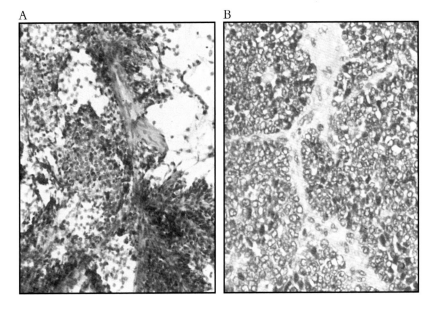

Image 14.19

A Low power of aspirate of Wilms' tumor showing few scattered branching complex tubules set in a loose mesenchymal stroma. (Papanicolaou).

B High power of stromal component of Wilms' tumor showing spindle shaped cells set in mesenchymal matrix. (Papanicolaou).

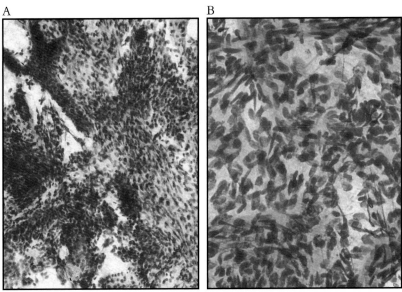

Image 14.20

Ultrastructure of aspirated cells from Wilms' tumor showing oligocilia.

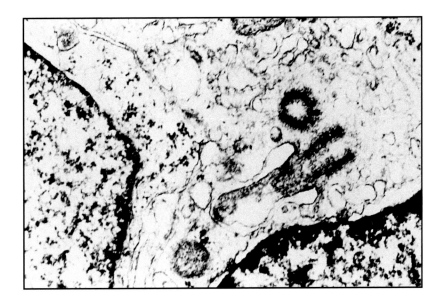

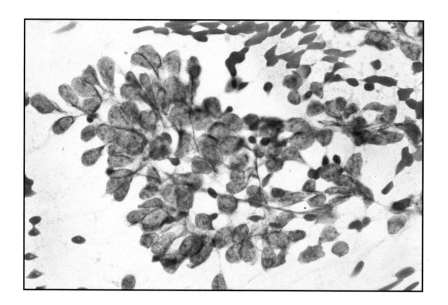

Image 14.21
Immunoperoxidase stain for cytokeratin performed on aspirated smear of Wilms' tumor demonstrating positive cytoplasmic staining of the cells.

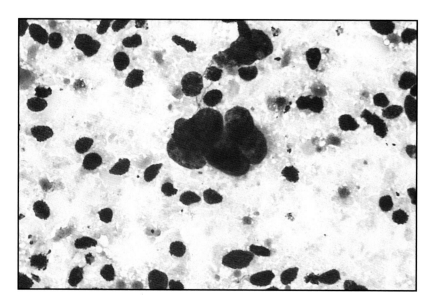

Image 14.22
FNA of recurrent Wilms' tumor showing anaplasia characterized by marked nuclear enlargement of some of the tumor cells as well as nuclear hyperchromasia. Multipolar mitotic figures are not seen in this field. (Romanowsky).

Image 14.23

A Aspirate of malignant rhabdoid tumor showing cluster of malignant cells having enlarged nuclei with vesicular chromatin pattern and prominent central nucleoli. A globular cytoplasmic structure is seen in some of the tumor cells. (Papanicolaou).

B EM of aspirate of malignant rhabdoid tumor showing tumor cells with large nuclei and prominent nucleoli as well as prominent whorled filamentous inclusions.

C Histology of primary rhabdoid tumor of kidney showing characteristic malignant cells having enlarged nuclei with vesicular chromatin pattern and prominent nucleoli as well as eosinophilic cytoplasmic inclusions. The histology corresponds quite well with the cytologic features noted in the aspirate. (H&E). A-C from Wakely PE, et al. Fine needle aspiration cytology of matastatic rhabdoid tumor. *Acta Cytol* 30:533-537, 1986 (with permission).

D FNA of clear cell sarcoma of kidney consisting of individually scattered polygonal to slightly spindle-shaped cells with clear cytoplasm and background mucoid matrix. (Romanowsky). From Akhtar M, et al. Fine needle aspiration biopsy of clear cell sarcoma of the kidney. Light and electron microscopic features. *Diagn Cytopathol* 5:181-187, 1989 (with permission).

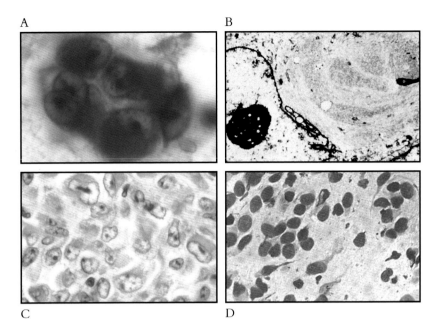

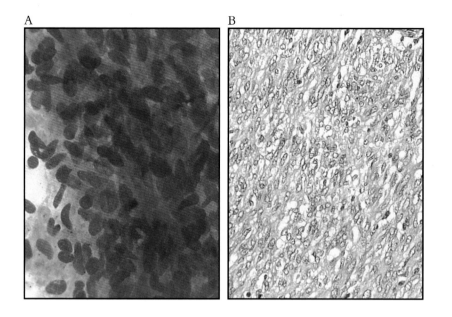

Image 14.24

A FNA of congenital mesoblastic nephroma showing loose clump of spindle-shaped cells demonstrating mild nuclear pleomorphism. (Romanowsky).

B Histologic section of mesoblastic nephroma revealing fascicles of spindle-shaped cells in which there is some mild nuclear pleomorphism and mitotic activity. (H&E). Slides courtesy of Dr Day, from Day P, et al. Fine-needle aspiration cytology of mesoblastic nephroma. A case report. *Acta Cytol* 36:404-406, 1992 (with permission).

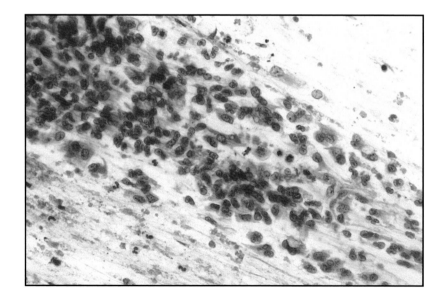

Image 14.25

This is an aspirate of a 10-year-old boy's renal neoplasm which subsequently proved to be a collecting duct carcinoma. The smears were moderately cellular and included many loosely cohesive cells. Most were mononucleated with only a thin rim of cytoplasm. Others had bizarrely shaped and/or multiple nuclei. Still others had greater volumes of cytoplasm some of which was highly vacuolated. (Papanicolaou).

Image 14.26
CT scan of Burkitt's lymphoma of abdomen showing bilateral involvement of the kidneys. From Gurley MA, et al. The utility of ancillary studies in pediatric FNA cytology. *Diagn Cytopathol* 8:137–146, 1992 (with permission).

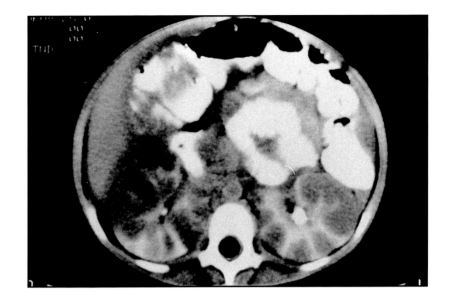

Image 14.27
Aspirate of Burkitt's lymphoma involving the kidney showing dispersed cell pattern with malignant lymphoid cells having high N/C ratio and multiple small cytoplasmic vacuoles. (Romanowsky). From *Diagn Cytopathol* 8:137–146, 1992 with permission.

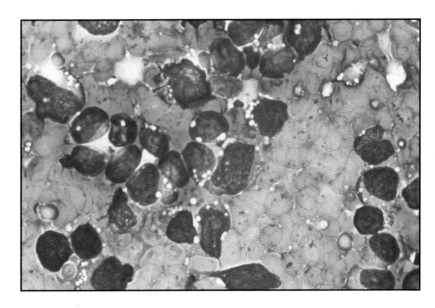

Image 14.28
Low power aspirate of Burkitt's lymphoma of kidney showing uniform population of malignant lymphoid cells having vesicular oval to round nuclei with multiple nucleoli. (Papanicolaou).

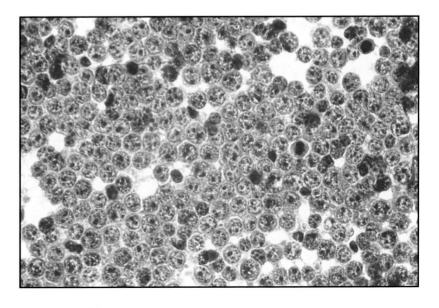

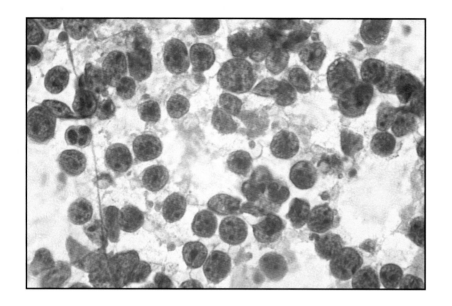

Image 14.29
Aspirate of Burkitt's lymphoma involving the kidney showing dispersed cell pattern of malignant cells having high N/C ratio. The nuclei contain multiple small nucleoli. (Papanicolaou).

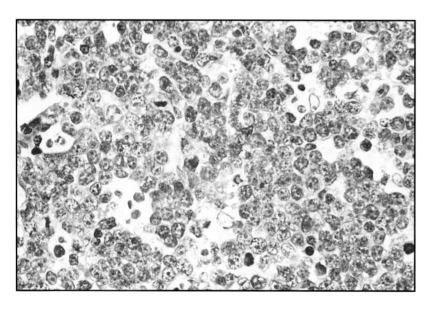

Image 14.30
Histology of Burkitt's lymphoma consisting of sheets of undifferentiated malignant lymphoid cells with scattered histiocytes. (H&E).

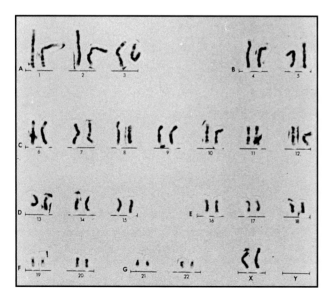

Image 14.31
The karyotype obtained from aspirated Burkitt's lymphoma involving the kidney revealing the characteristic (8:14) translocation. From Gurley MA, et al. The utility of ancillary studies in pediatric FNA cytology. *Diagn Cytopathol* 8:137-146, 1992 (with permission).

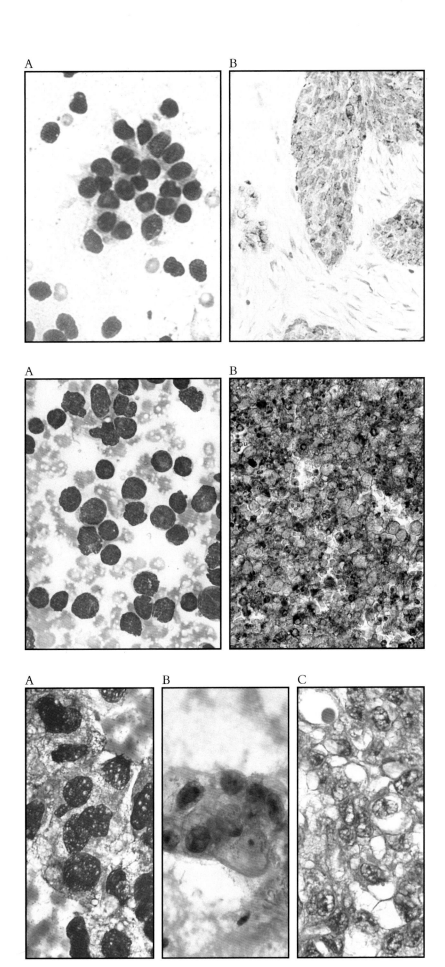

Image 14.32

A Cohesive and dispersed monomorphic tumor cells are present in this aspirate of an intraabdominal desmoplastic small round cell tumor in a 16 year old boy. Each cell has a single round nucleus with dense chromatin and a very high N/C ratio. (Romanowsky).

B The resected omentum was greatly expanded by nests of uniform neoplastic cells in well formed solid nests. The latter are set within a desmoplastic stroma. Many of the tumor cells are positive for desmin.

Image 14.33

A Aspirate of a retroperitoneal lymphoblastic lymphoma in a child showing dispersed pattern of markedly atypical lymphoid cells. (Romanowsky).

B Immunoperoxidase stain for leukocyte common antigen performed on the cell block from an aspirate of an undifferentiated retroperitoneal lymphoma in a child showing positive staining of the neoplastic lymphoid cells.

Image 14.34

A FNA of embryonal carcinoma of the ovary in a young child showing cluster of large malignant cells having pale vacuolated cytoplasm. Some faint intracytoplasmic globular material is noted. (Romanowsky).

B Cluster of malignant atypical cells having clear cytoplasm. (Papanicolaou).

C Cell block from aspirate of embryonal carcinoma of the ovary showing sheets of malignant cells having clear cytoplasm with occasional cells possessing eosinophilic globules. (H&E).

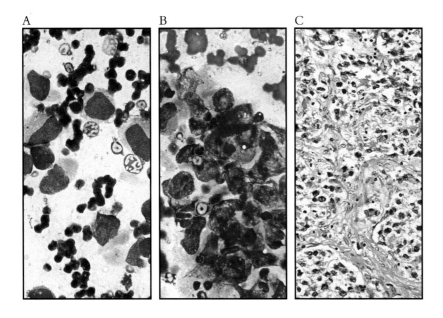

Image 14.35

A Transvaginal FNA of right adnexal mass in a 14-year-old girl with complete androgen insensitivity syndrome. Cytologic and histologic findings revealed a lesion consistent with seminoma. Individually scattered oval to irregular cells with a moderate amount of amphophilic cytoplasm was seen. Many of the cells possess prominent nucleoli. (Romanowsky).

B A cluster of poorly differentiated malignant cells showing considerable variation in nuclear size and shape as well as multiple prominent nucleoli is present. Note pale cytoplasm of the tumor cells. This seminoma lacked a "tigroid" background. (Romanowsky).

C Resected left adnexal mass showing characteristic histologic features of a seminoma. (H&E).

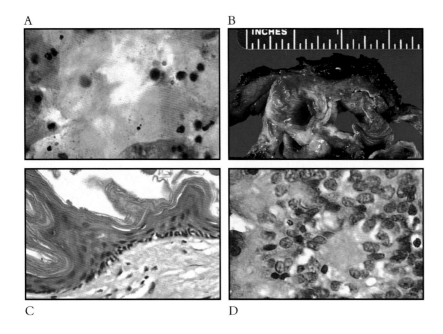

Image 14.36

A FNA of retrorectal cystic hamartoma (tailgut cyst) reveals numerous squamous cells and a few scattered inflammatory cells. (Papanicolaou).

B Resected large multiloculated cyst.

C Cysts lined by stratified squamous cells (H&E).

D Other portions of the resected retrorectal cystic hamartoma lined by ciliated columnar epithelial cells. (H&E). Slides courtesy of Dr NA Young, from *Diagn Cytopathol* 6:359-363, 1990 (with permission).

Image 14.37
CT scan of pancreatoblastoma in a young child showing large mass replacing most of the pancreas.

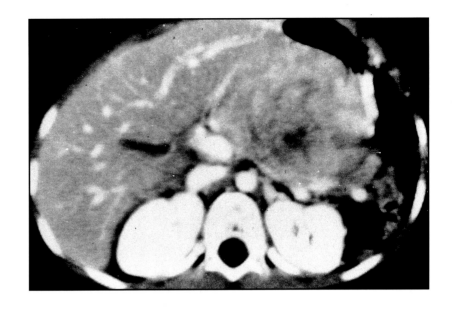

Image 14.38
Histologic examination of pancreatoblastoma reveals nests of cuboidal cells arranged in an organoid pattern with intervening dense bands of fibrous tissue. (H&E).

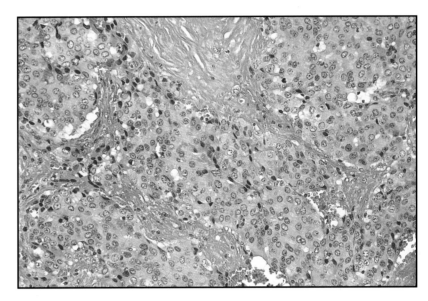

Image 14.39
Hypercellular smear of pancreatoblastoma revealing numerous oval to spindle to triangular-shaped cells having granular cytoplasm. The tumor cells are arranged in a dispersed fashion. (Papanicolaou).

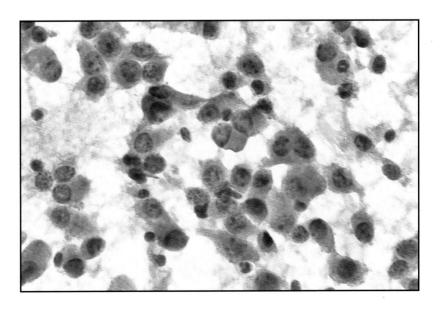

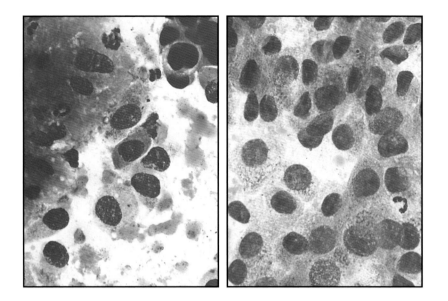

Image 14.40
Loose clusters of individually scattered cuboidal to spindle-shaped cells having a moderate amount of granular cytoplasm. (Romanowsky).

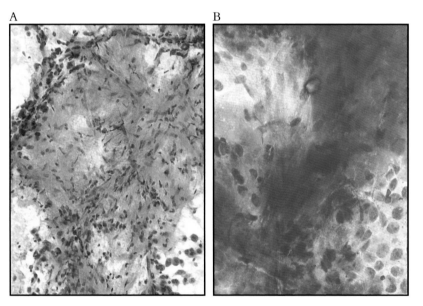

A

B

Image 14.41
A Low power of aspirate of pancreatoblastoma showing clumps of dense stroma with some interspersed capillaries and nearby tumor cells. (Papanicolaou).
B High power of FNA of pancreatoblastoma demonstrating dense amorphous fragments of stroma with some nearby peripherally arranged tumor cells. (Romanowsky).

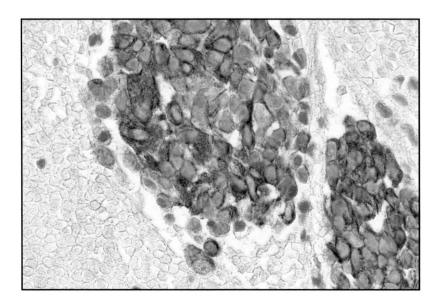

Image 14.42
Immunoperoxidase stain for NSE showing positive cytoplasmic staining of the tumor cells.

Image 14.43
Ultrastructure of pancreatoblastoma showing both smaller dense neuroendocrine type granules as well as larger zymogen-like granules.

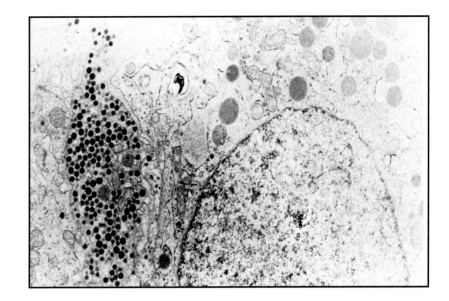

Image 14.44
A FNA of acinar cell carcinoma showing loose clusters of neoplastic cells having prominent nucleoli and granular cytoplasm. (Papanicolaou).
B Higher power of acinar cell tumor of the pancreas showing tight clusters of malignant acinar cells including some having a 3-dimensional configuration. (Courtesy of Dr G Thomas)

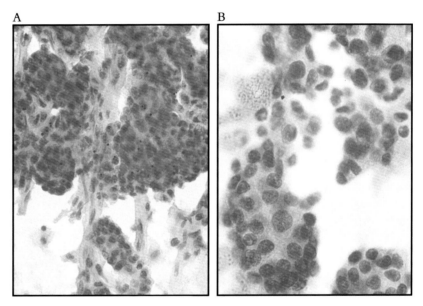

Image 14.45
This is an aspirate of a papillary cystic tumor (from a young adult woman). Branched papillae appear to fuse with more solid fragments of tumor cells. Each frond is lined by one or more rows of small uniform cells. (Papanicolaou).

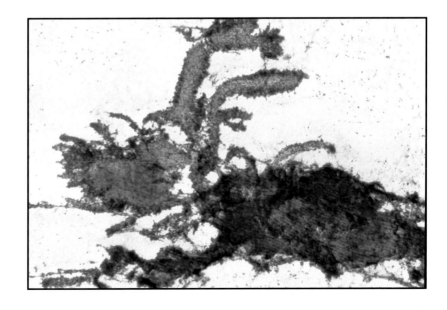

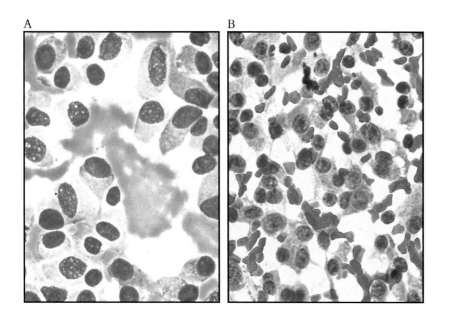

Image 14.46

A Numerous individually dispersed neoplastic cells are present in this aspirate of an islet cell tumor. Each cell has a round nucleus set eccentrically within basophilic cytoplasm. This creates the characteristic plasmacytoid appearance. (Romanowsky).

B With the Papanicolaou stain, chromatin is visualized as very finely granular and evenly dispersed. Small nucleoli are evident in a few nuclei. Several binucleated tumor cells are present.

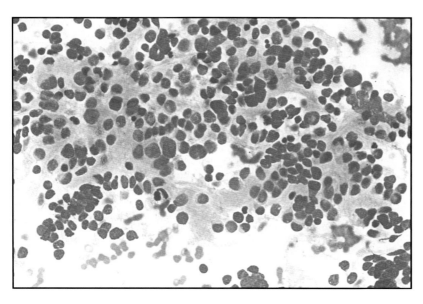

Image 14.47

Low power of aspirate of neuroblastoma showing numerous individually scattered neuroblastic cells along with some neuropil in the background. (Romanowsky).

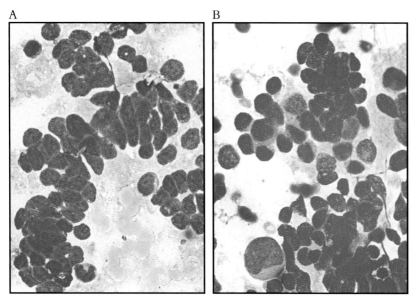

Image 14.48

A Aspirate of neuroblastoma showing prominent nuclear molding. (Romanowsky).

B Aspirate of neuroblastoma showing clumps of neuroblastic cells in which there is nuclear molding. Note also some larger differentiated neuroblasts. (Romanowsky).

Image 14.49
Binucleated to multinucleated ganglion cells are present as well as a few scattered neuroblasts. (Romanowsky).

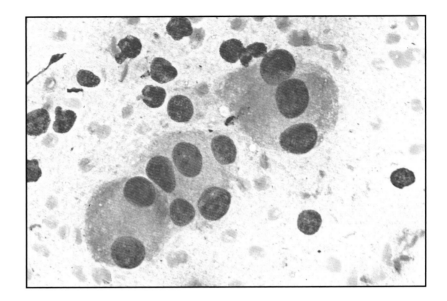

Image 14.50
A FNA of neuroblastoma showing a Homer-Wright rosette. The neuroblastic cells are arranged around some neuropil. (Papanicolaou).
B Hypercellular aspirate of neuroblastoma in which Homer-Wright rosettes are present. (Roman-owsky).

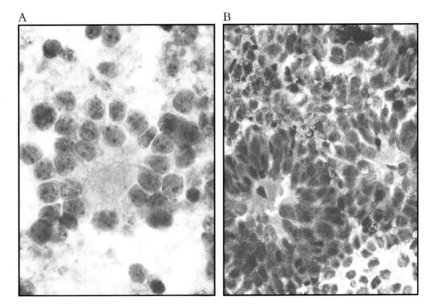

Image 14.51
The nuclei of neuroblastic cells vary from oval to slightly irregular and have characteristic evenly dispersed, finely granular chromatin with small to inconspicuous nucleoli. (Papanicolaou).

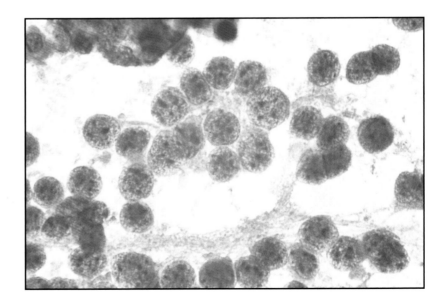

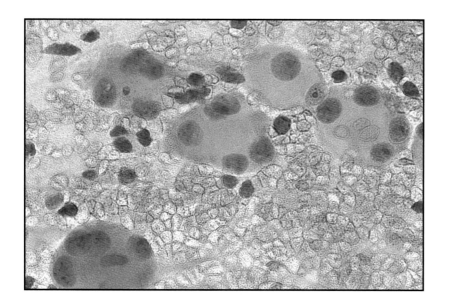

Image 14.52
Scattered ganglion cells and aspirate of ganglioneuroblastoma. Note that the ganglion cells are multinucleated and have larger and more vesicular chromatin with small but prominent nucleoli. (Papanicolaou).

A B

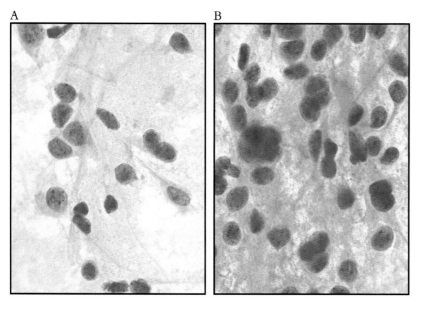

Image 14.53
A Scattered neuroblastic cells demonstrating delicate unipolar cell processes. (Papanicolaou).
B Aspirate of neuroblastoma showing few scattered neuroblastic cells having unipolar cytoplasmic processes. (Papanicolaou).

A B C

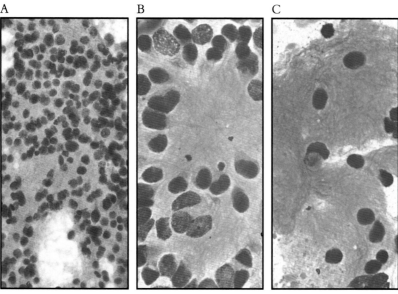

Image 14.54
A Low power of aspirate of neuroblastoma in which numerous scattered neuroblastic cells are seen enmeshed in a fibrillary neuropil. (Papanicolaou).
B High power of neuroblastoma showing scattered neuroblastic cells enmeshed in surrounding fibrillary neuropil. (Romanowsky).
C A clump of fibrillary neuropil associated with a few scattered neuroblastic cells is present. (Romanowsky).

Image 14.55
FNA of neuroblastoma in which a focus of mitotic-karyorrhectic cells are seen in the center of the field. (Papanicolaou).

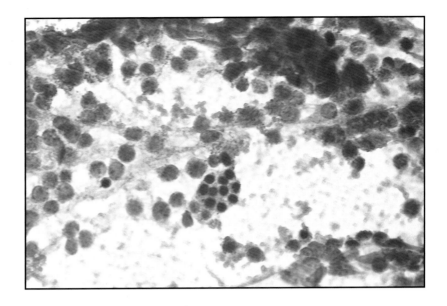

Image 14.56
Hypercellular aspirate of neuroblastoma in which scattered refractile clumps of calcified material are present. (Romanowsky).

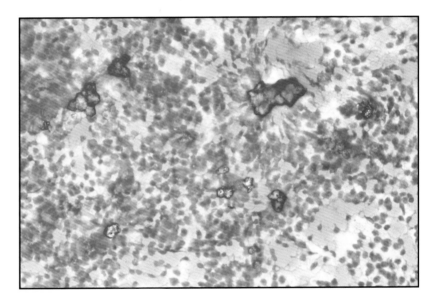

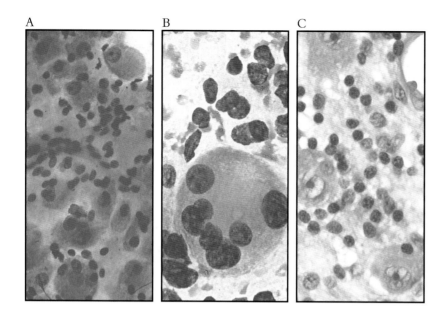

Image 14.57

A FNA of ganglioneuroblastoma in which scattered large, multinucleated large ganglion cells are seen associated with smaller neuroblastic cells in a background of neuromatous tissue. (Romanowsky).

B High power of ganglioneuroblastoma in which a few scattered multinucleated ganglion cells are seen with smaller dispersed neuroblastic cells. (Romanowsky).

C Resected ganglion neuroblastoma showing scattered ganglion cells having enlarged vesicular nuclei with prominent nucleoli along with nearby scattered neuroblastic cells. Neuromatous tissue is also present in the field. (H&E).

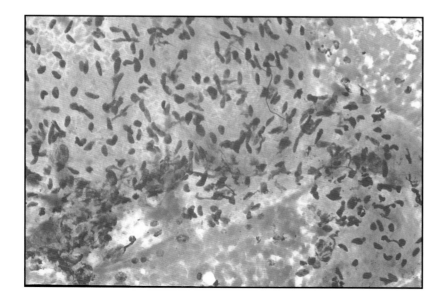

Image 14.58
Aspirate of ganglioneuroma in which neuronal fragments consist of spindle-shaped cells enmeshed in a pale fibrous staining stroma. (Romanowsky).

Image 14.59

A FNA cytologic findings of PNET consist of numerous malignant cells having high N/C ratios with scant amount of cytoplasm. Tumor cells have the prototypical neuroectodermal chromatin features characterized by evenly distributed "salt and pepper" type chromatin without prominent nucleoli. (Papanicolaou).

B Histologic correlate of PNET showing diffuse sheets of neuroblastic type cells having characteristic salt and pepper type chromatin. A few scattered degenerating cells are present having pyknotic nuclei. (H&E).

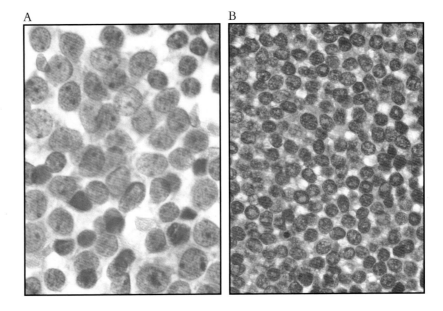

Image 14.60
Aspirate of PNET of chest wall showing neoplastic cells arranged in loose clusters and demonstrating prominent nuclear molding. (Romanowsky).

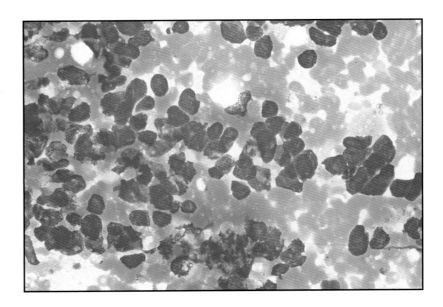

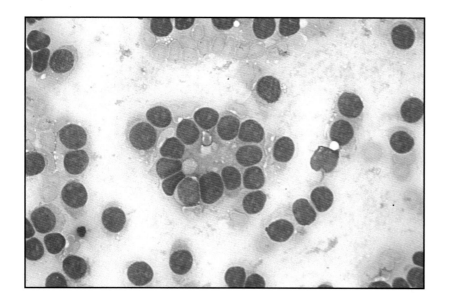

Image 14.61
Only occasionally, Homer-Wright rosettes can be appreciated in FNA of PNET. (Romanowsky).

A

B

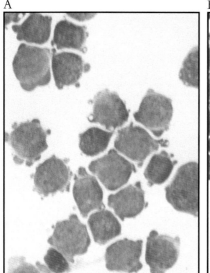

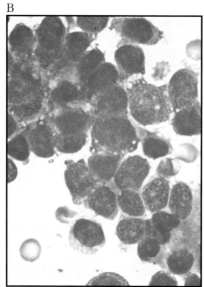

Image 14.62
A Dispersed malignant cells showing cytoplasmic vacuolization and blebs. (Romanowsky).
B Loose cluster of individually scattered neuroblastic cells in aspirate of PNET including some tumor cells showing fine cytoplasmic vacuolization. (Romanowsky). From Gurley AM, et al. *Diagn Cytopathol* 8:137-146, 1992 (with permission).

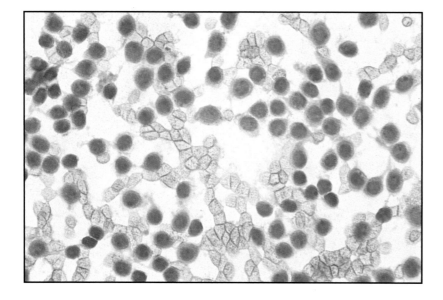

Image 14.63
FNA of PNET of soft tissue showing dispersed neuroblastic cells including many having unipolar cytoplasmic tags. (Papanicolaou).

Image 14.64
Aspirate of PNET showing pseudo-rosette formation characterized by neuroblastic cells adhering to branching blood vessels. (Romanowsky).

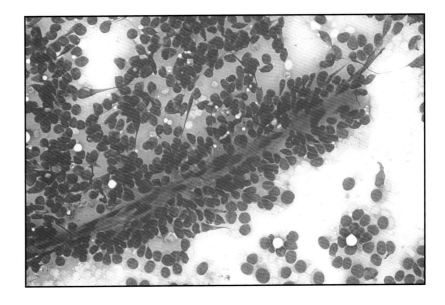

Image 14.65
Aspirate of PNET having a predominantly dispersed pattern which potentially could be confused with a malignant lymphoma. Helpful diagnostic features include the lack of lymphoglandular bodies in the background and neuroblastic quality of the nuclei characterized by evenly distributed "salt and pepper" chromatin pattern with the lack of prominent nucleoli. (Romanowsky).

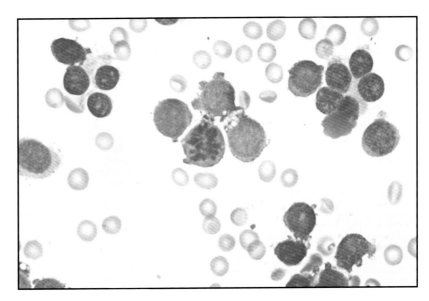

Image 14.66
A Immunoperoxidase stain for neuron specific enolase performed on aspirate of PNET.
B Immunoperoxidase stain for NSE performed on cell block of aspirate of neuroblastoma.
C Immunoperoxidase stain for neurofilaments demonstrating intense cytoplasmic staining of the ganglion cell.

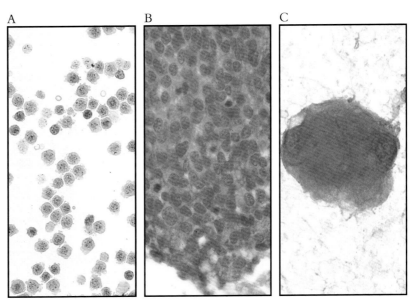

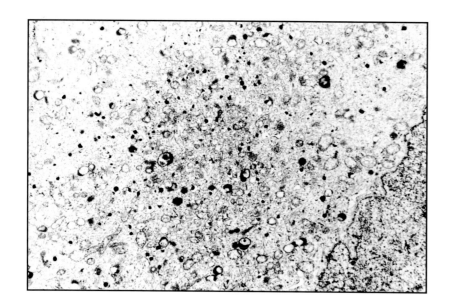

Image 14.67
Ultrastructural exam of neuroblastic cells obtained from FNA of adrenal mass. Note numerous neurosecretory type granules.

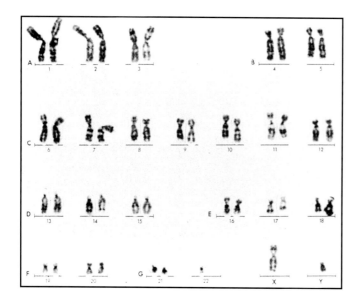

Image 14.68
Karyotype obtained from aspirate of PNET showing characteristic 11:22 translocation. From Gurley MA, et al. The utility of ancillary studies in pediatric FNA cytology. *Diagn Cytopathol* 8:137-146, 1992 (with permission).

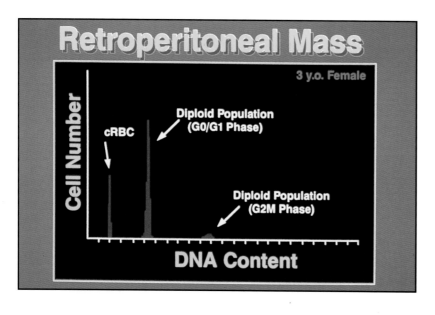

Image 14.69
Histogram of DNA studies by flow cytometry performed from aspirated material of neuroblastoma. Diploid results are associated with a poor prognosis.

Image 14.70
FNA of recurrent PNET involving pericardium. Note DNA streaking along with scattered benign histiocytic cells in addition to the malignant cells. Prominent tumor diathesis is seen in the background. (Romanowsky).

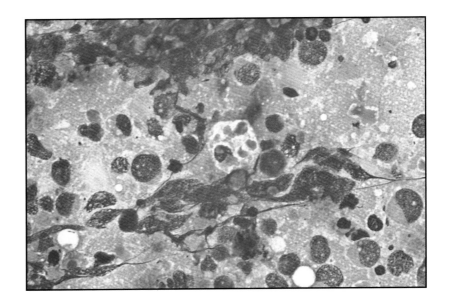

Image 14.71
CT scan of chest revealing mass lesion.

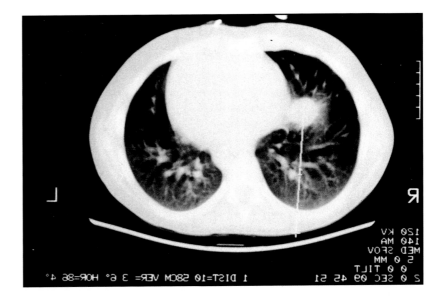

Image 14.72
Aspirate of chest mass demonstrates scattered histiocytes and a few neutrophils along with septated fungal hyphae. (Romanowsky).

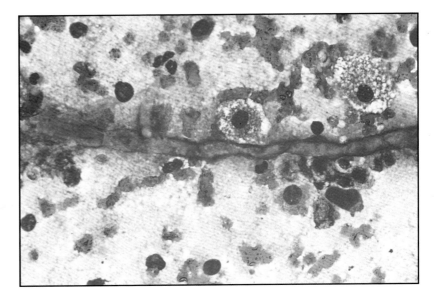

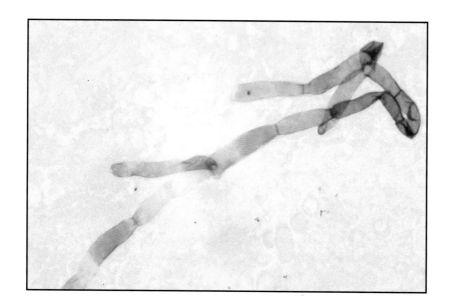

Image 14.73
GMS stain on aspirated smear shows characteristic branching septated hyphae of *Aspergillus*.

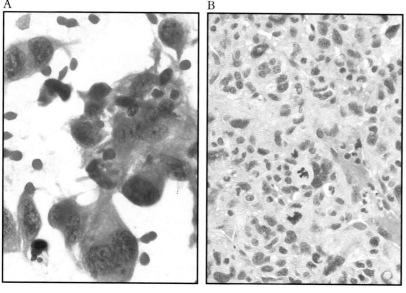

A   B

Image 14.74
A Aspirate of one of many lung nodules in a patient with metastatic osteogenic sarcoma of the femur. Scattered bizarre multinucleated tumor cells are present consistent with the aspirate from the bone primary. (Papanicolaou).
B Cell block from aspirate shows scattered bizarre malignant cells set within pale-staining osteoid. (H&E).

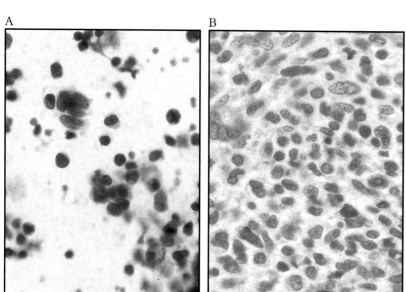

A   B

Image 14.75
A FNA of pulmonary blastoma consisting of scattered small malignant cells having a high N/C ratio. The nuclei vary from oval to spindle with a scant amount of surrounding cytoplasm. (Papanicolaou).
B Cell block from aspirate of pulmonary blastoma showing the presence of small malignant cells as well as scattered spindle-shaped cells. (H&E).

References

1. McGahey BE, Moriarty AT, Nelson WA, Hull MT. Fine-needle aspiration biopsy of small round blue cell tumors of childhood. *Cancer* 69:1067–1073, 1992.

2. Rajwanshi A, Rao KLN, Marwaha RK, Nijhawan VS, Gupta SK. Role of fine-needle aspiration cytology in childhood malignancies. *Diagn Cytopathol* 5:378–382, 1989.

3. Akhtar M, Ali A, Sabbah R, Bakry M, Nash JE. Fine needle aspiration biopsy diagnosis of round cell malignant tumors of childhood cancer. *Cancer* 55:1805–1817, 1985.

4. Akhtar M, Bedrossian CW, Ali MA, Bakry M. Fine-needle aspiration biopsy of pediatric neoplasms. Correlation between electron microscopy and immunocytochemistry in diagnosis and classification. *Diagn Cytopathol* 8:258–265, 1992.

5. Obers VJ, Phillips JI. Fine needle aspiration of pediatric abdominal masses. Cytologic and electron microscopic diagnosis. *Acta Cytol* 35:165–170, 1991.

6. Gorczyca W, Bedner E, Juszkiewicz P, Chosia M. Aspiration cytology in the diagnosis of malignant tumors in children. *Am J Pediatr Hematol Oncol* 14:129–135, 1992.

7. Layfield LJ, Reichman A. Fine needle aspiration cytology. Utilization in pediatric pathology. *Dis Markers* 8:301–315, 1990.

8. Layfield LJ, Glasgow B, Ostrzega N, Reynolds CP. Fine-needle aspiration cytology and the diagnosis of neoplasms in the pediatric age group. *Diagn Cytopathol* 7:451–461, 1991.

9. Valkov I, Bojikin B. Fine-needle aspiration biopsy of abdominal and retroperitoneal tumors in infants and children. *Diagn Cytopathol* 3:129–133, 1987.

10. Leiman G, Mair S. Aspiration cytology of neuroendocrine tumors below the diaphragm. *Diagn Cytopathol* 5:263–268, 1989.

11. Shakoor KA. Fine needle aspiration cytology in advanced pediatric tumors. *Pediatr Pathol* 9:713–718, 1989.

12. Silverman JF, Gurley AM, Holbrook CT, Joshi VV. Pediatric fine-needle aspiration biopsy. *Am J Clin Pathol* 95:653–659, 1991.

13. Gurley AM, Silverman JF, Lassaletta MM, Wiley JE, Holbrook CT, Joshi VV. The utility of ancillary studies in pediatric FNA cytology. *Diagn Cytopathol* 8:137–146, 1992.

14. Wakely PE Jr, Kardos TF, Frable WJ. Application of fine needle aspiration biopsy to pediatrics. *Hum Pathol* 19:1383–1386, 1988.

15. Dehner LP. Pediatric Surgical Pathology. 2nd ed. Williams & Wilkins, Baltimore, 1987.

16. Conran RM, Hitchcock CL, Waclawiw MA, Stocker JT, Ishak KG. Hepatoblastoma. The prognostic significance of histologic type. *Pediatr Pathol* 12:167–183, 1992.

17. Bhatia A, Mehrotra P. Fine needle aspiration cytology in a case of hepatoblastoma. *Acta Cytol* 30:439–441, 1986.

18. Dekmezian R, Sniege N, Popok S, Ordonez NF. Fine-needle aspiration cytology of pediatric patients with primary hepatic tumors. A comparative study of two hepatoblastomas and a liver cell carcinoma. *Diagn Cytopathol* 4:162–168, 1988.

19. Wakely PE Jr, Silverman JF, Geisinger KR, Frable WJ. Fine needle aspiration biopsy cytology of hepatoblastoma. *Mod Pathol* 3:688–693, 1990.

20. Suen KC. Diagnosis of primary hepatic neoplasms by fine-needle aspiration cytology. *Diagn Cytopathol* 2:99–109, 1986.

21. Diament MJ, Stanley P, Taylor S. Percutaneous fine needle biopsy in pediatrics. *Pediatr Radiol* 15:409–411, 1985.

22. Perez JS, Perez-Guillermo M, Bernal AB, Mercader JM. Hepatoblastoma. An attempt to apply histologic classification to aspirates obtained by fine needle aspiration cytology. *Acta Cytol* 38:175–182, 1994.

23. Suen KC, Magee JF, Halparin LS, Chan NH, Greene C. Fine needle aspiration cytology of fibrolamellar hepatocellular carcinoma. *Acta Cytol* 29:867–872, 1985.

24. Hajdu SI, Ehya H, Frable WJ, Geisinger K, Gompel C, Kern WH, Lowhagen T, Oertel YC, Ramzy I, Rilke FO, Saigo PE, Suprun HZ, Yazdi HM. The value and limitations of aspiration cytology in the diagnosis of primary tumors. A symposium. *Acta Cytol* 33:741–790, 1989.

25. Weinberg AG, Finegold MJ. Primary hepatic tumors of childhood. *Hum Pathol* 14:512–537, 1983.

26. Stocker JT, Ishak KG. Undifferentiated (embryonal) sarcoma of the liver. Report of 31 cases. *Cancer* 42:336–348, 1978.

27. Keating S, Taylor GP. Undifferentiated (embryonal) sarcoma of the liver. Ultrastructural and immunohistochemical similarities with malignant fibrous histiocytoma. *Hum Pathol* 16:693–699, 1985.

28. Parham DM, Kelly DR, Donnelly WH, Douglass EC. Immunohistochemical and ultrastructural spectrum of hepatic sarcomas of childhood. Evidence of a common histogenesis. *Mod Pathol* 4:648–653, 1991.

29. Silverman JF, Katz R. FNA of the adrenal gland. In: Cytopathology Annual. Williams and Wilkins, Baltimore (in press).

30. Wadih G, Nance KV, Silverman JF. Fine-needle aspiration of the adrenal gland. Fifty biopsies in 48 patients. *Arch Pathol Lab Med* 116:841–846, 1992.

31. Wakely PE Jr, Krummel TM, Johnson DE. Yolk sac tumor of the liver. *Mod Pathol* 4:121–125, 1991.

32. Domanski H, Dejmek A, Ljung R. Gaucher's disease in an infant diagnosed by fine needle aspiration of the liver and spleen. A case report. *Acta Cytol* 36:410–412, 1992.

33. Silverman JF, Singh HK, Joshi VV, Holbrook CT, Chauvenet AR, Harris LS, Geisinger KR. Cytomorphology of familial hemophagocytic syndrome (FHS). *Diagn Cytopathol* 9:404–410, 1993.

34. Silverman JF. Infectious and inflammatory diseases and other non-neoplastic disorders. Igaku-Shoin, New York, 1991, pp 245–253.

35. Frias-Hidvegi D. Liver and pancreas. Igaku-Shoin, New York, 1988, pp 43–62.

36. Silverman JF, Dabbs DJ, Ganick DJ, Holbrook CT, Geisinger KR. Fine needle aspiration cytology of neuroblastoma, including peripheral neuroectodermal tumor, with immunocytochemical and ultrastructural confirmation. *Acta Cytol* 32:367–376, 1988.

37. Drut R, Pollono D. Anaplastic Wilms' tumor. Initial diagnosis by fine needle aspiration. *Acta Cytol* 31:774-776, 1984.

38. Zuppan CW, Beckwith JB, Luckey DW. Anaplasia in unilateral Wilms' tumor. A report from the National Wilms' Tumor Study Pathology Center. *Hum Pathol* 19:1199-1209, 1988.

39. Akhtar M, Ali MA, Sackey K, Bakry M, Burgess A. Fine-needle aspiration biopsy diagnosis of malignant rhabdoid tumor of the kidney. *Diagn Cytopathol* 7:36-40, 1991.

40. Wakely PE Jr, Giacomantonio M. Fine needle aspiration cytology of metastatic rhabdoid tumor. *Acta Cytol* 30:533-537, 1986.

41. Perez JS, Perez-Guillermo M, Bernal AB, Lopez TM, Lopez FC. Malignant rhabdoid tumor of soft tissues. A cytopathological and immunohistochemical study. *Diagn Cytopathol* 8:369-373, 1992.

42. Drut R. Malignant rhabdoid tumor of the kidney diagnosed by fine-needle aspiration cytology. *Diagn Cytopathol* 6:124-126, 1990.

43. Weeks DA, Beckwith JB, Mierau GW. Rhabdoid tumor. An entity or a phenotype? *Arch Pathol Lab Med* 113:113-114, 1989.

44. Akhtar M, Ali MA, Sackey K, Burgess A. Fine-needle aspiration biopsy of clear-cell sarcoma of the kidney. Light and electron microscopic features. *Diagn Cytopathol* 5:181-187, 1989.

45. National Wilms' Tumor Study #4, Pediatric Oncology Group (POG) #8650, CCSG#461, NCI-INT-0070, pp 33-35, November 6, 1987.

46. Berg JW, Robbins GF. Late look at the safety of aspiration biopsy. *Cancer* 1962;15:826-827.

47. Schreeb T-V, Arner O, Skovsted G, Wikstad N. Renal adenocarcinoma. Is there a risk of spreading tumour cells in diagnostic puncture? *Scand J Urol Nephrol* 1:270-276, 1967.

48. Akhtar M, Ali MA, Sackey K, Sabbah R, Burgess A. Aspiration cytology of Wilms' tumor: Correlation of cytologic and histologic features. *Diagn Cytopathol* 5:269-274, 1989.

49. Sabbah RS, Aur RJA, Hanash K, El-Senoussi M. Management of the debilitated child with massive Wilms' tumor. *King Faisal Spec Hosp Med J* 2:77-83, 1982.

50. Bray GL, Pendergrass TW, Schaller RT Jr, Kiviat N, Beckwith JB. Preoperative chemotherapy in the treatment of Wilms' tumor diagnosed with the aid of fine needle aspiration biopsy. *Am J Pediatr Hematol Oncol* 8:75-78, 1986.

51. Saarinen UM, Wikstrom S, Koskimies O, Sariola H. Percutaneous needle biopsy preceding preoperative chemotherapy in the management of massive renal tumors in children. *J Clin Oncol* 9:406-415, 1991.

52. Geisinger KR, Wakely PE, Wofford MM. Unresectable stage IV nephroblastoma. A potential indication for fine-needle aspiration biopsy in children. *Diagn Cytopathol* 9:197-201, 1993.

53. Lemerle J, Vonte PA, Tournade MF, Delemarre JFM, Jereb B, Ahstrom L, Flamant R, Gerard-Marchant-R. Preoperative versus postoperative radiotherapy, single versus multiple courses of actinomycin D, in the treatment of Wilms' tumor. Preliminary results of a controlled clinical trial conducted by the International Society of Paediatric Oncology (S.I.O.P.). *Cancer* 38:647-654, 1976.

54. Lemerle J, Vonte PA, Tournade MF, Rodary C, Delemarre JFM, Sarrazin D, Burgers JM, Sandstedt B, Mildenberger H, Carli M, Jereb B, Moorman-Voestermans CGM. Effectiveness of preoperative chemotherapy in Wilms' tumor. Results of an International Society of Paediatric Oncology (SIOP) clinical trial. *J Clin Oncol* 1:604-609, 1983.

55. D'Angio GJ, Beckwith JB, Breslow N, Finklestein J, Green DM, Kelalis P. Wilms' tumor (nephroblastoma, renal embryoma). In: Pizzo PA, Poplack DG, eds. Principles and practices of pediatric oncology. JB Lippincott, Philadelphia, 1989, pp 583-606.

56. Zuppan CW, Beckwith JB, Weeks DA, Luckey DW, Pringle KC. The effects of preoperative therapy on the histologic features of Wilms' tumor. An analysis of cases from the Third National Wilms' Tumor Study. *Cancer* 68:385-394, 1991.

57. Hanash KA, Sackey K, Sabbah RS, Akhtar M, Aur RJA, Ali AM. Surgical treatment of bilateral synchronous Wilms' tumors. *J Surg Oncol* 34:172-175, 1987.

58. Montgomery BT, Kelalis PP, Blute ML, Bergstralh EJ, Beckwith JB, Norkook P, Green DM, D'Angio GJ. Extended followup of bilateral Wilms' tumor. Results of the National Wilms' Tumor Study. *J Urol* 146:514-518, 1991.

59. Geisinger KR, Hajdu SI, Helson L. Exfoliative cytology of non-lymphoreticular neoplasms in children. *Acta Cytol* 28:16-28, 1984.

60. Bracken RB, Sutow WW, Jaffe N, Ayala A, Guarda L. Preoperative chemotherapy for Wilms' tumor. *Urology* 19:55-60, 1982.

61. McLorie GA, McKenna PH, Greenberg M, Babyn P, Thorner P, Churchill BM, Weitzman S, Filler R, Khoury AE. Reduction in tumor burden allowing partial nephrectomy following preoperative chemotherapy in biopsy proved Wilms' tumor. *J Urol* 146:509-513, 1991.

62. Wakely PE Jr, Sprague RI, Kornstein MJ. Extrarenal Wilms' tumor. An analysis of four cases. *Hum Pathol* 20:691-695, 1989.

63. Dey P, Srinivasan R, Nijhawan R, Rajwanshi A, Banerjee CK, Rao KLN, Gupta SK. Fine needle aspiration cytology of mesoblastic nephroma. A case report. *Acta Cytol* 36:404-406, 1992.

64. Drut R. Cytologic characteristics of congenital mesoblastic nephroma in fine-needle aspiration cytology. A case report. *Diagn Cytopathol* 8:374-376, 1992.

65. Clark SP, Kung ITM, Tang SK. Fine-needle aspiration of cystic nephroma (multilocular cyst of the kidney). *Diagn Cytopathol* 8:349-351, 1992.

66. Drut R. Cystic nephroma. Cytologic findings in fine-needle aspiration biopsy. *Diagn Cytopathol* 18:593-595, 1992.

67. Fuzesi L, Cober M, Mittermayer C. Collecting duct carcinoma.Cytogenetic characterization. *Histopathology* 21:155-160, 1992.

68. Layfield LJ, Lenarsky C. Desmoplastic small cell tumors of the peritoneum coexpressing mesenchymal and epithelial markers. *Am J Clin Pathol* 96:536-543, 1991.

69. Setrakian S, Gupta PK, Heald J, Brooks JJ. Intraabdominal desmoplastic small round cell tumor. Report of a case diagnosed by fine needle aspiration cytology. *Acta Cytol* 36:373-376, 1992.

70. Caraway NP, Fanning TV, Bainbridge TC, Amato RJ, Katz RL. Fine needle aspiration of intraabdominal desmoplastic small cell tumors. *Acta Cytol* 36:599, 1992.

71. Thompson EN III, Teot LA, Geisinger KR. Exfoliative and aspiration cytomorphology of intraabdominal desmoplastic small round cell tumor. The first reported case. *Acta Cytol* 36:599, 1992.

72. Young NA, Neeson T, Bernal D, Hernandez E, Grotkowski CE. Retrorectal cystic hamartoma diagnosed by fine-needle aspiration biopsy. *Diagn Cytopathol* 6:359-363, 1990.

73. Cruickshank AH. Pathology of the Pancreas. Springer-Verlag, New York, 1986, pp 189-191.

74. Ichijima K, Akaishi K, Toyoda N, Kobashi Y, Ueda Y, Matsuo S, Yamabe H. Carcinoma of the pancreas with endocrine component in childhood. A case report. *Am J Clin Pathol* 83:95-100, 1985.

75. Kloppel, Heitz PU: Pancreatic Pathology. Churchill Livingstone, New York, 1985, pp 104-105.

76. Becker WF. Pancreatoduodenectomy for carcinoma of the pancreas in an infant. *Ann Surg* 145:864-872, 1957.

77. Benjamin E, Wright DH. Adenocarcinoma of the pancreas of childhood. A report of two cases. *Histopathology* 4:87-104, 1980.

78. Buchino JJ, Castello FM, Nagaraj HS. Pancreatoblastoma. A histochemical and ultrastructural analysis. *Cancer* 53:963-969, 1984.

79. Cubilla AL, Fitzgerald PJ. Classification of pancreatic cancer (nonendocrine). *Mayo Clin Proc* 54:449-458, 1979.

80. Frable WJ, Still WJS, Kay S. Carcinoma of the pancreas, infantile type. *Cancer* 27:667-673, 1971.

81. Horie A. Pancreatoblastoma: histopathologic criteria based on a review of six cases. In: Pancreatic Tumors in Children. GB Humphrey, GB Grindey, LP Dehner, RT Acton, TJ Pysher, eds. Martinus Nijhoff Publishers, Boston, 1982, pp 159-166.

82. Palosaari D, Clayton F, Seaman J. Pancreatoblastoma in an adult. *Arch Pathol Lab Med* 110:650-652, 1986.

83. Rich RH, Weber JL, Shandling B. Adenocarcinoma of the pancreas in a neonate managed by pancreatoduodenectomy. *J Pediatr Surg* 21:806-808, 1986.

84. Taxy JB. Adenocarcinoma of the pancreas in childhood. *Cancer* 37:1508-1518, 1976.

85. Mierau GW, Orsini EN. Diagnosis of human tumors. Case 2: Pancreatoblastoma mimicking fibrolamellar hepatocarcinoma. *Ultrastruct Pathol* 5:281-284, 1983.

86. Morohoshi T, Kanda M, Horie A, Chott A, Dreyer T, Kloppel G, Heitz PU. Immunocytochemical markers of uncommon pancreatic tumors. Acinar cell carcinoma, pancreatoblastoma, and solid cystic (papillary-cystic) tumor. *Cancer* 59:739-747, 1987.

87. Silverman JF, Holbrook CT, Pories WJ, Kodroff MB, Joshi VV. Fine needle aspiration cytology of pancreatoblastoma with immunocytochemical and ultrastructural studies. *Acta Cytol* 34:632-640, 1990.

88. Ishihara A, Sanda T, Takanari H, Yatani R, Liu PI. Elastase-1-secreting acinar cell carcinoma of the pancreas. A cytologic, electron microscopic and histochemical study. *Acta Cytol* 33:157-163, 1989.

89. Geisinger KR, Silverman JF. Fine-needle aspiration cytology of uncommon primary pancreatic neoplasms: A personal experience and review of the literature. In: Cytopathology Annual. WA Schmidt, ed. Williams and Wilkins, Baltimore, 1992, pp 23-48.

90. Shaw JA, Vance RP, Geisinger KR, Marshall RB. Islet cell neoplasms. A fine-needle aspiration cytology study with immunocytochemical correlations. *Am J Clin Pathol* 94:142-149, 1990.

91. Oertel JE, Heffess CS, Oertel YC. Pancreas. In: Diagnostic Surgical Pathology. Sternberg SS, ed. New York: Raven Press, 1989, pp 1057-1093.

92. Pettinato G, Manivel JC, Ravetto C, Terracciano LM, Gould EW, Tuoro AD, Jaszcz W, Albores-Saavedra J. Papillary cystic tumor of the pancreas. A clinicopathologic study of 20 cases with cytologic, immunohistochemical, ultrastructural, and flow cytometric observations, and a review of the literature. *Am J Clin Pathol* 98:478-488, 1992.

93. Cappellari JO, Geisinger KR, Albertson DA, Wolfman NT, Kute TE. Malignant papillary-cystic tumor of the pancreas. *Cancer* 66:193-198, 1990.

94. Bondeson L, Bondeson A-G, Genell S, Lindholm K, Thorstenson S. Aspiration cytology of a rare solid and papillary epithelial neoplasm of the pancreas. Light and electron microscopic study of a case. *Acta Cytol* 28:605-609, 1984.

95. Foote A, Simpson JS, Stewart RJ, Wakefield JSJ, Buchanan A, Gupta RK. Diagnosis of the rare solid and papillary epithelial neoplasm of the pancreas by fine needle aspiration cytology. Light and electron microscopic study of a case. *Acta Cytol* 30:519-522, 1986.

96. Al-Kaisi N, Weaver MG, Abdul-Karim FW, Siegler E. Fine needle aspiration cytology of neuroendocrine tumors of the pancreas. A cytologic, immunocytochemical and electron microscopic study. *Acta Cytol* 36:655-660, 1992.

97. Triche TJ, Askin FB, Kissane JM. Neuroblastoma, Ewing's sarcoma, and the differential diagnosis of small-, round-, blue-cell tumors. In: Pathology of Neoplasm in Children and Adolescents. M Finegold ed. In Major Problems in Pathology. 18th vol. WB Saunders, Philadelphia, 1986, pp 145-195.

98. Triche TJ, Askin FB. Neuroblastoma and the differential diagnosis of small-, round-, blue-cell tumors. *Hum Pathol* 14:569-595, 1983.

99. Shimada H, Chatten J, Newton WA Jr, Sachs N, Hamoudi AB, Chiba T, Marsden HB, Misugi K. Histopathologic prognostic factors in neuroblastic tumors. Definition of subtypes of ganglioneuroblastoma and an age-linked classification of neuroblastomas. *J Natl Cancer Inst* 73:405-416, 1984.

100. Joshi VV, Chatten J, Sather HN, Shimada H. Evaluation of the Shimada classification in advanced neuroblastoma with a special reference to the mitosis-karyorrhexis index. A report from the Children's Cancer Study Group. *Mod Pathol* 4:139-147, 1991.

101. Brodeur GM, Nakagawara A. Molecular basis of clinical heterogeneity in neuroblastoma. *Am J Pediatr Hematol Oncol* 14:111-116, 1992.

102. Lack EE, Travis WD, Oertel JE. Adrenal cortical nodules, hyperplasia, and hyperfunction. In: Pathology of the Adrenal Glands. Lack EE, ed. Churchill Livingstone, New York, 1990:75-113.

103. Joshi VV, Silverman JF, Altshuler G, Cantor AB, Larkin EW, Neill JSA, Norris HT, Shuster JJ, Holbrook CT, Hayes FA, Smith EI, Castleberry RP. Systematization of primary histopathologic and fine-needle aspiration cytologic features and description of unusual histopathologic features of neuroblastic tumors. A report from the Pediatric Oncology Group. *Hum Pathol* 24:493-504, 1993.

104. Palombini L, Vertrani A, Vecchione R, Del Basso, De Caro ML. The cytology of ganglioneuroma on fine needle aspiration smear. *Acta Cytol* 26;259-260, 1982.

105. Silverman JF, Berns LA, Holbrook CT, Neill JSA, Joshi VV. Fine needle aspiration cytology of primitive neuroectodermal tumors. A report of three cases. *Acta Cytol* 36:541-550, 1992.

106. Gonzalez-Campora R, Otal-Salaverri C, Panea-Flores P, Hevia-Vazquez A, Gomez-Pascual A, San-Martin-Diez V. Fine needle aspiration of peripheral neuroepithelioma of soft tissues. *Acta Cytol* 36:152-158, 1992.

107. Kushner BH, Hajdu SI, Gulati SC, Erlandson RA, Exelby PR, Lieberman PH. Extracranial primitive neuroectodermal tumors. The Memorial Sloan-Kettering Cancer Center experience. *Cancer* 67:1825-1829, 1991.

108. Coffin CM, Dehner LP. Peripheral neurogenic tumors of the soft tissues in children and adolescents. A clinicopathologic study of 139 cases. *Pediatr Pathol* 9:387-407, 1989.

109. Israel MA, Miser JS, Triche TJ, Kinsella T. Neuroepithelial tumors: In: Principles and Practice of Pediatric Oncology. Pizzo PA, Poplack DG. JB Lippincott Co, 1989, pp 623-634.

110. Marina NM, Etcubanas E, Parham DM, Bowman LC, Green A. Peripheral primitive neuroectodermal tumor (peripheral neuroepithelioma) in children. A review of the St. Jude experience and controversies in diagnosis and management. *Cancer* 64:1952-1960, 1989.

111. Askin FB, Rosai J, Sibley RK, Dehner LP. Malignant small cell tumor of the thoracopulmonary region in childhood. *Cancer* 43:2438-2451, 1979.

112. Linnoila RI, Tsokos M, Triche TJ, Marangos PJ, Chandra RS: Evidence for neural origin and PAS positive variants of the malignant cell tumor of thoracopulmonary region ("Askin tumor"). Am J Surg Pathol 10:124-133, 1986.

113. De Chadarevian JP, Vekemans M, Seemayer TA. Reciprocal translocation in small cell sarcomas. *N Engl J Med* 311:1702-1703, 1984.

114. Maletz N, McMorrow LE, Greco A, Wolman S. Ewing's sarcoma. Pathology, tissue culture, and cytogenetics. *Cancer* 58:252-257, 1986.

115. Whang-Peng J, Triche TJ, Knutsen T, Miser J, Douglas EC, Israel MA. Chromosome translocation in peripheral neuroepithelioma. *N Engl J Med* 311:584-585, 1984.

116. Kawaguchi K, Koike M. Neuron-specific enolase and Leu-7 immunoreactive small round cell neoplasm. The relationship to Ewing's sarcoma in bone and soft tissue. *Am J Clin Pathol* 86:79-83, 1986.

117. Dehner LP. Primitive neuroectodermal tumor and Ewing's sarcoma. *Am J Surg Path* 17:1-13, 1993.

118. Stephenson CF, Bridge JA, Sandberg AA. Cytogenetic and pathologic aspects of Ewing's sarcoma and neuroectodermal tumors. *Hum Pathol* 23:1270-1277, 1992.

119. Auger M, Bedard YC, Keating S. Diagnosis of a peripheral neuroectodermal tumour by fine needle aspiration. *Cytopathol* 1:243-249, 1990.

120. Neuhold N, Artlieb U, Wimmer M, Krisch I, Schratter M. Aspiration cytology, immunocytochemistry and electron microscopy of a malignant peripheral neuroectodermal tumor. A case report. *Acta Cytol* 33:74-79, 1989.

121. Tsokos M, Linnoila RI, Chandra RS, Triche TJ. Neuron-specific enolase in the diagnosis of neuroblastoma and other small, round cell tumors of childhood. *Hum Pathol* 15:575-584, 1984.

122. de Jong ASH, van Kessel-van Vark, van Heerde P. Fine needle aspiration biopsy diagnosis of rhabdomyosarcoma. An immunocytochemical study. *Acta Cytol* 31:573-577, 1987.

123. Kardos TF, Sprague RI, Wakely PE Jr, Frable WJ. Fine-needle aspiration biopsy of lymphoblastic lymphoma and leukemia. A clinical, cytologic, and immunologic study. *Cancer* 60:2448-2453, 1987.

124. Look AT, Hayes FA, Nitschke R, McWilliams NB, Green AA. Cellular DNA content as a predictor of response to chemotherapy in infants with unresectable neuroblastoma. *N Engl J Med* 311:231-235, 1984.

125. Kreiter SR, Geisinger KR, Chauvenet AR, Kute TE, Accettullo LA. DNA ploidy analysis in neuroblastoma: Flow cytometry versus image analysis cytometry. *Acta Cytol* 36:629, 1992.

126. Shimada H, Seeger R, Joshi V, Chatten J, Sather H, Hammond D. Histopathology and N-*myc* gene in advanced neuroblastomas: A report from the Children's Cancer Study group (CCSG). *Pediatr Pathol* 8:671-672, 1988.

127. Ganick DJ, Silverman JF, Holbrook CT, Dabbs DJ, Kodroff MB. Clinical utility of fine needle aspiration in the diagnosis and management of neuroblastoma. *Med Pediatr Oncol* 16:101-106, 1988.

128. Klein JO. Diagnostic lung puncture in the pneumonias of infants and children. *Pediatrics* 44:486-492, 1969.

129. Garcia de Olarte D, Trujillo H, Uribe A, Agudelo N. Lung puncture-aspiration as a bacteriologic diagnostic procedure in acute pneumonias of infants and children. *Clin Pediatr* 10:346-350, 1971.

130. Berger R, Arango L. The value and safety of percutaneous lung aspiration for children with serious pulmonary infections. *Pediatr Pulmonol* 1:309-313, 1985.

131. Hartman GE, Shochat SJ. Primary pulmonary neoplasms of childhood. A review. *Ann Thorac Surg* 36:108-119, 1983.

132. Weintraub J, Wenger RD, Vassilakos P. The application of immunocytochemical techniques to routinely-fixed and stained cytologic specimens. An aid in the differential diagnosis of undifferentiated malignant neoplasms. *Path Res Pract* 186:658-665, 1990.

133. Pettinato G, Swanson PE, Insabato L, De-Chiara A, Wick MR. Undifferentiated small round-cell tumors of childhood. The immunocytochemical demonstration of myogenic differentiation in fine-needle aspirates. *Diagn Cytopathol* 5:194-199, 1989.

134. Seidal T, Walaas L, Kindblom L-G, Angervall L. Cytology of embryonal rhabdomyosarcoma. A cytologic, light microscopic, electron microscopic, and immunohistochemical study of seven cases. *Diagn Cytopathol* 4:292-299, 1988.

135. Strausbauch PH, Neill JSA, Benning TL, Silverman JF. Applications of electron microscopy in fine-needle aspiration cytology. In: Cytopathology Annual. WA Schmidt, Series editor. Williams and Wilkins, Baltimore 1992: p173-195.

136. Akhtar M, Ali MA, Sabbah R. Aspiration cytology of Ewing's sarcoma. Light and electron microscopic correlations. *Cancer* 57:2051-2060, 1985.

137. Elsheikh T, Silverman JF, Wakely PE Jr, Holbrook CT, Joshi VV. Fine-needle aspiration cytology of Langerhan's cell histiocytosis (eosinophilic granuloma) of bone in children. *Diagn Cytopathol* 7:261-266, 1991.

138. Akhtar M, Ali MA, Sabbah R, Bakry M, Sackey K, Nash EJ. Aspiration cytology of neuroblastoma. Light and electron microscopic correlations. *Cancer* 57:797-803, 1986.

139. Akhtar M, Ali MA, Sabbah R, Sackey K, Bakry M. Aspiration cytology of retinoblastoma. Light and electron microscopic correlations. *Diagn Cytopathol* 4:306-311, 1988.

140. Akhtar M, Ali MA, Sackey K, Sabbah R, Bakry M. Aspiration cytology of neuroblastoma. Light microscopy with transmission and scanning electron microscopic correlations. *Diagn Cytopathol* 4:323-327, 1989.

141. Akhtar M, Ali MA, Owen EW. Application of electron microscopy in the interpretation of fine-needle aspiration biopsies. *Cancer* 48:2458-2463, 1981.

▣ Index

Numbers in **boldface** refer to pages on which images, tables, and figures appear.

B

Bacteria, staining in cerebrospinal fluid, **70-71**
Barrett's esophagus, cytomorphology, 154
Blastomyces, staining, **146**
Bone scintigraphy, metastatic disease, 177
Brain tumor, incidence in children, 2, 37
Branchial cleft cyst
  aspiration, 230
  clinical presentation, 230
  cytomorphology, 230, **240**
  diagnosis, 230
Breast
  carcinoma, 285-286
  cysts, 283-284
  inflammatory lesions, 283
  metastasis site, 286
Burkitt's lymphoma
  cerebrospinal fluid staining, **29**
  chromosomal translocation, 314
  clinical presentation, 214
  cytomorphology, 214, **223-224**, **327-328**
  incidence in children, 213-214
  metastasis in kidney, 302
  serous effusion analysis, **115**

C

Cancer
  characterization by cell size, 3-4, 104
  incidence in children, 1-2, 11, 173
  mortality in children, 1
Candida albicans
  Pap smear identification, 129
  staining in samples
    esophagus, 153
    lung, 140
    skin, 157, **162**
Cat-scratch disease. *See* Granulomatous lymphadenitis
Cellular lipid index, macrophage evaluation, 137
Central nervous system neoplasms
  imaging, 178-179, **196**
  incidence in children, 45
  sites of origin, 45
Cerebrospinal fluid
  acute leukemia staining, 24-29
  analysis
    astrocytoma, 48-49, **80-83**, **87-89**
    ependymoma, 50-51, **85**, **90**
    germinoma, 53-54
    glioblastoma, 49-50, **83-84**, **89-91**
    medulloblastoma, 46-47, **79-80**, **91-92**
    meningitis
      aseptic meningitis, 43
      histiocytes, 44
      traumatic tap comparison, 43
      white blood cell count, 42-43
    neuroblastoma, 56, **87**
    pineoblastoma, 54-55, **86**
    retinoblastoma, 55, **86**
    rhabdomyosarcoma, 56, **87**
    sickle cell anemia, **63**

cell counting, 38
collection, 38
contaminants
  blood, 18-19, **28**, 40
  epithelial cells, 40-41, **66**
  hematopoietic precursor cells, 41, **67**, **69-70**
  notochord material, 41-42, **68-69**
corrected total white cell count, 18-19
cytocentrifugation, 38-39
differential diagnosis of acute leukemias, 16-18
flow, 37
markers
  α-fetoprotein, 53-54
  human chorionic gonadotropin, 53-54
mechanism of tumor cell entry, 45-46
membrane filtration, 38-39
normal specimens
  erythrocytes, 40
  leukocyte count, 39
  ventricular surface cell characteristics, 39-40
origin, 37
Papanicolaou staining, 16-18, **26-29**, 39, **62-63**, **68-74**, **79-87**, **92**
sample preparation, 15-16, 38-39
storage, 38
Cervical cancer. *See also* Pap smear
  classification, 127
  cytomorphology, 128-**133**
  treatment, 128
Chlamydia
  Pap smear identification, 129, **133**
  staining in conjunctivitis, 157, **164**
Chondroblastoma
  calcium deposits, 253
  clinical presentation, 252
  cytomorphology, 253, **256**
  diagnosis, 253
Choroid plexus neoplasms
  cerebrospinal fluid evaluation, 52, **85**, **90**
  histologic features, 51-52, 59-60
  survival rates, 51
Chromatin
  effect of intrathecal chemotherapy, 19
  staining
    acute leukemias, **21-31**
    central nervous system tumors, **67**, **80-83**
    serous effusions, **109**, **111**, **117-118**
Chronic granulocytic leukemia, incidence in children, 19
Chronic lymphocytic thyroiditis
  clinical presentation, 233-234
  cytomorphology, 234, **241**
Clear cell sarcoma
  cytomorphology, 271, **278**
  immunostaining, 271
  incidence in children, 271
  prognosis, 271
Clofazine
  macrophage ingestion, 208
  staining of crystals, 208
CMV. *See* Cytomegalovirus
Computed tomography

classification, 211
cytomorphology, 155-156
gastrointestinal disease, 155
imaging, 180, **194**
large cell lymphoma cytomorphology, 215, **224**

O

Osteosarcoma
cytomorphology, 248-249, **254**
diagnosis, 249
exfoliative cytology, 105-106, **121-122**, **149**
imaging, 178, **192-193**
incidence in children, 2, 248
metastasis sites, 3
Ovarian cancer. *See also* Teratoma
cytomorphology, 303, **329-330**
incidence in children, 302

P

Pancreatoblastoma
cytomorphology, 303-305, **331-333**
differential diagnosis, 305
electron microscopy, 304-305
fine needle aspiration, 304
immunostaining, 304-305
incidence in children, 303
sites of origin, 303-304
Pap smear
application in children, 127
assessment of ovarian function, 129
cytomorphology, 128-129
microbe identification, 129
Papanicolaou stain. *See also* Pap smear
acute leukemias, **26-29**, **31**
bone tumors, **254-255**
central nervous system tumors, **62-63**, **68-74**, **79-87**, **92**
cervical cancer, **130-133**
epithelial disorders, **162-165**
evaluation of fine needle aspiration samples, 6
lymph node samples, **217-220**, **222-225**
serous effusions, **109**, **111-113**, **116-123**
Papillary-cystic tumor
cytomorphology, 306
incidence, 306
Parathyroid cyst, cytomorphology, 231
Peritonitis, serous effusion analysis, **109**
Pilomatrixoma
clinical presentation, 286
cytomorphology, 286-287, **289**
fine needle aspiration, 286-287
Pineal neoplasms
clinical presentation, 53
differential diagnosis, 53
parenchymal tumors, 54-55
types, 53
Pituitary adenoma, cytomorphology, 60
PNET. *See* Primitive neuroectodermal tumor
Pneumocystis carinii, staining, 140, **144-145**
Pneumonia

lipid-laden macrophages, 138
serous effusion analysis, **108**
Primitive neuroectodermal tumor
chromosomal translocation, 310, 314
cytomorphology, 309-312, **339-343**
diagnosis, 311-312
fine needle aspiration, 310
immunostaining, 311-312
peripheral, 309-310
sites of origin, 309
survival rates, 309

R

Reactive lymph node hyperplasia
cytomorphology, 205-206, **217**
diagnosis, 205-206
etiology, 205
Respiratory distress syndrome
diagnosis, 139
oxygen therapy
cellular alterations, 138-140
complications, 138-139
surfactant deficiency, 138
Respiratory syncytial virus, effect on lung cells, 140-141
Retinoblastoma
cerebrospinal fluid examination, 55, **86**, 238
clinical presentation, 238
cytomorphology, 238-239, **244**
diagnosis, 55, 239
heredity, 238
immunostaining, 239
incidence in children, 2, 238
Rhabdomyosarcoma
cerebrospinal fluid evaluation, 56, **87**
chromosomal analysis, 267
classification, 4, 266
cytomorphology, 266-267, **275-276**
diagnosis, 267
exfoliative cytology, 104-105, **120**
fine needle aspiration, 266
imaging, **190**
immunotyping, 267
incidence in children, 265-266
metastasis in cerebrospinal fluid, 56
urinary cytology, **165**
Romanowsky stain
acute leukemias, **21-32**
bone tumors, **254-256**
central nervous system tumors, **63-69**, **72-78**, **80-82**, **88**, **92**
evaluation of fine needle aspiration samples, 6
lymph node samples, **217-221**, **223-225**
serous effusions, **108**, **110**, **112-117**,
Rosai-Dorfman disease
cytomorphology, 209, **220**
diagnosis, 209-210
Salivary gland
adenoma, 237
carcinoma, 237-238
cytomorphology of tumors, 237-238, **243-244**